Mood Disorders: Diagnosis and Treatment

Mood Disorders: Diagnosis and Treatment

Editor: Peter Garner

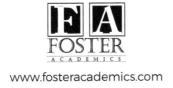

www.fosteracademics.com

www.fosteracademics.com

Cataloging-in-Publication Data

Mood disorders : diagnosis and treatment / edited by Peter Garner.
     p. cm.
Includes bibliographical references and index.
ISBN 978-1-63242-501-0
1. Affective disorders. 2. Affective disorders--Diagnosis. 3. Affective disorders--Treatment.
4. Psychology, Pathological. I. Garner, Peter.
RC537 .M66 2017
616.852 7--dc23

Foster Academics,
118-35 Queens Blvd., Suite 400,
Forest Hills, NY 11375, USA

ISBN 978-1-63242-501-0 (Hardback)

Printed and bound in the United States of America.

Contents

Preface IX

Chapter 1 **Medial prefrontal cortex serotonin 1A and 2A receptor binding interacts to predict threat-related amygdala reactivity**...................................1
Patrick M Fisher, Julie C Price, Carolyn C Meltzer, Eydie L Moses-Kolko, Carl Becker, Sarah L Berga and Ahmad R Hariri

Chapter 2 **Social stimulation and corticolimbic reactivity in premenstrual dysphoric disorder**..12
Malin Gingnell, Victoria Ahlstedt, Elin Bannbers, Johan Wikström, Inger Sundström-Poromaa and Mats Fredrikson

Chapter 3 **Meta-analytic methods for neuroimaging data explained**...........................22
Joaquim Radua and David Mataix-Cols

Chapter 4 **Epigenetic modifications associated with suicide and common mood and anxiety disorders**..33
Abdulrahman M El-Sayed, Michelle R Haloossim, Sandro Galea and Karestan C Koenen

Chapter 5 **Contextual modulation of medial prefrontal cortex to neutral faces in anxious adolescents**..47
Tara S Peris and Adriana Galván

Chapter 6 **Facial emotion processing in major depression: a systematic review of neuroimaging findings**..54
Anja Stuhrmann, Thomas Suslow and Udo Dannlowski

Chapter 7 **The Behavioural Inhibition System, anxiety and hippocampal volume in a non-clinical population**..71
Liat Levita, Catherine Bois, Andrew Healey, Emily Smyllie, Evelina Papakonstantinou, Tom Hartley and Colin Lever

Chapter 8 **Individual differences in cognitive reappraisal usage modulate the time course of brain activation during symptom provocation in specific phobia**..81
Andrea Hermann, Verena Leutgeb, Wilfried Scharmüller, Dieter Vaitl, Anne Schienle and Rudolf Stark

Chapter 9 **Area-dependent time courses of brain activation during video-induced symptom provocation in social anxiety disorder**.................................92
Stephanie Boehme, Alexander Mohr, Michael PI Becker, Wolfgang HR Miltner and Thomas Straube

Chapter 10   **Sex differences in the neurobiology of fear conditioning and extinction: a preliminary FMRI study of shared sex differences with stress-arousal circuitry**..**101**
Kelimer Lebron-Milad, Brandon Abbs, Mohammed R Milad, Clas Linnman, Ansgar Rougemount-Bücking, Mohammed A Zeidan, Daphne J Holt and Jill M Goldstein

Chapter 11   **Event-related potential studies of post-traumatic stress disorder**............................**111**
Arash Javanbakht, Israel Liberzon, Alireza Amirsadri, Klevest Gjini and Nash N Boutros

Chapter 12   **Reduced hippocampal and medial prefrontal gray matter mediate the association between reported childhood maltreatment and trait anxiety in adulthood and predict sensitivity to future life stress**............................**123**
Adam X Gorka, Jamie L Hanson, Spenser R Radtke and Ahmad R Hariri

Chapter 13   **Quantitative meta-analysis of neural activity in posttraumatic stress disorder**..**133**
Jasmeet P Hayes, Scott M Hayes and Amanda M Mikedis

Chapter 14   **Amygdala activation to threat under attentional load in individuals with anxiety disorder**..**146**
Thomas Straube, Judith Lipka, Andreas Sauer, Martin Mothes-Lasch and Wolfgang HR Miltner

Chapter 15   **Brain white matter microstructure alterations in adolescent rhesus monkeys exposed to early life stress: associations with high cortisol during infancy**..**156**
Brittany R Howell, Kai M McCormack, Alison P Grand, Nikki T Sawyer, Xiaodong Zhang, Dario Maestripieri, Xiaoping Hu and Mar M Sanchez

Chapter 16   **Functional anomalies in healthy individuals with a first degree family history of major depressive disorder**..**170**
Francesco Amico, Angela Carballedo, Danuta Lisiecka, Andrew J Fagan, Gerard Boyle and Thomas Frodl

Chapter 17   **Resting state amygdala prefrontal connectivity predicts symptom change after cognitive behavioral therapy in generalized social anxiety disorder**..**178**
Heide Klumpp, Michael K Keutmann, Daniel A Fitzgerald, Stewart A Shankman and K Luan Phan

Chapter 18   **Intolerance of uncertainty predicts fear extinction in amygdala-ventromedial prefrontal cortical circuitry**..**185**
Jayne Morriss, Anastasia Christakou and Carien M. van Reekum

Chapter 19   **Current understanding of the bi-directional relationship of major depression with inflammations**...198

Berhane Messay, Alvin Lim and Anna L Marsland

Permissions

List of Contributors

Index

Preface

Every book is a source of knowledge and this one is no exception. The idea that led to the conceptualization of this book was the fact that the world is advancing rapidly; which makes it crucial to document the progress in every field. I am aware that a lot of data is already available, yet, there is a lot more to learn. Hence, I accepted the responsibility of editing this book and contributing my knowledge to the community.

Mood disorder is a psychological disorder characterized by the elevation or lowering of a person's mood, such as depression or bipolar disorder. This book is a valuable compilation of topics, ranging from the basic to the most complex advancements in the field of mood disorders. The text focuses on the treatment of this disease with utmost detail. Some of the commonly used treatments like behavioral therapy, cognitive behavior therapy, mood stabilizers, etc. are discussed through case studies for better understanding. In this book, using case studies and examples, constant effort has been made to make the understanding of the difficult concepts of mood disorders as easy and informative as possible, for the readers.

While editing this book, I had multiple visions for it. Then I finally narrowed down to make every chapter a sole standing text explaining a particular topic, so that they can be used independently. However, the umbrella subject sinews them into a common theme. This makes the book a unique platform of knowledge.

I would like to give the major credit of this book to the experts from every corner of the world, who took the time to share their expertise with us. Also, I owe the completion of this book to the never-ending support of my family, who supported me throughout the project.

Editor

Medial prefrontal cortex serotonin 1A and 2A receptor binding interacts to predict threat-related amygdala reactivity

Patrick M Fisher[1,2*], Julie C Price[2,3], Carolyn C Meltzer[4], Eydie L Moses-Kolko[5], Carl Becker[3], Sarah L Berga[6] and Ahmad R Hariri[7,8]

Abstract

Background: The amygdala and medial prefrontal cortex (mPFC) comprise a key corticolimbic circuit that helps shape individual differences in sensitivity to threat and the related risk for psychopathology. Although serotonin (5-HT) is known to be a key modulator of this circuit, the specific receptors mediating this modulation are unclear. The colocalization of 5-HT_{1A} and 5-HT_{2A} receptors on mPFC glutamatergic neurons suggests that their functional interactions may mediate 5-HT effects on this circuit through top-down regulation of amygdala reactivity. Using a multimodal neuroimaging strategy in 39 healthy volunteers, we determined whether threat-related amygdala reactivity, assessed with blood oxygen level-dependent functional magnetic resonance imaging, was significantly predicted by the interaction between mPFC 5-HT_{1A} and 5-HT_{2A} receptor levels, assessed by positron emission tomography.

Results: 5-HT_{1A} binding in the mPFC significantly moderated an inverse correlation between mPFC 5-HT_{2A} binding and threat-related amygdala reactivity. Specifically, mPFC 5-HT_{2A} binding was significantly inversely correlated with amygdala reactivity only when mPFC 5-HT_{1A} binding was relatively low.

Conclusions: Our findings provide evidence that 5-HT_{1A} and 5-HT_{2A} receptors interact to shape serotonergic modulation of a functional circuit between the amygdala and mPFC. The effect of the interaction between mPFC 5-HT_{1A} and 5-HT_{2A} binding and amygdala reactivity is consistent with the colocalization of these receptors on glutamatergic neurons in the mPFC.

Background

Research in human and non-human animal models implicates a corticolimbic circuitry composed of structural and functional connections between the amygdala and regions of the medial prefrontal cortex (mPFC) including the anterior cingulate cortex (ACC) in generating and regulating behavioral and physiological responses to threat-related stimuli [1-4]. Regions of the mPFC are crucially involved in the integration and subsequent regulation of stimulus-driven amygdala response, partly via glutamatergic projections to populations of GABAergic neurons within the amygdala [5-7]. Variability in the structure and function of this corticolimbic circuitry has been associated with interindividual differences in personality measures, reflecting sensitivity to environmental threat and related risk for psychopathology [2,8-11].

Serotonin (5-hydroxytryptamine, 5-HT) exerts potent modulatory effects on mood, affect, and responsiveness to stress and threat [12]. Neuroimaging studies in humans have mapped interindividual differences in amygdala reactivity to biologically salient environmental stimuli (for example, facial expressions of threat) onto variability in 5-HT signaling within this corticolimbic circuitry [2,13-21]. However, the role of specific 5-HT-receptor signaling pathways in mediating these effects are not fully understood [12]. Previous work in humans using positron emission tomography (PET) has implicated 5-HT_{1A} and 5-HT_{2A} receptors in modulating mood, affect and threat responsiveness, and in the

* Correspondence: patrick.fisher@gmail.com
[1]Center for Neuroscience, University of Pittsburgh, Pittsburgh, Pennsylvania 15260, USA
Full list of author information is available at the end of the article

corticolimbic circuitry supporting these behaviors [22-26]. Importantly, the anatomical localization of these two receptors within prefrontal cortex positions them to mediate effectively the observed effects of 5-HT signaling on corticolimbic circuit dynamics.

In the mPFC, the excitatory 5-HT$_{2A}$ and inhibitory 5-HT$_{1A}$ receptors are colocalized on glutamatergic pyramidal neurons [27]. The 5-HT$_{2A}$ receptor is specifically localized to proximal portions of apical dendrites [28,29], where convergent inputs are integrated, and is therefore positioned to facilitate mPFC function through second-messenger signaling cascades, resulting in membrane depolarization [27,30]. By contrast, the 5-HT$_{1A}$ receptor is localized to the initial segment of the axon, where action potentials are typically generated [27-29,31-34], thus this receptor is positioned to exert an inhibitory effect on mPFC function through 'gating' glutamatergic output via membrane hyperpolarization. Collectively, these two receptors are crucially positioned to mediate effects of 5-HT on glutamatergic neuronal activity and mPFC function, including top-down regulation of amygdala reactivity [27,35].

In one previous study, we identified an inverse correlation between mPFC 5-HT$_{2A}$ binding and threat-related amygdala reactivity [14]. In another, we reported that 5-H$_{1A}$ autoreceptor binding in the dorsal raphe nucleus was inversely correlated with amygdala reactivity [15]. However, the effects of mPFC 5-HT$_{1A}$ binding on threat-related amygdala reactivity were not explored in either of these studies. More importantly, whether mPFC 5-HT$_{1A}$ binding moderates the previously observed inverse association between mPFC 5-HT$_{2A}$ binding and threat-related amygdala reactivity, as suggested by the aforementioned colocalization of these receptors within the mPFC, has not yet been determined.

In the current study we explored this hypothetical functional interaction using multimodal PET/functional magnetic resonance imaging (fMRI) neuroimaging data in a sample of 39 healthy adult volunteers that partially overlaps with those of our two previous reports [14,15]. We hypothesized that mPFC 5-HT$_{1A}$ binding would be positively correlated with threat-related amygdala reactivity, reflecting the inhibitory effects of the 5-HT$_{1A}$ receptor on prefrontal pyramidal neurons, which are positioned to exert an inhibitory effect on the amygdala. Consistent with our previous report, we further hypothesized that mPFC 5-HT$_{2A}$ binding would be inversely correlated with amygdala reactivity. Finally, in light of the molecular interactions predicted from the colocalization of 5-HT$_{1A}$ and 5-HT$_{2A}$ receptors, we hypothesized that mPFC 5-HT$_{1A}$ binding would significantly interact with mPFC 5-HT$_{2A}$ binding, so that 5-HT$_{2A}$ binding would

be inversely correlated with amygdala reactivity only at relatively low levels of 5-HT$_{1A}$ binding.

Results

Amygdala reactivity

Consistent with previous reports, we observed robust threat-related reactivity in the bilateral amygdala across all participants [36,37] (Figure 1). The magnitude of right amygdala reactivity, but not left amygdala reactivity, was inversely correlated with age (right amygdala: r^2 = 0.19, P = 0.005; left amygdala: r^2 = 0.02, P = 0.35). Neither right nor left amygdala reactivity was correlated with gender (r^2 values < 0.03, P values > 0.3).

Serotonin receptor binding

We focused on quantifying 5-HT$_{1A}$ and 5-HT$_{2A}$ binding within the pregenual and subgenual prefrontal cortex (pgPFC and sgPFC, respectively) because of previous reports supporting an integral structural and functional relationship between the amygdala and these mPFC regions in the context of processing threat that is modulated by 5-HT signaling [1,2,6,14,38,39].

Reflecting 5-HT$_{1A}$ binding, we observed specific [^{11}C] WAY100635 binding within both pgPFC (mean ± SD binding potential, non-displaceable (BP$_{ND}$) = 4.32 ± 1.18) and sgPFC (BP$_{ND}$ = 4.86 ± 1.41) for all subjects. Reflecting 5-HT$_{2A}$ binding, we observed specific [^{18}F] altanserin binding within both pgPFC (BP$_{ND}$ = 1.06 ± 0.37) and sgPFC (BP$_{ND}$ = 1.19 ± 0.46). 5-HT$_{1A}$ and 5-HT$_{2A}$ binding between the pgPFC and sgPFC were significantly correlated (5-HT$_{1A}$ BP$_{ND}$: r^2 = 0.69, P = 5.87

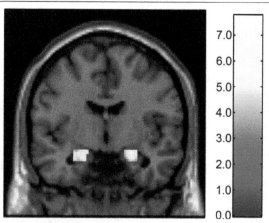

Figure 1 Amygdala reactivity to perceptual processing of fearful and angry facial expressions. Statistical parametric map representing bilateral amygdala clusters exhibiting a significant response to task (faces > shapes; right amygdala: (24, -6, -11), z = 6.28, k = 145 voxels (P < 0.05, corrected); left amygdala: (-18, -7, -15), z = 5.77, k = 146 voxels (P < 0.05, corrected). Color bar indicates t-scores.

$\times 10^{-11}$; 5-HT$_{2A}$ BP$_{ND}$: $r^2 = 0.63$, $P = 1.80 \times 10^{-9}$). However, within regions, 5-HT$_{1A}$ binding was not significantly correlated with 5-HT$_{2A}$ binding (pgPFC: $r^2 = 3.28 \times 10^{-5}$, $P = 0.97$; sgPFC: $r^2 = 0.001$, $P = 0.88$). 5-HT$_{2A}$ binding was significantly inversely correlated with age (pgPFC: $r^2 = 0.41$, $P = 1.30 \times 10^{-5}$; sgPFC: $r^2 = 0.41$, $P = 1.29 \times 10^{-5}$), but 5-HT$_{1A}$ binding did not have a significant correlation with age (pgPFC: $r^2 = 0.01$, $P = 0.53$, sgPFC: $r^2 = 0.003$, $P = 0.73$). Neither 5-HT$_{1A}$ nor 5-HT$_{2A}$ binding was significantly correlated with gender (r^2 values < 0.01, P values > 0.5).

5-HT$_{1A}$ binding and amygdala reactivity
Regional 5-HT$_{1A}$ binding was not significantly correlated with amygdala reactivity in either pgPFC nor sgPFC (right amygdala versus pgPFC 5-HT$_{1A}$ BP$_{ND}$: $t_{36} = -0.76$, $P = 0.94$; right amygdala versus sgPFC 5-HT$_{1A}$ BP$_{ND}$: $t_{36} = 0.54$, $P = 0.60$; left amygdala versus pgPFC 5-HT$_{1A}$ BP$_{ND}$: $t_{36} = 0.16$, $P = 0.88$; left amygdala versus sgPFC 5-HT$_{1A}$ BP$_{ND}$: $t_{36} = -0.09$, $P = 0.93$) (Figure 2A,B).

5-HT$_{2A}$ binding and amygdala reactivity
Regional 5-HT$_{2A}$ binding was significantly inversely correlated with amygdala reactivity [14]. Specifically, right amygdala reactivity was inversely correlated with 5-HT$_{2A}$ binding within both pgPFC ($t_{36} = -3.44$, $P = 0.002$; Figure 2D) and sgPFC ($t_{36} = -2.49$, $P = 0.02$). There was no significant correlation between left amygdala reactivity and 5-HT$_{2A}$ binding within either pgPFC ($t_{36} = -0.61$, $P = 0.55$; Figure 2C) or sgPFC ($t_{36} = 0.72$, $P = 0.47$). Thus, we focused our analyses on the effects of interaction between 5-HT$_{1A}$ and 5-HT$_{2A}$ binding on right amygdala reactivity.

Interaction between 5-HT$_{1A}$ and 5-HT$_{2A}$ binding and amygdala reactivity
Consistent with our hypothesis, there was a significant interaction between 5-HT$_{1A}$ and 5-HT$_{2A}$ binding in both the pgPFC ($t_{34} = 2.18$, $P = 0.03$) and sgPFC ($t_{34} = 2.72$, $P = 0.01$) in predicting threat-related right amygdala reactivity (Figure 3). Further examination of this interaction effect showed that 5-HT$_{2A}$ binding was significantly inversely correlated with right amygdala reactivity when 5-HT$_{1A}$ binding was < 4.99 (0.6 SDs above the mean) in the pgPFC or < 5.48 (0.4 SDs above the mean) in the sgPFC. It should be noted that the inverse correlations between 5-HT$_{2A}$ binding and right amygdala reactivity remained significant when 5-HT$_{1A}$ binding, the interaction term and age were included in the models (pgPFC: $t_{34} = -3.55$, $P = 0.001$; sgPFC: $t_{34} = -2.72$, $P = 0.006$).

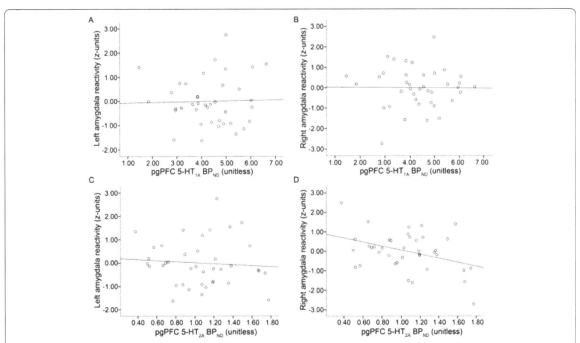

Figure 2 Association between amygdala reactivity and 5-HT$_{1A}$ BP$_{ND}$ and 5-HT$_{2A}$ BP$_{ND}$. (A,B) Plot of non-significant correlation between left and right amygdala reactivity and pgPFC 5-HT$_{1A}$ BP$_{ND}$. **(C)** Plot of non-significant correlation between left amygdala reactivity and pgPFC 5-HT$_{2A}$ BP$_{ND}$. **(D)** Plot of significant inverse correlation between right amygdala reactivity and pgPFC 5-HT$_{2A}$ BP$_{ND}$. 5-HT = serotonin; BP$_{ND}$ = binding potential, non-displaceable; pgPFC = pregenual prefrontal cortex; sgPFC = subgenual prefrontal cortex.

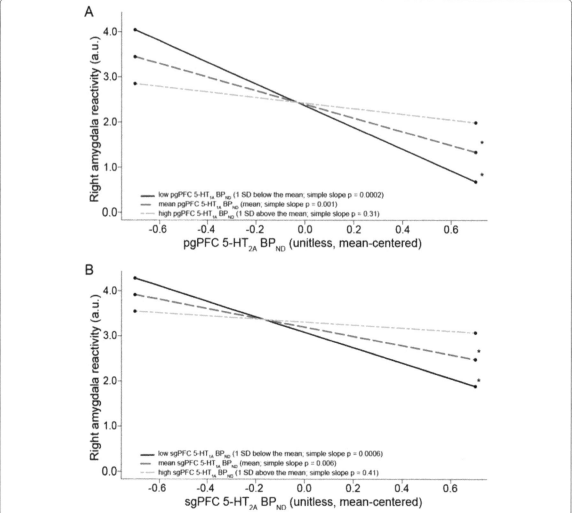

Figure 3 5-HT$_{1A}$ BP$_{ND}$ **significantly moderated the correlation between 5-HT$_{2A}$ BP$_{ND}$ and right amygdala reactivity**. **(A)** pgPFC 5-HT$_{1A}$ BP$_{ND}$ moderated the correlation between pgPFC 5-HT$_{2A}$ BP$_{ND}$ and right amygdala reactivity. Lines indicate simple slope between pgPFC 5-HT$_{2A}$ BP$_{ND}$ and right amygdala reactivity at three arbitrarily chosen pgPFC 5-HT$_{1A}$ BP$_{ND}$ values: low (1 SD below mean (-1 SD), solid black line), mean (equivalent to mean, red dotted line) and high (1 SD above mean (+1 SD), green dotted line). **(B)** sgPFC 5-HT$_{1A}$ BP$_{ND}$ significantly moderated the association between sgPFC 5-HT$_{2A}$ BP$_{ND}$ and right amygdala reactivity. Lines indicate simple slope between sgPFC 5-HT$_{2A}$ BP$_{ND}$ and right amygdala reactivity at three arbitrarily chosen sgPFC 5-HT$_{1A}$ BP$_{ND}$ values: low (-1 SD, solid black line), mean (red dotted line) and high (+1 SD, green dotted line). *Indicates simple slope, $P < 0.05$; 5-HT = serotonin; a.u. = arbitrary units; BP$_{ND}$ = binding potential, non-displaceable; pgPFC = pregenual prefrontal cortex; sgPFC = subgenual prefrontal cortex.

Discussion

Results from our current analyses indicate that the interaction between 5-HT$_{1A}$ and 5-HT$_{2A}$ receptors in the mPFC is crucial for shaping the response of the human amygdala to threat. Specifically, 5-HT$_{2A}$ binding was inversely correlated with threat-related amygdala reactivity, but only when 5-HT$_{1A}$ binding was at mean or relatively low levels. Importantly, these patterns were independent of age and gender, suggesting the general importance and widespread effects that the interaction between mPFC 5-HT$_{1A}$ and 5-HT$_{2A}$ receptors may have on amygdala reactivity. The right lateralized nature of this interaction effect may reflect relatively greater involvement of the right amygdala in the perceptual processing of facial stimuli and, subsequently, greater 5-HT modulation of reactivity in this hemisphere. Although a number of studies have reported asymmetries in monoaminergic modulation of cortical and subcortical circuits

[40-43], the biological mechanisms mediating such lateralized effects are difficult to ascertain on the basis of the existing literature.

We explicitly tested for an interaction effect (that is, moderation) between 5-HT$_{1A}$ and 5-HT$_{2A}$ binding because we believe that this represents the most straightforward approach for interpreting how these two systems potentially interact to modulate threat-related amygdala reactivity. Although conceptually and intuitively appealing, we did not employ a metric reflecting the ratio of 5-HT$_{1A}$ and 5-HT$_{2A}$ binding for two reasons: 1) its association with amygdala reactivity would be arbitrarily dependent upon how the ratio term is constructed and 2) testing for the effect of a ratio term (that is, X_1 multiplied by the inverse of X_2) is essentially a test for an interaction effect in which one of the variables is transformed, which we believe would render interpretation difficult at best. Consequently, we believe our test for an interaction between 5-HT$_{1A}$ and 5-HT$_{2A}$ binding represents the most appropriate and parsimonious statistical test.

These findings are remarkably consistent with the predominant anatomical localization of 5-HT$_{1A}$ and 5-HT$_{2A}$ receptors to the axon hillock and apical dendrites of prefrontal glutamatergic pyramidal neurons, respectively. Given its principal localization on apical dendrites proximal to the soma, the excitatory 5-HT$_{2A}$ receptor is situated to mediate 5-HT depolarization of prefrontal glutamatergic neurons. By contrast, the localization of the inhibitory 5-HT$_{1A}$ receptor to the initial portion of the axon hillock positions it to mediate 5-HT hyperpolarization of these same neurons. Considering the high coexpression of 5-HT$_{1A}$ and 5-HT$_{2A}$ receptors on most prefrontal glutamatergic neurons, this arrangement suggests that the 5-HT$_{1A}$ receptor can effectively (and negatively) gate the depolarizing effects of the 5-HT$_{2A}$ receptors on prefrontal output. In turn, such serotonergic modulation of prefrontal neuron output may shape the capacity of this circuitry to exert an inhibitory effect on amygdala reactivity (Figure 4). We interpret our current findings of an inverse correlation of mPFC 5-HT$_{2A}$ binding with amygdala reactivity but only at mean and low levels of 5-HT$_{1A}$ binding as reflecting the coexpression of these receptors and their role in mediating serotonergic modulation of this circuitry. The absence of a main effect of mPFC 5-HT$_{1A}$ binding on amygdala reactivity is further consistent with this gating model, with the capacity for mPFC 5-HT$_{1A}$ receptors to modulate threat-related amygdala reactivity being dependent upon additional signaling mechanisms such as, but not necessarily limited to, mPFC 5-HT$_{2A}$ receptors. Although interpretation of our findings is consistent with the previously described localization of the 5-HT$_{1A}$ and 5-HT$_{2A}$ receptors within prefrontal cortex, our results reflect only statistical correlation, and do not establish causality. Future studies aimed at establishing a causal link between 5-HT$_{1A}$ and 5-HT$_{2A}$ receptor interactions on prefrontal pyramidal neuron excitability and the

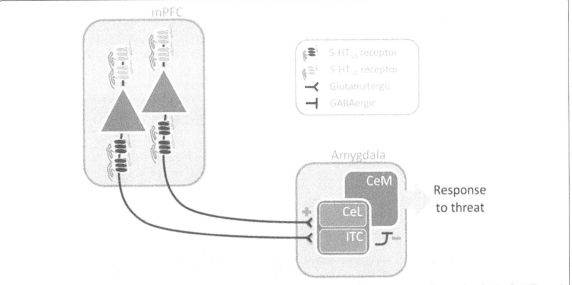

Figure 4 Schematic illustrating mPFC projection neurons that act to regulate amygdala response to threat-related stimuli. 5-HT$_{1A}$ and 5-HT$_{2A}$ in mPFC are positioned to modulate this circuitry by biasing excitability of these mPFC neurons, thereby affecting the capacity to regulate amygdala reactivity. 5-HT = serotonin; mPFC = medial prefrontal cortex; CeL = lateral central nucleus of the amygdala; CeM = medial central nucleus of the amygdala; ITC = intercalated cells.

response of the amygdala in the context of threat are necessary.

There is strong evidence suggesting that 5-HT signaling within the amygdala plays an important role in modulating threat-related amygdala reactivity [13,20,44], and both 5-HT$_{1A}$ and 5-HT$_{2A}$ receptors are expressed in the amygdala [45-47]. However, we did not observe a significant correlation between either 5-HT$_{1A}$ or 5-HT$_{2A}$ binding in the amygdala and amygdala reactivity (data not shown). Unlike in the mPFC, 5-HT$_{1A}$ and 5-HT$_{2A}$ receptors may be more evenly distributed on both glutamatergic and GABAergic neurons within the amygdala [47,48]. This potential for both receptor subtypes to cause inhibitory and excitatory modulation of the amygdala complicate efforts to map correlations between estimates of local binding and reactivity in the absence of cell-type specific values, which are beyond the scope of current PET techniques. Finally, additional 5-HT receptor signaling mechanisms within the amygdala, such as the 5-HT$_3$ and 5-HT$_{2C}$ receptors, have been implicated in anxiety-related behavioral phenotypes in animal models, and may have a greater role in mediating the effects of local 5-HT signaling on amygdala function [44,49-51].

There are important limitations to our study. Our blood oxygen level-dependent (BOLD) fMRI challenge paradigm was explicitly designed to elicit threat-related amygdala reactivity associated with driving behavioral and physiologic arousal in response to environmental stimulation. Our task did not engage any mPFC region involved in regulating amygdala reactivity and overlapping with our PET region of interest (ROI). Thus, we were not able to explore the effects of mPFC 5-HT$_{1A}$ and 5-HT$_{2A}$ binding on mPFC function related to the top-down regulation of amygdala reactivity. Alternative paradigms such as those involving emotion regulation or extinction of conditioned fear responses may help to determine effects of 5-HT$_{1A}$ and 5-HT$_{2A}$ signaling on related mPFC and amygdala reactivity.

BOLD fMRI and PET receptor imaging provide only indirect metrics of amygdala excitation and 5-HT receptor signaling, respectively. The small sample size in our study limited our power to model interaction effects, thus our findings must be interpreted with caution. The interpretation that our findings reflect the interactive effects of 5-HT$_{1A}$ and 5-HT$_{2A}$ receptors on glutamatergic neurons is based on evidence that 1) each of these receptors is predominantly localized to glutamatergic neurons [28,32], 2) colocalization of 5-HT$_{1A}$ and 5-HT$_{2A}$ receptors within the mPFC is predominantly observed on glutamatergic neurons [27], and 3) projections from the mPFC to the amygdala are composed of glutamatergic neurons [52,53]. Despite this, the PET technique does not allow identification of binding associated only with neurons that directly innervate the

amygdala, thus we could not confirm the causality of this association using methods currently available. Future studies examining these associations in the context of pharmacological challenge (that is, receptor-specific antagonism) could provide more direct evidence implicating the interaction between mPFC 5-HT$_{1A}$ and 5-HT$_{2A}$ receptors in mediating the effects of 5-HT signaling on threat-related amygdala reactivity.

Conclusions
Our current findings provide unique *in vivo* evidence that 5-HT receptors in the mPFC play an important role in shaping interindividual variability in threat-related amygdala reactivity. Specifically, the data reveal that mPFC 5-HT$_{1A}$ receptors effectively gate the capacity for mPFC 5-HT$_{2A}$ receptors to drive prefrontal pyramidal neuron excitability related to the regulation of threat-related amygdala reactivity. The current work further highlights the effectiveness of multimodal neuroimaging in identifying molecular signaling pathways that modulate neurobiological circuits in humans, and specifically implicates the interaction between mPFC 5-HT$_{1A}$ and 5-HT$_{2A}$ receptors in modulating the response of the human amygdala and possibly mediating the effects of altered 5-HT signaling on mood, affect and related psychopathology.

Methods
The study was approved by the institutional review board of the University of Pittsburgh, and written informed consent was obtained from all participants.

Participants
In total, 39 healthy adult volunteers participated in the study (20 men, 19 women, mean ± SD age 39.1 ± 12.7 years). Subjects were recruited through local advertisements, referrals and ongoing studies. Subjects were generally healthy. Exclusion criteria included 1) current or lifetime mood, anxiety and psychotic disorder as assessed by the Structured Clinical Interview of the fourth edition of the *Diagnostic and Statistical Manual* (DSM-I) [54], 2) family psychiatric history, 3) history of substance abuse or use of antidepressants, 4) early dementia or mild cognitive impairment according to the Mini Mental State Examination [55], 5) reversed sleep-wake cycle, 6) positive test of urine sample for drugs of abuse assessed on the day of scanning. The association between mPFC 5-HT$_{2A}$ binding and amygdala reactivity has been described previously involving a subset of this cohort (35 people) [14]. Most subjects completed the fMRI and two PET scan sessions on the same day (n = 33). Those subjects who did not complete all three scan sessions on the same day (n = 6) completed them within 1 month.

fMRI

Protocol

The experimental fMRI paradigm consisted of four blocks of a face-processing task interleaved with five blocks of a sensorimotor control task [14,15]. During the face-processing task, subjects viewed a trio of faces (expressing either anger or fear) and selected one of two faces (bottom) identical to a target face (top). Angry and fearful facial expressions can represent honest indicators of ecologically valid threat, especially that related to conspecific challengers [56]. Based on this, we interpreted the amygdala activation elicited by our task as being threat-related. Subject performance (accuracy and reaction time) was monitored during all scans.

Each sensorimotor control block consisted of six different shapes (circles and vertical and horizontal ellipses) trios. Subjects viewed a shapes trio and selected one of two shapes (bottom) identical to a target shape (top). Each of the six shape trios was presented for 4 seconds with a fixed interstimulus interval (ISI) of 2 seconds, giving a total block length of 36 seconds. Each face-processing block consisted of six face trios, balanced for gender and representing one target affect (angry or fearful) derived from a standard set of pictures of facial affect [57]. Each of the six face trios was presented for 4 seconds with a variable ISI of 2-6 seconds (mean ISI = 4 seconds) for a total block length of 48 seconds. All blocks were preceded by a brief instruction (''Match faces'' or ''Match shapes'') lasting 2 seconds. Total protocol time was 390 seconds.

As we were not interested in neural networks associated with face-specific processing *per se*, but rather in eliciting a maximal amygdala response across all subjects, we chose not to use neutral faces as control stimuli because neutral faces can be subjectively experienced as affectively laden or ambiguous, and thus engage the amygdala [58,59].

Acquisition parameters

The acquisition parameters have been described previously [14,15,60]. Briefly, each subject was scanned using a head-only scanner (GE Signa 1.5-T; GE Medical Systems, Milwaukee, WI, USA). BOLD functional images were acquired using a reverse spiral sequence covering 28 slices, each 3.8 mm thick, encompassing the entire cerebrum and most of the cerebellum (repetition time (TR) = 2000 ms, echo time (TE) = 35 ms, field of view (FOV) = 240 mm, matrix = 64 × 64, 195 whole-brain volumes acquired). The first two functional volumes acquired were discarded to allow the scanner to reach equilibrium. Scanning parameters were selected to optimize BOLD signal while maintaining enough slices to acquire whole-brain data. Before the acquisition of fMRI data for each subject, localizer scans were acquired and visually inspected for artifacts such as

ghosting, and to ensure good signal across the entire volume of acquisition. Before the acquisition of BOLD data, an auto-shimming procedure was conducted in each subject to minimize field inhomogeneities. The fMRI data for all 39 subjects included in this study were cleared of any related problems.

Data analysis

Whole-brain image analysis was completed using the general linear model (GLM) of SPM8 http://www.fil.ion. ucl.ac.uk/spm. Images for each subject were realigned to the first volume in the time series to correct for head motion, spatially normalized into a standard stereotactic space (Montreal Neurological Institute template) using a 12-parameter affine model (final resolution of functional images = 2 mm isotropic voxels), and smoothed to minimize noise and residual difference in gyral anatomy with a Gaussian filter, set at 6-mm full-width at half-maximum. Voxel-wise signal intensities were ratio-normalized to the whole-brain global mean. Preprocessed data sets were analyzed using second-level random-effects models that account for both scan-to-scan and participant-to-participant variability to determine task-specific regional responses.

Variability in single-subject whole-brain functional volumes was determined using the software program Artifact Recognition Toolbox http://www.nitrc.org/projects/artifact_detect. Individual whole-brain BOLD fMRI volumes meeting at least one of the following two criteria were excluded from determination of task-specific effects: 1) significant mean volume signal intensity variation (that is, within-volume mean signal greater or less 4 SDs of mean signal of all volumes in time series); and 2) individual volumes with scan-to-scan movement exceeding 2 mm translation or two degrees of rotation in any direction. On average, 2.1 volumes per subject were excluded because of significant variation in mean volume signal intensity (range of volumes excluded per subject = 0-17), and across all subjects, no volumes were excluded because of excessive motion. Only 1% of all volumes were excluded, thus we believe that this approach enhanced our capacity to determine task-specific effects by excluding volumes with substantial variability without compromising our power to detect task-specific effects by excluding a large number of volumes. We believe this method effectively balances the use of available functional neuroimaging data with a reasonable approach towards accounting for effects due to artifacts or movement.

After preprocessing, our GLM, employing canonical hemodynamic response functions, was used to estimate condition-specific and task-specific BOLD activation for each individual (β weights and contrast images, respectively). Individual contrast images (that is, the weighted sum of the β images) were used in second-level random-effects models to determine mean task-specific amygdala reactivity using one-sample t-tests. Group-level effects for our contrast of interest (that is, faces > shapes) were assessed within the amygdala using an ROI constructed from the WFU Pickatlas (version 1.04) [61,62].

To address the issue of multiple voxel-level comparisons, AlphaSim, a software program within AFNI http://afni.nimh.nih/gov/afni that uses a Monte Carlo simulation method, was used to determine that a voxel-wise statistical threshold of $P < 0.05$, uncorrected, combined with a cluster extent threshold of $k > 56$ voxels within our amygdala search volume was sufficiently unlikely ($\alpha < 0.05$) to have occurred by chance [63]. This threshold was used to assess our main effect of task within the amygdala. Single-subject amygdala-reactivity values for our contrast of interest were extracted from SPM8 using Marsbar (version 0.42) [64]. A sphere of 5 mm radius was centered on the voxel exhibiting the maximal response to our task across all subjects within both the right and left amygdala. Regional 5-HT receptor binding and other variables were regressed against these extracted BOLD values. Neuroimaging data are reported using the coordinate system of Talairach and Tournoux.

General PET methods

Details concerning the MR and PET imaging procedures related to both [^{11}C]WAY100635 and [^{18}F]altanserin are described below, and have also been described previously [14,15,65-67] (see previous reports for discussion about the limitations, challenges and methodological attempts to minimize potential artifacts and biases related to these radioligands [25,67-71]).

Structural MR images (GE Signa 1.5-T scanner) were acquired for each subject using a spoiled-gradient (SPGR) recalled sequence (TR = 25 ms, TE = 5 ms, FOV = 240 mm, slice thickness = 1.5 mm, matrix = 256 × 192) with parameters optimized for contrast between gray matter, white matter and cerebrospinal fluid (CSF).

Catheters were placed in an antecubital vein for radioligand injection and in a radial artery for arterial blood sampling. PET scans were acquired using a PET scanner (ECAT HR+; CTI PET systems, Knoxville, TN) in 3D imaging mode (63 transaxial planes, 2.4 mm thickness, 152 mm FOV). Head movement was minimized by use of a thermoplastic mask immobilization system. A 10 minute transmission scan (rotating ^{68}Ge/^{68}Ga rods) was acquired for attenuation correction of emission data. PET data were further corrected for dead time and scatter.

Each radioligand was administered as a slow bolus over 20 seconds. PET data acquisition and arterial blood sampling was initiated at the start of radioligand injection. The total radioactivity concentration in plasma was determined from approximately 35 0.5-ml hand-drawn blood samples collected over the scanning interval. Additional blood samples were acquired at five to six timepoints during the scan duration for determination of the fraction of the total radioactivity resulting from radiolabeled metabolites of the parent radioligand. Total plasma radioactivity concentration was corrected for radiolabeled metabolites and this 'metabolite-corrected' arterial input function was used for data analysis [69,71].

Image reconstruction was performed using filtered back-projection for a final image resolution of about 6 mm. ROIs were drawn on resliced MR images for each subject, and applied to their respective, co-registered PET images (ROIs drawn by SZ and CB). Bilateral ROIs were identified for the sgPFC, pgPFC, amygdala and cerebellum (Figure 5). The cerebellum was used as the reference region for non-displaceable radiotracer uptake (that is, free and nonspecific concentrations, V_{ND}) for both [^{11}C]WAY 100635 and [^{18}F]altanserin.

PET data for both radioligands were analyzed using the Logan graphical method [72] to obtain regional volume of distribution values (V_T). Regional V_T values were used to determine the non-displaceable binding potential, BP_{ND}, a measure of specific binding. The BP_{ND} is directly proportional to B_{avail}/K_d, where B_{avail} is the concentration of receptors available for radiotracer binding (that is, not occupied by endogenous 5-HT), and K_d is the equilibrium dissociation rate constant (that is, inversely related to binding affinity). The PET binding measures were corrected for partial volume effects that arise from atrophy-related CSF dilution using a previously validated two-component MR-based atrophy correction algorithm [66,73,74].

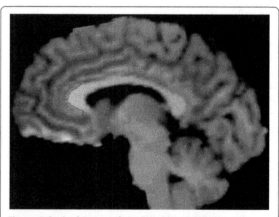

Figure 5 Sagittal image of single-subject magnetic resonance image with pgPFC (top) and sgPFC (bottom) ROIs outlined. Despite its appearance, pgPFC and sgPFC ROIs are drawn on consecutive transaxial slices. pgPFC = pregenual prefrontal cortex; ROIs = regions of interest; sgPFC = subgenual prefrontal cortex.

[^{18}F]Altanserin specific methods

The radiosynthesis of [^{18}F]altanserin was performed using a modification of the original method [75] that has been used in several studies in our laboratory [14,67,76-78]. [^{18}F]Altanserin was administered via intravenous injection (7.23 ± 0.31 mCi), and PET scanning was performed over 90 minutes. The Logan analysis regression was performed over the 12-90 minute post-injection integration intervals (10 points) to obtain regional [^{18}F]altanserin V_T and BP_{ND} values.

[^{11}C]WAY100635 specific methods

The radiosynthesis of [^{11}C]WAY 100635 was performed as previously described [79], and has been used in several previous studies in our laboratory [15,65,71]. [^{11}C]WAY100635 was administered via intravenous injection (14.01 ± 2.10 mCi), and PET scanning was performed over 90 minutes. The Logan analysis regressions were performed over the 14-90 minute post-injection integration interval (13 points) to obtain regional [^{11}C]WAY100635 V_T and BP_{ND} values.

Regression analyses

The association between threat-related amygdala reactivity and 5-HT$_{1A}$ and 5-HT$_{2A}$ binding was determined using a linear regression analysis between extracted single-subject amygdala BOLD values and ROI-specific 5-HT$_{1A}$ or 5-HT$_{2A}$ binding values in SPSS (version 17.0; SPSS Inc., Chicago, IL, USA). We previously reported within a subset of this cohort that both amygdala reactivity and mPFC 5-HT$_{2A}$ binding are inversely correlated with age [14], and this is consistent with other previous studies [76,78,80]. To account for age-related variability in these two measures, age was included as a covariate in all analyses. Consequently, plots indicate the amygdala reactivity values standardized for age effects. These values are the standardized residuals of amygdala reactivity after accounting for effects of age. This procedure was adopted to illustrate more clearly the relationship between regional 5-HT receptor binding and amygdala reactivity, independent of age. The statistics reported reflect the regression analysis results between observed BOLD and binding values including age as a covariate. As gender was not significantly correlated with our neuroimaging data, it was not included in any analyses determining the relationship between prefrontal 5-HT$_{1A}$ or 5-HT$_{2A}$ binding and amygdala reactivity.

The association of the interaction between mPFC 5-HT$_{1A}$, 5-HT$_{2A}$ binding and threat-related amygdala reactivity was determined using SPSS software and a linear regression model including 5-HT$_{1A}$ binding, 5-HT$_{2A}$ binding, age and the interaction term as covariates. Additional statistics related to the interaction effects were calculated using a previously validated approach http://www.people.ku.edu/~preacher/interact/mlr2.htm that incorporates parameters estimated from our statistical model (for example, regression coefficients, coefficient covariances) [81]. These additional statistics included simple slopes at specified 5-HT$_{1A}$ binding values, significance of simple slopes, and range of 5-HT$_{1A}$ binding values over which association between 5-HT$_{2A}$ binding and amygdala reactivity was significant.

Acknowledgements
We thank S. Ziolko, R. Coleman, S. Hulland, M. Lightfoot and A. Saul for technical assistance. We also thank the University of Pittsburgh Medical Center PET facility and Magnetic Resonance Research Center for imaging resources. We are grateful to our funding sources including the Multi-modal neuroimaging training program fellowship from the National Institute of Drug Addiction (R90 DA023420 to PMF), National Institute of Mental Health (MH067602 and MH064625 to CCM and MH072837 to ARH) and National Alliance for Research on Schizophrenia and Depression (Young Investigator Award to ARH).

Author details
^{1}Center for Neuroscience, University of Pittsburgh, Pittsburgh, Pennsylvania 15260, USA. ^{2}Center for the Neural Basis of Cognition, University of Pittsburgh, Pittsburgh, Pennsylvania 15260, USA. ^{3}Department of Radiology, University of Pittsburgh, Pittsburgh, Pennsylvania 15260, USA. ^{4}Department of Radiology, Emory University, Atlanta, Georgia 30322, USA. ^{5}Department of Psychiatry, University of Pittsburgh, Pittsburgh, Pennsylvania 15260, USA. ^{6}Department of Gynecology & Obstetrics, Emory University, Atlanta, Georgia 30322, USA. ^{7}Department of Neuroscience & Psychology, Duke University, Durham, North Carolina 27710, USA. ^{8}Institute for Genome Sciences & Policy, Duke University, Durham, North Carolina 27710, USA.

Authors' contributions
PMF designed the study, and participated in data collection, analysis and interpretation and drafting of manuscript. JCP participated in data analysis, interpretation and drafting of manuscript. CCM acquired related funding and participated in interpretation of data. ELMK acquired related funding and participated in interpretation of data. CB participated in data analysis. SLB acquired related funding. ARH designed the study, acquired related funding, and participated in data analysis, interpretation and drafting of manuscript. All authors provided comments and suggestions during manuscript preparation. All authors read and approved the final manuscript.

Competing interests
The authors declare that they have no competing interests.

References
1. Hariri AR, Drabant EM, Weinberger DR: Imaging genetics: perspectives from studies of genetically driven variation in serotonin function and corticolimbic affective processing. *Biological Psychiatry* 2006, **59**(10):888.
2. Pezawas L, Meyer-Lindenberg A, Drabant EM, Verchinski BA, Munoz KE, Kolachana BS, Egan MF, Mattay VS, Hariri AR, Weinberger DR: **5-HTTLPR polymorphism impacts human cingulate-amygdala interactions: a genetic susceptibility mechanism for depression.** *Nat Neurosci* 2005, **8**(6):828-34.
3. Phelps EA, Delgado MR, Nearing KI, LeDoux JE: **Extinction Learning in Humans: Role of the Amygdala and vmPFC.** *Neuron* 2004, **43**(6):897.
4. Quirk GJ, Mueller D: **Neural mechanisms of extinction learning and retrieval.** *Neuropsychopharmacology* 2008, **33**(1):56-72.
5. Likhtik E, Pelletier JG, Paz R, Pare D: **Prefrontal control of the amygdala.** *J Neurosci* 2005, **25**(32):7429-37.
6. Quirk GJ, Likhtik E, Pelletier JG, Pare D: **Stimulation of medial prefrontal cortex decreases the responsiveness of central amygdala output neurons.** *J Neurosci* 2003, **23**(25):8800-7.

7. Sesack SR, Deutch AY, Roth RH, Bunney BS: Topographical organization of the efferent projections of the medial prefrontal cortex in the rat: an anterograde tract-tracing study with Phaseolus vulgaris leucoagglutinin. *J Comp Neurol* 1989, 290(2):213-42.

8. Shin LM, Wright CI, Cannistraro PA, Wedig MM, McMullin K, Martis B, Macklin ML, Lasko NB, Cavanagh SR, Krangel TS, Orr SP, Pitman RK, Whalen PJ, Rauch SL: A functional magnetic resonance imaging study of amygdala and medial prefrontal cortex responses to overtly presented fearful faces in posttraumatic stress disorder. *Arch Gen Psychiatry* 2005, 62(3):273-81.

9. Fakra E, Hyde LW, Gorka A, Fisher PM, Munoz KE, Kimak M, Halder I, Ferrell RE, Manuck SB, Hariri AR: Effects of HTR1A C(-1019)G on amygdala reactivity and trait anxiety. *Arch Gen Psychiatry* 2009, 66(1):33-40.

10. Buckholtz JW, Callicott JH, Kolachana B, Hariri AR, Goldberg TE, Genderson M, Egan MF, Mattay VS, Weinberger DR, Meyer-Lindenberg A: Genetic variation in MAOA modulates ventromedial prefrontal circuitry mediating individual differences in human personality. *Mol Psychiatry* 2008, 13(3):313-24.

11. Etkin A, Klemenhagen KC, Dudman JT, Rogan MT, Hen R, Kandel ER, Hirsch J: Individual differences in trait anxiety predict the response of the basolateral amygdala to unconsciously processed fearful faces. *Neuron* 2004, 44(6):1043-55.

12. Holmes A: Genetic variation in cortico-amygdala serotonin function and risk for stress-related disease. *Neuroscience & Biobehavioral Reviews* 2008, 32(7):1293-1314.

13. Bigos KL, Pollock BG, Aizenstein HJ, Fisher PM, Bies RR, Hariri AR: Acute 5-HT reuptake blockade potentiates human amygdala reactivity. *Neuropsychopharmacology* 2008, 33(13):3221-5, Epub 2008 May 7.

14. Fisher PM, Meltzer CC, Price JC, Coleman RL, Ziolko SK, Becker C, Moses-Kolko EL, Berga SL, Hariri AR: Medial prefrontal cortex 5-HT2A density is correlated with amygdala reactivity, response habituation, and functional coupling. *Cereb Cortex* 2009, bhp022.

15. Fisher PM, Meltzer CC, Ziolko SK, Price JC, Hariri AR: Capacity for 5-HT1A-mediated autoregulation predicts amygdala reactivity. *Nature Neuroscience* 2006, 9(11):1362-3.

16. Hariri AR, Mattay VS, Tessitore A, Kolachana B, Fera F, Goldman D, Egan MF, Weinberger DR: Serotonin transporter genetic variation and the response of the human amygdala. *Science* 2002, 297(5580):400-3.

17. Heinz A, Braus DF, Smolka MN, Wrase J, Puls I, Hermann D, Klein S, Grusser SM, Flor H, Schumann G, Mann K, Buchel C: Amygdala-prefrontal coupling depends on a genetic variation of the serotonin transporter. *Nat Neurosci* 2005, 8(1):20-1.

18. Heinz A, Jones DW, Mazzanti C, Goldman D, Ragan P, Hommer D, Linnoila M, Weinberger DR: A relationship between serotonin transporter genotype and in vivo protein expression and alcohol neurotoxicity. *Biol Psychiatry* 2000, 47(7):643-9.

19. Munafo MR, Brown SM, Hariri AR: Serotonin transporter (5-HTTLPR) genotype and amygdala activation: a meta-analysis. *Biol Psychiatry* 2008, 63(9):852-7.

20. Rhodes RA, Murthy NV, Dresner MA, Selvaraj S, Stavrakakis N, Babar S, Cowen PJ, Grasby PM: Human 5-HT transporter availability predicts amygdala reactivity in vivo. *J Neurosci* 2007, 27(34):9233-9237.

21. Harmer CJ, Mackay CE, Reid CB, Cowen PJ, Goodwin GM: Antidepressant drug treatment modifies the neural processing of nonconscious threat cues. *Biological Psychiatry* 2006, 59(9):816.

22. Frokjaer VG, Mortensen EL, Nielsen FÅ, Haugbol S, Pinborg LH, Adams KH, Svarer C, Hasselbalch SG, Holm S, Paulson OB, Knudsen GM: Frontolimbic serotonin 2A receptor binding in healthy subjects is associated with personality risk factors for affective disorder. *Biological Psychiatry* 2008, 63(6):569.

23. Bhagwagar Z, Hinz R, Taylor M, Fancy S, Cowen P, Grasby P: Increased 5-HT2A receptor binding in euthymic, medication-free patients recovered from depression: a positron emission study with [11C]MDL 100,907. *Am J Psychiatry* 2006, 163(9):1580-1587.

24. Tauscher J, Bagby RM, Javanmard M, Christensen BK, Kasper S, Kapur S: Inverse relationship between serotonin 5-HT(1A) receptor binding and anxiety: a [(11)C]WAY-100635 PET investigation in healthy volunteers. *Am J Psychiatry* 2001, 158(8):1326-8.

25. Parsey RV, Olvet DM, Oquendo MA, Huang YY, Ogden RT, Mann JJ: Higher 5-HT1A receptor binding potential during a major depressive episode

predicts poor treatment response: preliminary data from a naturalistic study. *Neuropsychopharmacology* 2006, 31(8):1745-9.

26. Szewczyk B, Albert PR, Burns AM, Czesak M, Overholser JC, Jurjus GJ, Meltzer HY, Konick LC, Dieter L, Herbst N, May W, Rajkowska G, Stockmeier CA, Austin MC: Gender-specific decrease in NUDR and 5-HT1A receptor proteins in the prefrontal cortex of subjects with major depressive disorder. *Int J Neuropsychopharmacol* 2009, 12(2):155-68.

27. Amargos-Bosch M, Bortolozzi A, Puig MV, Serrats J, Adell A, Celada P, Toth M, Mengod G, Artigas F: Co-expression and in vivo interaction of serotonin1A and serotonin2A receptors in pyramidal neurons of prefrontal cortex. *Cereb Cortex* 2004, 14(3):281-99.

28. Jakab RL, Goldman-Rakic PS: 5-Hydroxytryptamine2A serotonin receptors in the primate cerebral cortex: possible site of action of hallucinogenic and antipsychotic drugs in pyramidal cell apical dendrites. *Proceedings of the National Academy of Sciences of the United States of America* 1998, 95(2):735-40.

29. de Almeida J, Mengod G: Quantitative analysis of glutamatergic and GABAergic neurons expressing 5-HT2A receptors in human and monkey prefrontal cortex. *Journal of Neurochemistry* 2007, 103(2):475-486.

30. Puig MV, Artigas F, Celada P: Modulation of the activity of pyramidal neurons in rat prefrontal cortex by raphe stimulation in vivo: involvement of serotonin and GABA. *Cereb Cortex* 2005, 15(1):1-14.

31. Azmitia EC, Gannon PJ, Kheck NM, Whitaker-Azmitia PM: Cellular localization of the 5-HT1A receptor in primate brain neurons and glial cells. *Neuropsychopharmacology* 1996, 14(1):35-46.

32. Cruz DA, Eggan SM, Azmitia EC, Lewis DA: Serotonin1A receptors at the axon initial segment of prefrontal pyramidal neurons in schizophrenia. *Am J Psychiatry* 2004, 161(4):739-42.

33. de Almeida J, Mengod G: Serotonin 1A receptors in human and monkey prefrontal cortex are mainly expressed in pyramidal neurons and in a GABAergic interneuron subpopulation: implications for schizophrenia and its treatment. *J Neurochem* 2008, 107(2):488-96.

34. Miner LAH, Backstrom JR, Sanders-Bush E, Sesack SR: Ultrastructural localization of serotonin2A receptors in the middle layers of the rat prelimbic prefrontal cortex. *Neuroscience* 2003, 116(1):107.

35. Puig MV, Celada P, Diaz-Mataix L, Artigas F: In vivo modulation of the activity of pyramidal neurons in the rat medial prefrontal cortex by 5-HT2A receptors: relationship to thalamocortical afferents. *Cereb Cortex* 2003, 13(8):870-82.

36. Hariri AR, Drabant EM, Munoz KE, Kolachana BS, Mattay VS, Egan MF, Weinberger DR: A susceptibility gene for affective disorders and the response of the human amygdala. *Arch Gen Psychiatry* 2005, 62(2):146-52.

37. Hariri AR, Tessitore A, Mattay VS, Fera F, Weinberger DR: The amygdala response to emotional stimuli: a comparison of faces and scenes. *Neuroimage* 2002, 17(1):317-23.

38. Barbas H: Anatomic basis of cognitive-emotional interactions in the primate prefrontal cortex. *Neurosci Biobehav Rev* 1995, 19(3):499-510.

39. Kim MJ, Whalen PJ: The structural integrity of an amygdala-prefrontal pathway predicts trait anxiety. *J Neurosci* 2009, 29(37):11614-8.

40. Besson C, Louilot A: Asymmetrical involvement of mesolimbic dopaminergic neurons in affective perception. *Neuroscience* 1995, 68(4):963-8.

41. Merali Z, McIntosh J, Anisman H: Anticipatory cues differentially provoke in vivo peptidergic and monoaminergic release at the medial prefrontal cortex. *Neuropsychopharmacology* 2004, 29(8):1409-18.

42. Sullivan RM, Dufresne MM: Mesocortical dopamine and HPA axis regulation: role of laterality and early environment. *Brain Res* 2006, 1076(1):49-59.

43. Young EJ, Williams CL: Valence dependent asymmetric release of norepinephrine in the basolateral amygdala. *Behav Neurosci* 2010, 124(5):633-44.

44. Christianson JP, Ragole T, Amat J, Greenwood BN, Strong PV, Paul ED, Fleshner M, Watkins LR, Maier SF: 5-Hydroxytryptamine 2C receptors in the basolateral amygdala are involved in the expression of anxiety after uncontrollable traumatic stress. *Biological Psychiatry* 2010, 67(4):339-345.

45. Kia HK, Miquel MC, Brisorgueil MJ, Daval G, Riad M, El Mestikawy S, Hamon M, Verge D: Immunocytochemical localization of serotonin1A receptors in the rat central nervous system. *J Comp Neurol* 1996, 365(2):289-305.

46. Barnes NM, Sharp T: A review of central 5-HT receptors and their function. *Neuropharmacology* 1999, 38(8):1083.

47. McDonald AJ, Mascagni F: Neuronal localization of 5-HT type 2A receptor immunoreactivity in the rat basolateral amygdala. *Neuroscience* 2007, 146(1):306.

48. Aznar S, Qian Z, Shah R, Rahbek B, Knudsen GM: The 5-HT1A serotonin receptor is located on calbindin- and parvalbumin-containing neurons in the rat brain. *Brain Research* 2003, 959(1):58.

49. Burghardt NS, Bush DEA, McEwen BS, LeDoux JE: Acute selective serotonin reuptake inhibitors increase conditioned fear expression: blockade with a 5-HT2C receptor antagonist. *Biological Psychiatry* 2007, 62(10):1111.

50. Bhatnagar S, Sun LM, Raber J, Maren S, Julius D, Dallman MF: Changes in anxiety-related behaviors and hypothalamic-pituitary-adrenal activity in mice lacking the 5-HT-3A receptor. *Physiol Behav* 2004, 81(4):545-55.

51. Clark MS, Vincow ES, Sexton TJ, Neumaier JF: Increased expression of 5-HT1B receptor in dorsal raphe nucleus decreases fear-potentiated startle in a stress dependent manner. *Brain Res* 2004, 1007(1-2):86-97.

52. Smith Y, Pare JF, Pare D: Differential innervation of parvalbumin-immunoreactive interneurons of the basolateral amygdaloid complex by cortical and intrinsic inputs. *Journal of Comparative Neurology* 2000, 416(4):496-508.

53. Ghashghaei HT, Barbas H: Pathways for emotion: interactions of prefrontal and anterior temporal pathways in the amygdala of the rhesus monkey. *Neuroscience* 2002, 115(4):1261-79.

54. First MB, Spitzer RL, Gibbon M, Williams JBM: *Structured Clinical Interview for DSM-IV Axis I Disorders: Research Version, Non-Patient Edition* 1996.

55. Folstein MF, Folstein SE, McHugh PR: "Mini-mental state". A practical method for grading the cognitive state of patients for the clinician. *Journal of Psychiatric Research* 1975, 12(3):189-98.

56. Darwin C, Ekman P: In *The expression of the emotions in man and animals. Volume xxxvi..* 3 edition. New York: Oxford University Press; 1998:472.

57. Ekman P, Friesen WV: *Pictures of Facial Affect* Palo Alto: Consulting Psychologists Press; 1976.

58. Schwartz CE, Wright CI, Shin LM, Kagan J, Rauch SL: Inhibited and uninhibited infants "grown up": adult amygdalar response to novelty. *Science* 2003, 300(5627):1952-3.

59. Wright CI, Martis B, Schwartz CE, Shin LM, Fischer HH, McMullin K, Rauch SL: Novelty responses and differential effects of order in the amygdala, substantia innominata, and inferior temporal cortex. *Neuroimage* 2003, 18(3):660-9.

60. Schwartz CE, Wright CI, Shin LM, Kagan J, Whalen PJ, McMullin KG, Rauch SL: Differential amygdalar response to novel versus newly familiar neutral faces: a functional MRI probe developed for studying inhibited temperament. *Biol Psychiatry* 2003, 53(10):854-62.

61. Lancaster JL, Woldorff MG, Parsons LM, Liotti M, Freitas CS, Rainey L, Kochunov PV, Nickerson D, Mikiten SA, Fox PT: Automated Talairach atlas labels for functional brain mapping. *Hum Brain Mapp* 2000, 10(3):120-31.

62. Maldjian JA, Laurienti PJ, Kraft RA, Burdette JH: An automated method for neuroanatomic and cytoarchitectonic atlas-based interrogation of fMRI data sets. *Neuroimage* 2003, 19(3):1233-9.

63. Forman SD, Cohen JD, Fitzgerald M, Eddy WF, Mintun MA, Noll DC: Improved assessment of significant activation in functional magnetic resonance imaging (fMRI): use of a cluster-size threshold. *Magnetic Resonance in Medicine* 1995, 33(5):636-647.

64. Brett M, Anton J, Valabregue R, Poline J: Region of interest analysis using an SPM toolbox. *NeuroImage* 2002, 16(2):S497.

65. Bailer UF, Frank GK, Henry SE, Price JC, Meltzer CC, Mathis CA, Wagner A, Thornton L, Hoge J, Ziolko SK, Becker CR, McConaha CW, Kaye WH: Exaggerated 5-HT1A but normal 5-HT2A receptor activity in individuals ill with anorexia nervosa. *Biological Psychiatry* 2007, 61(9):1090.

66. Cidis Meltzer C, Drevets WC, Price JC, Mathis CA, Lopresti B, Greer PJ, Villemagne VL, Holt D, Mason NS, Houck PR, Reynolds CF, DeKosky ST: Gender-specific aging effects on the serotonin 1A receptor. *Brain Research* 2001, 895(1-2):9-17.

67. Soloff PH, Price JC, Mason NS, Becker C, Meltzer CC: Gender, personality, and serotonin-2A receptor binding in healthy subjects. *Psychiatry Res* 2010, 181(1):77-84.

68. Price JC, Lopresti BJ, Mason NS, Holt DP, Huang Y, Mathis CA: Analyses of [18F]altanserin bolus injection PET data. I. Consideration of radiolabeled metabolites in baboons. *Synapse* 2001, 41(1):1-10.

69. Price JC, Lopresti BJ, Meltzer CC, Smith GS, Mason NS, Huang Y, Holt DP, Gunn RN, Mathis CA: Analyses of [18F]altanserin bolus injection PET data.

70. Parsey RV, Slifstein M, Hwang DR, Abi-Dargham A, Simpson N, Mawlawi O, Guo NN, Van Heertum R, Mann JJ, Laruelle M: Validation and reproducibility of measurement of 5-HT1A receptor parameters with [carbonyl-11C]WAY-100635 in humans: comparison of arterial and reference tisssue input functions. *J Cereb Blood Flow Metab* 2000, 20(7):1111-33.

71. Meltzer CC, Price JC, Mathis CA, Butters MA, Ziolko SK, Moses-Kolko E, Mazumdar S, Mulsant BH, Houck PR, Lopresti BJ, Weissfeld LA, Reynolds CF: Serotonin 1A receptor binding and treatment response in late-life depression. *Neuropsychopharmacology* 2004, 29(12):2258-65.

72. Logan J, Fowler JS, Volkow ND, Wolf AP, Dewey SL, Schlyer DJ, MacGregor RR, Hitzemann R, Bendriem B, Gatley SJ, et al: Graphical analysis of reversible radioligand binding from time-activity measurements applied to [N-11C-methyl]-(-)-cocaine PET studies in human subjects. *Journal of Cerebral Blood Flow & Metabolism* 1990, 10(5):740-7.

73. Meltzer CC, Kinahan PE, Greer PJ, Nichols TE, Comtat C, Cantwell MN, Lin MP, Price JC: Comparative evaluation of MR-based partial-volume correction schemes for PET. *Journal of Nuclear Medicine* 1999, 40(12):2053-65.

74. Meltzer CC, Leal JP, Mayberg HS, Wagner HN Jr, Frost JJ: Correction of PET data for partial volume effects in human cerebral cortex by MR imaging. *Journal of Computer Assisted Tomography* 1990, 14(4):561-70.

75. Lemaire C, Cantineau R, Guillaume M, Plenevaux A, Christiaens L: Fluorine-18-Altanserin: A Radioligand for the Study of Serotonin Receptors with PET: Radiolabeling and In Vivo Biologic Behavior in Rats. *J Nucl Med* 1991, 32(12):2266-2272.

76. Meltzer CC, Smith G, Price JC, Reynolds CF, Mathis CA, Greer P, Lopresti B, Mintun MA, Pollock BG, Ben-Eliezer D, Cantwell MN, Kaye W, DeKosky ST: Reduced binding of altanserin to serotonin type 2A receptors in aging: persistence of effect after partial volume correction. *Brain Research* 1998, 813(1):167.

77. Smith GS, Price JC, Lopresti BJ, Huang Y, Simpson N, Holt D, Mason NS, Meltzer CC, Sweet RA, Nichols T, Sashin D, Mathis CA: Test-retest variability of serotonin 5-HT2A receptor binding measured with positron emission tomography and [18F]altanserin in the human brain. *Synapse* 1998, 30(4):380-392.

78. Bailer UF, Price JC, Meltzer CC, Mathis CA, Frank GK, Weissfeld L, McConaha CW, Henry SE, Brooks-Achenbach S, Barbarich NC, Kaye WH: Altered 5-HT(2A) receptor binding after recovery from bulimia-type anorexia nervosa: relationships to harm avoidance and drive for thinness. *Neuropsychopharmacology* 2004, 29(6):1143-55.

79. McCarron JA, Turton DR, Pike VW, Poole KG: Remotely-controlled production of the 5-HT(1A) receptor radioligand, [carbonyl-11C]WAY-100635, via 11C-carboxylation of an immobilized Grignard reagent. *Journal of Labelled Compounds and Radiopharmaceuticals* 1996, 38(10):941.

80. Tessitore A, Hariri AR, Fera F, Smith WG, Das S, Weinberger DR, Mattay VS: Functional changes in the activity of brain regions underlying emotion processing in the elderly. *Psychiatry Research: Neuroimaging* 2005, 139(1):9.

81. Preacher KJ, Curran PJ, Bauer DJ: Computational tool for probing interaction effects in multiple linear regression, multilevel modeling, and latent curve analysis. *Journal of Educational and Behavioral Statistics* 2006, 31(4):437-448.

Social stimulation and corticolimbic reactivity in premenstrual dysphoric disorder: a preliminary study

Malin Gingnell[1,2*], Victoria Ahlstedt[1], Elin Bannbers[1], Johan Wikström[3], Inger Sundström-Poromaa[1†] and Mats Fredrikson[2†]

Abstract

Background: Premenstrual dysphoric disorder (PMDD), characterized by luteal phase-induced negative affect and loss of impulse control, often results in compromised social interactions. Although amygdala activation is generally linked to negative affect, increased amygdala reactivity to aversive stimuli in the luteal phase has not been consistently reported in PMDD. We tested the hypothesis that amygdala hyper-reactivity in PMDD is symptom specific, rather than generalized, and linked to socially relevant stimuli. Blood oxygenation level dependent signal changes during exposure to negative images with social and non-social content were evaluated in the mid-follicular and late luteal phase of the menstrual cycle. Fourteen women with PMDD and 13 healthy controls participated.

Results: When compared with healthy controls, women with PMDD in the luteal phase had enhanced reactivity to social stimuli compared to non-social stimuli in the amygdala and insula, but attenuated reactivity in the anterior cingulate cortex. Functional couplings between emotion processing and controlling areas were significantly different, being positive in women with PMDD and negative in healthy controls. Changes in progesterone levels in women with PMDD correlated positively with altered amygdala reactivity.

Conclusions: Socially relevant aversive stimulation elicited enhanced activity in affective processing brain regions that were functionally coupled to compromised activity in cognitive control areas. Because increased reactivity correlated positively with alterations in ovarian steroid levels, data preliminary support the hypothesis that enhanced progesterone sensitivity in PMDD affects corticolimbic processing of social emotions.

Background

Premenstrual dysphoric disorder (PMDD), characterized by luteal phase-induced anxious and depressive symptoms as well as emotional lability [1], affects around 5% of women of reproductive age [2]. The symptomatology compromises quality of life, including social interactions [3]. Because the core symptoms of PMDD are affective in nature, it has been suggested that brain areas in the fear circuit [4], particularly the amygdala, mediate PMDD symptoms [5]. The amygdala, insula and anterior cingulate cortex (ACC) form a hypothesized corticolimbic emotion processing network [4,6], with the amygdala and insula activated by bottom-up emotional processes, and the ACC involved in top-down regulation [4,7]. Although increased amygdala reactivity characterizes negative affective states like anxiety and depression [8-15], studies on amygdala reactivity in PMDD are inconsistent [16-18]. Protopopescu et al. [16] reported increased amygdala reactivity in response to emotional words, but their results reflected alterations in reactivity over the menstrual cycle in healthy controls rather than in women with PMDD. Gingnell et al. [17] also reported a luteal phase-induced increase in amygdala reactivity to emotional faces, but only among a subgroup of patients with PMDD with high trait anxiety [17]. Furthermore, Gingnell et al. [18] observed increased reactivity to negative emotional stimuli in the amygdala and insula, but no differences between patients and controls and with no menstrual phase modulation.

* Correspondence: malin.gingnell@psyk.uu.se
†Equal contributors
[1]Department of Women's and Children's Health, Uppsala University, Uppsala, Sweden
[2]Department of Psychology, Uppsala University, Uppsala, Sweden
Full list of author information is available at the end of the article

Some anxiety disorders are characterized by a generally altered emotional reactivity. In post-traumatic stress disorder (PTSD), for example, increased amygdala reactivity and decreased activity in emotion controlling areas is observed not only in response to trauma-related challenge but also to non-symptomatic stimulation such as aversive emotional faces, even outside awareness [19-21]. By contrast, in other disorders like specific phobia, amygdala hyper-reactivity is circumscribed to phobic cues and absent in response to other emotionally relevant situations [22]. It has not been determined if amygdala reactivity in women with PMDD reflects a generally altered emotional responsivity or whether exaggerated amygdala reactivity is specific to symptomatic challenges. PMDD symptoms compromise everyday social functions both at work and at home, resulting in frequent reports of disrupted interpersonal interactions [23]. Although it is uncertain if partner violence is a significant risk factor for PMDD [24-26], both women with a history of trauma and with PTSD are more likely to experience PMDD, especially when trauma exposure involves interpersonal violence [27,28]. In addition, women with PMDD with a history of trauma have abnormal neuroendocrine stress responses compared to women with PMDD without a trauma history [24-26,29].

Because PMDD symptoms affect social interactions and perceived social threat might be crucial for the development of the disorder, it is conceivable that enhanced amygdala reactivity is elicited mainly by socially relevant stimuli. Emotional words and general emotional stimuli [16,17] might not tap into PMDD symptomatology, and therefore not increase amygdala reactivity. If so, mixing generally emotion-arousing stimulation with more focused symptomatic challenges may produce inconsistent results, such as those previously reported [16-18]. Furthermore, even though the amygdala has a key role in anxiety and negative affect, both theoretical reasoning [30] and empirical results [8,15] support that other areas in the fear circuit [4], such as the insula, and cognitive control areas, like the ACC, are involved in emotional processing.

We hypothesized that socially relevant stimulation is a prime elicitor of negative affect in PMDD, reflected in corticolimbic circuit functions with increased brain reactivity in the affective processing regions of the amygdala and insula [4,6-8,15,30], as well as decreased reactivity in the regulatory ACC region [31] and an altered functional coupling between the processing and regulatory areas [31]. Because PMDD symptoms include negative emotional symptoms that are experienced in the luteal but not the follicular phase of the menstrual cycle, altered reactivity and connectivity should be evident predominantly in the luteal phase and possibly coupled to variations in ovarian steroid hormones [5,32]. This hypothesis was tested by evaluating brain reactivity and connectivity using

functional magnetic resonance imaging (fMRI) of blood oxygenation level-dependent (BOLD) activity to social and non-social negative stimuli in the follicular and luteal phase of the menstrual cycle in women with PMDD and healthy controls. We also explored if ovarian steroid hormones correlated with corticolimbic circuit functions.

Methods
We re-analyzed data from a study including social and non-social aversive emotional pictures [18]. The original paradigm included exposure to emotional images of negative or positive valence. All emotional-image slides were proceeded either by a red cue, signaling negative affect, or a green, associated with positive pictures. The timing was such that the color cue was displayed 5 s before a 2 s exposure of the social slide, and followed by a 2.5 to 3.5 s black screen with a inter-trial interval of 9 to 11 seconds.

The emotional stimuli, 15 negative and 15 positive pictures, were selected from the International Affective Pictures System (IAPS) [33]. For an example of the paradigm see Additional file 1. We analyzed BOLD responses to socially relevant and irrelevant negative emotional stimuli. Negative stimuli were chosen because PMDD mainly comprises negative emotional symptoms [1].

Participants
Seventeen women with PMDD and 16 asymptomatic controls were recruited through a newspaper advertisement and from women with a PMDD diagnosis.

PMDD was diagnosed according to the definitions in the Diagnostic and Statistical Manual of Mental Disorders IV [1]. Details of the diagnostic procedure have been described previously [34]. Briefly, prospective ratings of daily symptoms using the Cyclicity Diagnoser (CD-scale) were completed to confirm the presence of PMDD and to estimate the severity of PMDD symptoms. The number of days during the 10 days before menses when participants reported a score of 2 or more on the CD-scale for each of the the four core symptoms of PMDD (irritability, depression, anxiety and mood swings) (i.e. a scale 0–40) [35], and number of days when social interaction was avoided (0 to 10) were used as measures of PMDD severity. The asymptomatic controls were physically healthy women with regular menstrual cycles and no history of premenstrual dysphoric symptoms. None of the controls reported premenstrual dysphoric symptoms on daily ratings. The study was approved by the Ethical Review Board of Uppsala, Sweden, and all participants gave written informed consent.

Exclusion criteria were pregnancy; treatment with hormonal compounds or psychotropic drugs; or presence of any ongoing psychiatric disorder. Absence of other psychiatric disorders was confirmed using the structured psychiatric interview, Mini International Neuropsychiatry

Interview [36]. Furthermore, participants with pacemakers, cardiac defibrillators, aneurysm clips, cochlear implants or other implants including magnets, batteries or wires were excluded. One woman with PMDD and one healthy control dropped out after the first scanning session due to personal reasons, and two healthy controls and three women with PMDD were excluded due to movement artifacts (peaks of movement in the x/y/z-axis of more than 3 mm or more than 2 degrees of rotation), or incomplete scanning sessions due to hardware problems. There were no significant differences in demographic or behavioral data between excluded and remaining participants. Fourteen women with PMDD and 13 healthy controls were analyzed.

Timing according to the menstrual cycle

fMRI scanning was performed twice, once in the mid-follicular phase (6 to 12 days after the onset of menstrual bleeding) and once to coincide with the late luteal phase (postovulatory day 8 to 13), according to a positive luteinizing hormone assay (Clearplan, Unipath, Bedford, UK). Monitoring of the luteal phase was confirmed by progesterone serum concentrations and records of the next menstrual bleeding. The study was counterbalanced across the menstrual cycle with half of the participants scanned first in the follicular phase and then in the luteal phase, and the other half scanned in the reverse order.

Hormonal analyses

Blood samples were drawn before each scanning. Estradiol and progesterone serum concentrations were determined by competitive immunometric electrochemistry luminescence detection at the Department of Clinical Chemistry, Uppsala University Hospital. The samples were run on a Roche Cobas e601 with Cobas Elecsys reagent kits (Roche Diagnostics, Bromma, Sweden). The measurement interval was 0.1 to 191 nmol/l for progesterone and 18.4 to 15,781 pmol/l for estradiol. The progesterone intra-assay coefficient of variation was 2.21% at 2.39 nmol/l and 2.82% at 31.56 nmol/l. The estradiol intra-assay coefficient of variation was 6.8% at 85.5 pmol/l and 2.8% at 1,640 pmol/l.

Mood and anxiety scales

Prior to each fMRI scan, participants completed the self-rated version of the Montgomery-Åsberg Depression Rating Scale (MADRS-S) [37] and the state portion of the Spielberger State-Trait Anxiety Inventory (STAI-S) [38].

Functional magnetic resonance imaging - scans and paradigm

fMRI was performed using a 3 T whole body scanner (Achieva 3 T X Philips scanner Philips Medical Systems, Best, The Netherlands) equipped with an eight-channel head coil. At the beginning of each scanning session, an anatomical T_1-weighted reference data set to a voxel size of $0.8 \times 1.0 \times 2.0$ mm^3 and 60 slices were acquired. During stimulus presentations, BOLD imaging was performed using a single shot echo-planar imaging sequence with parameters echo time/repetition time 35/3,000 ms, flip angle 90°, acquisition matrix 76×77, acquired voxel size $3.0 \times 3.0 \times 3.0$ mm^3 and 30 slices.

The participants lay facing upwards in the scanner with their heads lightly fixated. Visual stimuli were presented through goggles mounted on the head coil (VisualSystem, NordicNeuroLab, Bergen, Norway). The stimulus paradigm was implemented using the commercial software package E-prime (Psychology Software Tools, Sharpsburg, PA, USA). To synchronize the paradigm and the MR sequence, a SyncBox (NordicNeuroLab) was used. The paradigm included 15 negative pictures selected from the IAPS [33] preceded by a color cue indicating the valence. We compared the eight slides displaying negative social situations (for example, injured humans, abduction of a young female; IAPS: 3320, 2710, 3051, 3160, 6312, 6570, 8230, 9042) with the seven pictures containing negative, but non-social stimuli (for example, snakes, threatening dogs; IAPS: 1050, 1052, 1111, 1201, 1274, 1525, 9620). After scanning, participants again viewed and rated pictures for valence and arousal using the Self-Assessment Manikin used in the IAPS material [33]. Arousal ratings are available in Additional file 2 but are not included here, as we did not test any arousal-related hypotheses. The valence ratings for social and non-social stimuli were analyzed in a Group by Phase analysis of variance, with additional follow-up t-tests.

Functional magnetic resonance imaging - preprocessing and analysis

The Digital Imaging and Communications in Medicine images from the scanner were converted to Neuroimaging Informatics Technology Initiative files using the freeware package MRicron [39]. The data were then analyzed in MatLab (MathWorks, Natick, MA, USA) using SPM5 [40]. The individual BOLD images were realigned to a mean image for the session, slice timed to the middle slice of each whole brain volume, co-registered with the individual anatomic scan, normalized into Montreal Neurological Institute (MNI) coordinates space using normalization parameters obtained from a segmentation into the white matter, grey matter and cerebrospinal fluid of the individual anatomical scan, and smoothing was performed using an 8 mm kernel.

For each individual, BOLD signal changes in the fMRI time series were regressed on to social and non-social negative images. Onsets and durations for stimuli included in the paradigm but not analyzed in the present study (that is, anticipatory periods, positive emotional stimuli) and the six movement parameters obtained in the realignment step were included in the model. Contrast maps were calculated for each individual of the contrast between social and non-social negative images. These contrast maps were then used for group comparisons. Analyses of group differences were first performed to compare women with PMDD and healthy controls during the luteal phase. Regions of interest (ROIs) were generated using the automatic anatomical labeling definitions in the Wake Forest University School of Medicine PickAtlas [41-43] and included the bilateral amygdala, insula and ACC. Then, a ROI defined by the group differences observed in the luteal phase was used for between-group comparisons in the follicular phase and for within-group comparisons between phases. To test the *a priori* hypothesis of increased reactivity in the amygdala and insula as well as attenuated reactivity in the ACC in PMDD during the luteal phase, an uncorrected p-value of 0.05 with $k \geq 5$, corrected for the search volume of each ROI, was used. Functional couplings during the luteal phase between the amygdala and the insula, respectively, to the ACC, were evaluated with extracted data from the significant clusters, as defined by the between-participants effects in the luteal phase, used as seeds for correlations. These analyses were performed in each group separately. The relatively lenient statistical threshold was deliberately chosen as we restricted analyses only to ROIs where specific hypotheses were advanced. This approach does not only focus on type I errors but also gives a balance between type I and type II errors [44,45].

Self-reports and affective picture ratings were compared by paired and independent t-tests, respectively. Estradiol and progesterone levels were compared using Mann-Whitney U test and Wilcoxon signed rank tests, respectively. Symptom severity and number of days when social interaction was avoided were evaluated using Student's t-tests. In addition, partial correlations adjusted for affective ratings were performed between alterations in brain reactivity and change in ovarian steroid hormone levels (follicular to luteal phase) to evaluate if brain activity was tied primarily to changes in hormonal activity or subjective ratings.

Results
Demographics and hormonal results
No significant group differences emerged for age (PMDD 35.0 ± 8.9 years; healthy controls 33.1 ± 7.8 years; $t(25) = 0.6$; $p = 0.56$), day of testing in the follicular phase (PMDD 8.5 ± 1.9; healthy controls 10.1 ± 3.5; $t(25) = 1.8$; $p = 0.084$), or luteal phase (PMDD -4.6 ± 3.8, healthy controls -4.4 ± 2.7; $t(25) = 0.35$; $p = 0.73$). Similarly, hormonal levels did not differ between groups for follicular phase progesterone ($U = 52.5$, $p = 0.062$), luteal phase progesterone ($U = 68.0$, $p = 0.28$), follicular phase estradiol ($U = 75.0$, $z = -0.77$, $p = 0.44$) and luteal phase estradiol ($U = 77.5$, $z = -0.66$, $p = 0.51$). Estradiol levels were similar in the follicular

and luteal phase in both groups (for both groups $Z < 0.87$, $p > 0.38$). However, progesterone increased significantly from the follicular to the luteal phase in both groups (healthy controls $Z = 2.9$, $p = 0.004$; and PMDD $Z = 3.3$; $p = 0.001$; Figure 1).

Behavioral results
Women with PMDD had higher MADRS-S and STAI-S scores during the luteal compared to the follicular phase ($t(13) = 2.7$, $p = 0.017$ and $t(13) = 2.5$, $p = 0.027$, respectively) whereas in healthy controls luteal phase ratings did not differ from the follicular phase (for both measures $t(13) < 1.1$, $p > 0.27$). When compared to healthy controls, women with PMDD scored higher on MADRS-S ($t(25) = 5.4$, $p < 0.0001$) and STAI-S ($t(25) = 5.7$, $p < 0.0001$) in the luteal phase but not in the follicular phase (for both measures $t(25) < 1.8$, $p > 0.078$; Figure 2). Women with PMDD had a symptom severity of 27.9 ± 2.3 (range 0 to 40) [35] and avoided social interaction during 5.1 ± 1.0 out of 10 premenstrual days. Corresponding values for healthy controls were 8.1 ± 2.5 and 1.3 ± 0.6, respectively. The group differences were statistically significant for both measures (symptom severity: $t(25) = 5.6$, $p < 0.0001$; avoiding social interaction: $t(25) = 3.2$, $p = 0.003$.

For valence ratings, the only significant difference was found for ratings of social stimuli in the luteal phase ($F = 6.62$, $p = 0.017$). Women with PMDD rated the social images significantly more negative than healthy controls during the luteal phase ($t(24) = 2.5$, $p = 0.021$; Figure 3) but not in the follicular phase ($t(25) = 1.2$, $p = 0.24$). Also, women with PMDD rated the social stimuli as more negative than the non-social stimuli both in the follicular ($t(13) = 3.4$, $p = 0.005$) and the luteal phase ($t(13) = 4.3$, $p = 0.001$; Figure 3), whereas healthy controls gave similar ratings for social and non-social stimuli during both phases (both phases $t(13) < 1.6$, $p > 0.14$). Arousal ratings are available in the Additional file 2: Table S1.

Brain results
Between group comparisons of reactivity
During the luteal phase, women with PMDD had higher reactivity to social stimuli than healthy controls in the amygdala (-21, 2, -15; $k = 11$; $z = 2.18$; $p = 0.015$) and insula (45, -9, -2; $k = 10$; $z = 2.13$; $p = 0.016$), but lower reactivity in the ACC (two clusters: 9, 33, 23; $k = 12$; $z = 2.22$; $p = 0.013$; and 3, 50, 11; $k = 27$; $z = 3.23$; $p = 0.001$) (Figure 4). No group differences were observed in the follicular phase. The contrast between non-social and social images revealed no group differences in either phase.

Within group comparisons of reactivity
In women with PMDD, There was higher amygdala reactivity to social than non-social stimuli in the luteal as compared to the follicular phase (-21, 2, -15; $k = 5$;

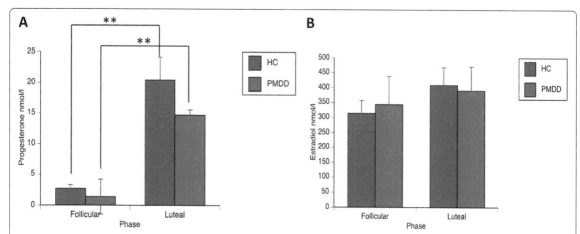

Figure 1 Hormone levels. (A) Progesterone and **(B)** estradiol levels in women with PMDD and healthy controls during the follicular and luteal phase of the menstrual cycle. In both groups, progesterone increased significantly in the luteal phase whereas estradiol was similar across phases. No significant group differences emerged in either phase. *******p* <0.001. HC, healthy controls; PMDD, premenstrual dysphoric disorder.

z = 1.94; *p* = 0.015). No phase differences were observed in healthy controls.

Connectivity
Connectivity analyses revealed a pattern of positive connectivity between BOLD reactivity in emotion processing and controlling areas in PMDD (amygdala and ACC: 6, 45, 23; k = 5; z = 2.39; *p* = 0.008; and insula and ACC: 9, 33, 23; k = 6; z = 2.62; *p* = 0.004) whereas there was a trend towards a negative relation between the ACC and insula in healthy controls (6, 33, 23; k = 1; z = 1.74; *p* = 0.041). The pattern was identical when three outliers in BOLD reactivity (>2 SD from mean of group) were removed

(Figure 5). The correlation strength between the insula and the ACC differed significantly between PMDD and healthy controls (z = 2.99; *p* = 0.0027).

Correlations with brain reactivity, ovarian steroids and affective ratings
For women with PMDD, the phase-related increase in amygdala reactivity to social as compared to non-social stimuli correlated positively with the corresponding change in progesterone level (r_{xy} = 0.61, *P* = 0.020). When partializing out the valence ratings, the correlation between progesterone and amygdala remained (r_{xy} = 0.63, *P* = 0.020).

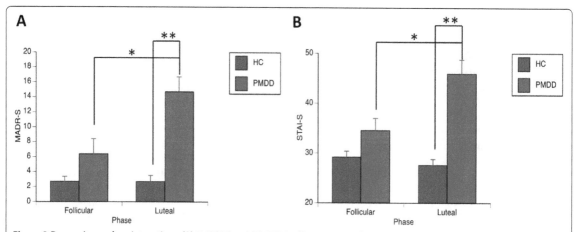

Figure 2 Depression and anxiety ratings. (A) MADRS-S and **(B)** STAI-S self-report ratings for women with PMDD and healthy controls during the follicular and luteal phase of the menstrual cycle. Women with PMDD had higher scores than healthy controls during the luteal phase and higher in the luteal than the follicular phase. No significant group differences were present in the follicular phase or for healthy controls between phases. ******p* <0.05; *******p* <0.001. MADRS-S, Montgomery-Åsberg Depression Rating Scale - self-rated version; STAI-S, State-Trait Anxiety Inventory - self-rated version PMDD, premenstrual dysphoric disorder; HC, healthy controls.

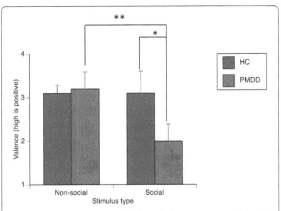

Figure 3 Valence ratings in the luteal phase. Women with PMDD rated images with social content as more negatively valenced than images with a non-social content, and rated social stimuli as more negative than did healthy controls. There were no group differences for ratings of non-social stimuli. *p <0.05, **p <0.001. HC, healthy controls; PMDD, premenstrual dysphoric disorder.

Discussion

We tested the hypothesis that women with PMDD are overly sensitive to negative social stimulation rather than generally affected by negative emotional stimuli and that this would be reflected in altered corticolimbic processing. Subjective reports confirmed an anxious and depressive state of mind, and sensitivity to social stimulation, in women with PMDD during the luteal phase. The negative feeling state was coupled to exaggerated reactivity in the amygdala and insula and attenuated reactivity in ACC regions projecting to the amygdala [46]. Amygdala reactivity was also higher in the luteal than the follicular phase. Collectively, data preliminary support the hypothesis that increased sensitivity to social stimulation characterizes PMDD and that corticolimbic circuit activity is altered more by socially relevant than irrelevant stimuli. Thus, previous inconsistent results on amygdala reactivity in PMDD [16-18] may reflect the use of a mixture of social and non-social stimuli.

The connectivity pattern must be regarded as preliminary due to the small sample size. Previous studies have reported functional couplings between the amygdala and the ACC [46] as well as between the ACC and insula [47,48]. The theoretically predicted negative functional couplings with enhanced reactivity in emotion processing areas associated with reduced reactivity in emotion regulating areas [31], consistent with top-down emotional control, was observed in healthy controls. By contrast, and in line with the hypothesis, women with PMDD displayed an aberrant connectivity pattern with positive couplings between both amygdala and insula reactivity on the one hand and ACC on the other, indicating the primacy of bottom-up processes. In social

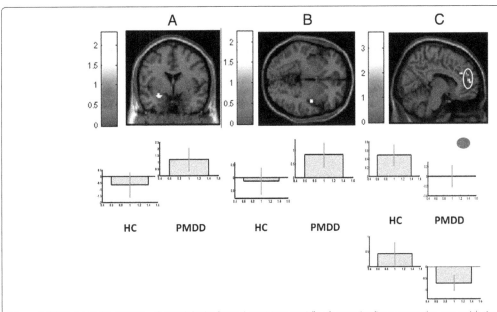

Figure 4 BOLD reactivity. Patients with PMDD had enhanced reactivity to socially relevant stimuli as compared to non-social stimuli in two regions of interest, the **(A)** left amygdala (−21, 2, −15; k = 11; z = 2.18; P = 0.015) and **(B)** the right insula (45, −9, −2, k = 10, z = 2.13, p = 0.016) when compared to healthy controls in the luteal phase. **(C)** Women with PMDD also had attenuated reactivity to social stimuli in the midline ACC in two clusters marked in red and yellow respectively (9, 33, 23; k = 12; z = 2.22; p = 0.013; and 3, 50, 11; k = 27; z = 3.23; p = 0.001). All anatomic localizations are given in Talairach coordinates. Brighter colors represent higher t scores. Below the brain images, contrast estimate plots are given for the peak voxel of each cluster. Healthy controls are given in the left panels and PMDD to the right. ACC, anterior cingulate cortex; PMDD, premenstrual dysphoric disorder.

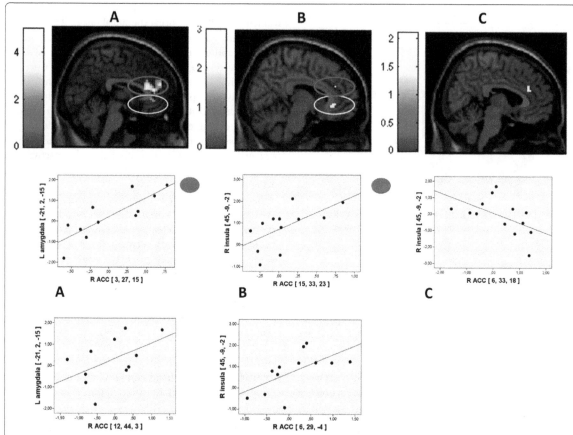

Figure 5 Connectivity. Connectivity analyses revealed a pattern of positive connectivity between BOLD reactivity in emotion processing and controlling areas in PMDD between the **(A)** amygdala and ACC (two clusters marked in red and yellow respectively: 3, 27, 15; k = 90; z = 3.53; p <0.001; and 12, 44, 3; k = 29; z = 2.68; p <0.016) and the **(B)** insula and ACC (two clusters marked in red and yellow respectively: 15, 33, 23; k = 7; z = 2.45; p = 0.008; and 6, 29, −4; k = 11; z = 2.46; p = 0.007). **(C)** For healthy controls there was a trend towards a negative relation between the ACC and insula (6, 33, 18; k = 9; z = 1.89; p = 0.029). All anatomic localizations are given in Talairach coordinates. Brighter colors represent higher t scores. Below the brain images, schematic representations of the connectivity are given for each cluster. Three outliers with BOLD reactivity >2 SD from mean of group were excluded from analyses. ACC, anterior cingulate cortex; PMDD, premenstrual dysphoric disorder.

anxiety disorder, Klumpp and coworkers [49] recently reported that increased insula activation occurred simultaneously as ACC activity decreased, supporting an intrinsic relationship between the insula and the ACC. Conceptually similar results were reported for patients with social anxiety disorder, with decreased connectivity between the amygdala and rostral parts of the ACC to disorder-relevant stimuli [50], while studies in major depression report both reduced and enhanced connectivity between the ACC and amygdala [51]. The ACC areas with attenuated reactivity and compromised connectivity that was observed in our study are associated both with voluntary efforts to suppress emotional reactions [5] and with more automated regulatory processes [52,53]. Based on the present results, we cannot determine if voluntary or automated processes are implicated. Collectively, however, data

support the bottom-up initiation of emotional reactions, rather than top-down control, in response to negative social stimulation in PMDD.

We did not seek to define the mechanisms through which luteal phase-determined corticolimbic processes to social stimuli in PMDD are altered. However, it could be that the subjective experience of social as compared to non-social stimuli in PMDD *per se* is of greater relevance to the patients and thus determines the increased amygdala reactivity. In support of this, we observed significant differences in subjective distress elicited by social but not non-social stimuli in the luteal phase between women with PMDD and healthy controls. However, patients with PMDD consistently rated social stimuli as more negative than non-social stimuli across both cycle phases, making it unlikely that alteration in experience is the sole mechanism driving the change in corticolimbic processing. In addition, amygdala reactivity over the course of the menstrual cycle did not correlate with alterations in affective ratings, but with progesterone levels. It is possible that amygdala reactivity in PMDD is a more sensitive measure than subjective ratings. This is in parallel to increased amygdala reactivity to emotional stimuli, without any relation to subjective reports, previously observed for carriers of the short version of the serotonin transporter promoter length polymorphism [54,55]. Our study may implicate that an overly sensitive threat detection system directed towards social stimuli could be a prerequisite for negative social interactions in PMDD during the luteal phase.

Another potential mechanism that may influence amygdala sensitivity over the menstrual cycle is alterations in progesterone levels [5,32]. Progesterone increased to a similar extent between the follicular and luteal phase both in women with PMDD and in healthy controls, but the increase in amygdala reactivity and the corresponding change in progesterone levels were positively correlated only in women with PMDD. Analyses disentangling phase-determined alterations in affective ratings from progesterone changes further supported the notion that hormonal alterations and not subjective experiences were coupled to amygdala reactivity. This indicates that individual differences in central nervous system activity over the menstrual phase are linked to ovarian steroid hormones rather than subjective experiences. As progesterone levels did not increase more in PMDD than healthy controls and since no change in ACC reactivity was observed across phases, data support the theory that PMDD symptomatology reflects increased amygdala sensitivity to progesterone [56].

Limitations of this study included the relatively few participants and the lenient statistical threshold, warranting replication in a larger sample before the hypothesis of socially determined corticolimbic alterations in PMDD can be confirmed. Furthermore, only the contrast between social and non-social images with negative valence was analyzed, and future studies could disentangle the effect of each stimulus type by contrasting both types of images to more neutral slides. Strengths include the careful diagnostic procedure with prospective ratings of PMDD symptoms and direct estimates of progesterone as well as a methodology focusing on a theoretically defined brain territory with corresponding statistical small volume corrections for multiple comparisons.

Conclusions

This pilot study indicates that aversive and socially relevant stimuli as compared to non-social aversive stimuli enhanced activity in affective processing brain regions that were functionally coupled to cognitive control areas with compromised activity. We therefore argue that patients with PMDD are characterized by altered corticolimbic

circuit processing specifically in response to social emotions, and that progesterone in part influences corticolimbic processing by tuning emotion processing areas.

Additional files

Additional file 1: A schematic example of the used paradigm. The paradigm included exposure to emotional images of negative or positive valence that were preceded by a cue indicating the upcoming valence. In our study, only BOLD reactivity while viewing images of negative valence with social and non-social content was studied.

Additional file 2: Table S1. Valence and arousal ratings. A table including the ratings of pictorial stimuli on the IAPS nine-point visual analog scale for women with PMDD and healthy controls across the menstrual cycle.

Abbreviations
ACC: anterior cingulate cortex; BOLD: blood oxygenation level-dependent; fMRI: functional magnetic resonance imaging; IAPS: International Affective Pictures System; MADRS-S: Montgomery-Åsberg Depression Rating Scale -self rated; PMDD: premenstrual dysphoric disorder; PTSD: post-traumatic disorder; ROI: region of interest; STAI-S: State-Trait Anxiety Inventory -self-rated.

Competing interests
ISP serves occasionally on advisory boards or acts as invited speaker at scientific meetings for MSD, Novo Nordisk, Bayer Health Care, and Lundbeck A/S. The other authors declare that they have no competing interests.

Authors' contributions
MG: design of study, data collection, statistical analyses, manuscript writing and final approval of the manuscript. VA: statistical analyses and final approval of the manuscript. EB: data collection and final approval of the manuscript. JW: data collection and final approval of the manuscript. ISP: design of study, financial support, data collection, critical revision and final approval of the manuscript. MF: design of study, financial support, statistical analyses, manuscript writing and final approval of the manuscript. All authors have read and approved the final manuscript.

Acknowledgements
Supported by the Swedish Council for Working Life and Social Research (ISP, MF); and the Swedish Research Council and the Swedish Brain Foundation (MF). The sponsors had no role in collection, analysis or interpretation of data.

Author details
[1]Department of Women's and Children's Health, Uppsala University, Uppsala, Sweden. [2]Department of Psychology, Uppsala University, Uppsala, Sweden. [3]Department of Radiology, Oncology and Radiation Science, Uppsala University, Uppsala, Sweden.

References
1. American Psychiatric Association: In *Diagnostic and Statistical Manual of Mental Disorders, Text Revision.* 4th edition. Washington, DC, USA: American Psychiatric Publishing, Inc; 2000.
2. Sveindóttir H, Bäckström T: **Prevalence of menstrual cycle symptom cyclicity and premenstrual dysphoric disorder in a random sample of women using and not using oral contraceptives.** *Acta Obstet Gynecol Scand* 2000, **79:**405–413.
3. Robinson R, Swindle RW: **Premenstrual symptom severity: impact on social functioning and treatment-seeking behaviours.** *J Womens Health Gend Based Med* 2000, **9:**757–768.
4. Shin LM, Liberzon I: **The neurocircuitry of fear, stress, and anxiety disorders.** *Neuropsychopharmacology* 2010, **35:**169–191.
5. van Wingen GA, van Broekhoven F, Verkes RJ, Petersson KM, Bäckström T, Buitelaar JK, Fernández G: **Progesterone selectively increases amygdala reactivity in women.** *Mol Psychiatry* 2008, **13:**325–333.

6.   Davidson R, Putnam K, Larson C: **Dysfunction in the neural circuitry of emotion regulation – a possible prelude to violence.** *Science* 2000, 258:591–594.

7.   Bush G, Luu P, Posner MI: **Cognitive and emotional influences in anterior cingulate cortex.** *Trends Cogn Sci* 2000, 4:215–222.

8.   Etkin A, Wager T: **Functional neuroimaging of anxiety: a meta-analysis of emotional processing in PTSD, social anxiety disorder, and specific phobia.** *Am J Psychiatry* 2007, 164:1476–1488.

9.   Ressler K, Mayberg H: **Targeting abnormal neural circuits in mood and anxiety disorders: from the laboratory to the clinic.** *Nat Neurosci* 2007, 10:1116–1124.

10. Freitas-Ferrari MC, Hallak JE, Trzesniak C, Filho AS, Machado-de-Sousa JP, Chagas MH, Nardi AE, Crippa JA: **Neuroimaging in social anxiety disorder: a systematic review of the literature.** *Prog Neuropsychopharmacol Biol Psychiatry* 2010, 30:565–580.

11. Del Casale A, Ferracuti S, Rapinesi C, Serata D, Piccirilli M, Savoja V, Kotzalidis GD, Manfredi G, Angeletti G, Tatarelli R, Girardi P: **Functional neuroimaging in specific phobia.** *Psychiatry Res* 2012, 30:181–197.

12. Hayes JP, Hayes SM, Mikedis AM: **Quantitative meta-analysis of neural activity in posttraumatic stress disorder.** *Biol Mood Anxiety Disord* 2012, 2:2–9.

13. Linares IM, Trzesniak C, Chagas MH, Hallak JE, Nardi AE, Crippa JA: **Neuroimaging in specific phobia disorder: a systematic review of the literature.** *Rev Bras Psiquiatr* 2012, 1:101–111.

14. Patel R, Spreng RN, Shin LM, Girard TA: **Neurocircuitry models of posttraumatic stress disorder and beyond: a meta-analysis of functional neuroimaging studies.** *Neurosci Biobehav Rev* 2012, 36:2130–2142.

15. Fredrikson M, Faria V: **Neuroimaging in anxiety disorders.** In *Modern Trends in Pharmacopsychiatry: anxiety disorders.* Edited by Baldwin D, Leonard B. Basel: Karger; 2013.

16. Protopopescu X, Tuescher O, Pan H, Epstein J, Root J, Chang L, Altemus M, Polanecsky M, McEwen B, Stern E, Silbersweig D: **Toward a functional neuroanatomy of premenstrual dysphoric disorder.** *J Affect Disord* 2008, 108:87–94.

17. Gingnell M, Morell A, Bannbers E, Wikström J, Sundström Poromaa I: **Menstrual cycle effects on amygdala reactivity to emotional stimulation in premenstrual dysphoric disorder.** *Horm Behav* 2012, 62:400–406.

18. Gingnell M, Bannbers E, Wikström J, Fredrikson M, Sundström-Poromaa I: **Premenstrual dysphoric disorder and prefrontal reactivity during anticipation of emotional stimuli.** *Eur Neuropsychopharmacol* 2013, 23:1471–1483.

19. Rauch SL, Shin LM, Phelps EA: **Neurocircuitry models of posttraumatic stress disorder and extinction: human neuroimaging research, past, present, and future.** *Biol Psychiatry* 2006, 60:376–382.

20. Shin LM, Whalen PJ, Pitman RK, Bush G, Macklin ML, Lasko NB, Orr SP, McInerney SC, Rauch SL: **An fMRI study of anterior cingulate function in posttraumatic stress disorder.** *Biol Psychiatry* 2001, 50:932–942.

21. Shin LM, Wright CI, Cannistraro PA, Wedig MM, McMullin KB, Martis B, Macklin ML, Lasko NB, Cavanagh SR, Krangel TS, Orr SP, Pitman RK, Whalen PJ, Rauch SL: **A functional magnetic resonance imaging study of amygdala and medial prefrontal cortex responses to overtly presented fearful faces in posttraumatic stress disorder.** *Arch Gen Psychiatry* 2005, 62:273–281.

22. Wright CI, Martis B, McMullin K, Shin LM, Rauch SL: **Amygdala and insular responses to emotionally valenced human faces in small animal specific phobia.** *Biol Psychiatry* 2003, 54:1067–1076.

23. Heinemann LA, Do Minh T, Filonenko A, Uhl-Hochgraber K: **Explorative evaluation of the impact of premenstrual disorder on daily functioning and quality of life.** *Patient* 2010, 3:125–132.

24. Girdler SS, Leserman J, Bunevicius R, Klatzkin R, Pedersen CA, Light KC: **Persistent alterations in biological profiles in women with abuse histories: influence of premenstrual dysphoric disorder.** *Health Psychol* 2007, 26:201–213.

25. Girdler SS, Pedersen CA, Straneva PA, Leserman J, Stanwyck CL, Benjamin S, Light KC: **Dysregulation of cardiovascular and neuroendocrine responses to stress in premenstrual dysphoric disorder.** *Psychiatry Res* 1998, 81:163–178.

26. Segebladh B, Bannbers E, Kask K, Nyberg S, Bixo M, Heimer G, Sundström-Poromaa I: **Prevalence of violence exposure in women with premenstrual dysphoric disorder in comparison with other gynecological patients and asymptomatic controls.** *Acta Obstet Gynecol Scand* 2011, 90:746–752.

27. Pilver CE, Levy BR, Libby DJ, Desai RA: **Posttraumatic stress disorder and trauma characteristics are correlates of premenstrual dysphoric disorder.** *Arch Womens Ment Health* 2011, 14:383–393.

28. Wittchen HU, Perkonigg A, Pfister H: **Trauma and PTSD - an overlooked pathogenic pathway for premenstrual dysphoric disorder?** *Arch Womens Ment Health* 2003, 6:293–297.

29. Girdler SS, Sherwood A, Hinderliter AL, Leserman J, Costello NL, Straneva PA, Pedersen CA, Light KC: **Biological correlates of abuse in women with premenstrual dysphoric disorder and healthy controls.** *Psychosom Med* 2003, 65:849–856.

30. Paulus MP, Stein MB: **An insular view of anxiety.** *Biol Psychiatry* 2006, 60:383–387.

31. Ochsner KN, Silvers JA, Buhle JT: **Functional imaging studies of emotion regulation: a synthetic review and evolving model of the cognitive control of emotion.** *Ann N Y Acad Sci* 2012, 1251:1–24.

32. Andreano JM, Cahill L: **Menstrual cycle modulation of medial temporal activity evoked by negative emotion.** *Neuroimage* 2010, 53:1286–1293.

33. Lang PJ, Bradley MM, Cuthbert BN: In *International Affective Picture System (IAPS): Affective Ratings of Pictures and Instruction Manual*, Technical Report A-6. Gainsville, USA: University of Florida; 2005.

34. Gingnell M, Comasco E, Oreland L, Fredrikson M, Sundström-Poromaa I: **Neuroticism-related personality traits are related to symptom severity in patients with premenstrual dysphoric disorder and to the serotonin transporter gene-linked polymorphism 5-HTTPLPR.** *Arch Womens Ment Health* 2010, 13:417–423.

35. Wang M, Seippel L, Purdy RH, Backstrom T: **Relationship between symptom severity and steroid variation in women with premenstrual syndrome: study on serum pregnenolone, pregnenolone sulfate, 5 alpha-pregnane-3,20-dione and 3 alpha-hydroxy-5 alpha-pregnan-20-one.** *J Clin Endocrinol Metab* 1996, 3:1076–1082.

36. Sheehan D, Lecrubier Y, Sheehan KH, Amorim P, Janavs J, Weiller E, Hergueta T, Baker R, Dunbar GC: **The Mini-International Neuropsyciatric interview (M.I.N.I.): the development and validation of a structured diagnostic psychiatric interview for DSM-IV and ICD-10.** *J Clin Psychiatry* 1998, 59:22–33.

37. Montgomery SA, Asberg M: **A new depression scale designed to be sensitive to change.** *Br J Psychiatry* 1979, 134:382–389.

38. Spielberger CD, Gorusch RL, Lushene R: *Manual for the State-Trait Anxiety (STAI Form Y).* Palo Alto, CA: Consulting Psychologist Press; 1983.

39. mrICRON. [http://neuro.debian.net/pkgs/mricron.html]

40. SPM 5. [http://www.fil.ion.ucl.ac.uk/spm/software/spm5/]

41. Lancaster J, Summerlin J, Rainey L, Freitas C, Fox P: **The Talairach Daemon, a database server for Talairach Atlas Labels.** *Neuroimage* 1997, 5(4, Part 2 of 4 Parts):S633.

42. Lancaster J, Woldorff M, Parsons L, Liotti M, Freitas C, Rainey L, Kuchunov PV, Nickerson D, Mikiten SA, Fox PT: **Automated Talairach atlas labels for functional brain mapping.** *Hum Brain Mapp* 2000, 10:120–131.

43. Maldjian J, Laurienti P, Kraft R, Burdette J: **An automated method for neuroanatomic and cytoarchitectonic atlas-based interrogation of fMRI data sets.** *Neuroimage* 2003, 19:1233–1239.

44. Forman SD, Cohen JD, Fitzgerald M, Eddy WF, Mintun MA, Noll DC: **Improved assessment of significant activation in functional magnetic resonance imaging (fMRI): use of a cluster-size threshold.** *Magn Reson Med* 1995, 33:636–647.

45. Hariri AR, Tessitore A, Mattay VS, Fera F, Weinberger DR: **The amygdala response to emotional stimuli: a comparison of faces and scenes.** *Neuroimage* 2002, 17:317–323.

46. Roy AK, Shehzad Z, Margulies DS, Kelly AM, Uddin LQ, Gotimer K, Biswal BB, Castellanos FX, Milham MP: **Functional connectivity of the human amygdala using resting state fMRI.** *Neuroimage* 2008, 45:614–626.

47. Taylor KS, Seminowicz DA, Davis KD: **Two systems of resting state connectivity between the insula and cingulate cortex.** *Hum Brain Mapp* 2009, 30:2731–2745.

48. Cauda F, D'Agata F, Sacco K, Duca S, Geminiani G, Vercelli A: **Functional connectivity of the insula in the resting brain.** *Neuroimage* 2011, 55:8–23.

49. Klumpp H, Post D, Angstadt M, Fitzgerald DA, Phan KL: **Anterior cingulate cortex and insula response during indirect and direct processing of emotional faces in generalized social anxiety disorder.** *Biol Mood Anxiety Disord* 2013, 3:7.

50. Prater KE, Hosanagar A, Klumpp H, Angstadt M, Phan KL: **Aberrant amygdala-frontal cortex connectivity during perception of fearful faces and at rest in generalized social anxiety disorder.** *Depress Anxiety* 2013, 30:234–241.

51. Carballedo A, Scheuerecker J, Meisenzahl E, Schoepf V, Bokde A, Möller HJ, Doyle M, Wiesmann M, Frodl T: **Functional connectivity of emotional processing in depression.** *J Affect Disord* 2011, 134:272–279.

52. Milad MR, Wright CI, Orr SP, Pitman RK, Quirk GJ, Rauch SL: **Recall of fear extinction in humans activates the ventromedial prefrontal cortex and hippocampus in concert.** *Biol Psychiatry* 2007, **62**:446–454.

53. Phelps EA, Delgado MR, Nearing KI, LeDoux JE: **Extinction learning in humans: role of the amygdala and vmPFC.** *Neuron* 2004, **43**:897–905.

54. Fakra E, Hyde LW, Gorka A, Fisher PM, Muñoz KE, Kimak M, Halder I, Ferell RE, Manuck SB, Hariri AR: **Effects of HTR1A C(−1019)G on amygdala reactivity and trait anxiety.** *Arch Gen Psychiatry* 2009, **66**:33–40.

55. Hariri AR, Mattay VS, Tessitore A, Kolachana B, Fera F, Goldman D, Egan MF, Weinberger DR: **Serotonin transporter genetic variation and the response of the human amygdala.** *Science* 2002, **297**:400–403.

56. Bäckström T, Andreen L, Brizniece V, Björn I, Johansson IM, Nordenstam-Haghjo M, Nyberg S, Sundström-Poromaa I, Wahlström G, Wang M, Zhu D: **The role of hormones and hormonal treatments in premenstrual syndrome.** *CNS Drugs* 2003, **17**:325–342.

3

Meta-analytic methods for neuroimaging data explained

Joaquim Radua[1,2*] and David Mataix-Cols[1]

Abstract

The number of neuroimaging studies has grown exponentially in recent years and their results are not always consistent. Meta-analyses are helpful to summarize this vast literature and also offer insights that are not apparent from the individual studies. In this review, we describe the main methods used for meta-analyzing neuroimaging data, with special emphasis on their relative advantages and disadvantages. We describe and discuss meta-analytical methods for global brain volumes, methods based on regions of interest, label-based reviews, voxel-based meta-analytic methods and online databases. Regions of interest-based methods allow for optimal statistical analyses but are affected by a limited and potentially biased inclusion of brain regions, whilst voxel-based methods benefit from a more exhaustive and unbiased inclusion of studies but are statistically more limited. There are also relevant differences between the different available voxel-based meta-analytic methods, and the field is rapidly evolving to develop more accurate and robust methods. We suggest that in any meta-analysis of neuroimaging data, authors should aim to: only include studies exploring the whole brain; ensure that the same threshold throughout the whole brain is used within each included study; and explore the robustness of the findings via complementary analyses to minimize the risk of false positives.

Keywords: activation likelihood estimation, effect-size signed differential mapping, functional magnetic resonance imaging, kernel density analysis, meta-analysis, magnetic resonance imaging, multilevel kernel density analysis, parametric voxel-based meta-analysis, region of interest, signed differential mapping, voxel-based morphometry

Introduction

The number of neuroimaging studies has grown exponentially in recent years. However, findings from different studies may sometimes be difficult to integrate into a coherent picture. Inconsistent results are not uncommon. Furthermore, a few influential studies might often eclipse robust findings from other studies. In other words, we may at times not see the forest for the trees. In this context, meta-analyses are helpful to combine and summarize the data of interest and potentially offer insights that are not immediately apparent from the individual studies.

The present paper aims to describe the main methods which have been used for the meta-analysis of neuroimaging data, as well as their advantages and drawbacks, with some examples of application to mood and anxiety disorders. The first section of the paper introduces how a standard meta-analysis is conducted, that is, when there is only one variable of interest, with an example from a meta-analysis of global brain volumes. This is important for a better appreciation of the pros and cons of the meta-analytic methods that we review later. The second section of the paper describes the meta-analyses of neuroimaging studies based on regions of interest (ROI) and their particular issues. The third section introduces the various available voxel-based meta-analytic methods, which aim to overcome some of the limitations of the ROI-based methods but have, in turn, their own limitations. The similarities and differences between the various voxel-based methods are also discussed in depth. Finally, we describe the available online databases of neuroimaging studies. This paper is meant to be accessible for the applied researcher in the fields of psychiatry, neurology and allied disciplines. Other excellent, more technical, reviews of meta-analytical methods can be found elsewhere [1,2].

* Correspondence: Joaquim.Radua@kcl.ac.uk
[1]Institute of Psychiatry, King's College London, De Crespigny Park, London, UK
Full list of author information is available at the end of the article

Standard meta-analyses

Prior to any meta-analytic calculation, researchers conduct an exhaustive and critical literature search, often including contact with the authors of the original studies in order to retrieve important pieces of missing information. Then, researchers conduct a mathematical summary of the findings of the included studies (that is, the meta-analysis proper). Finally, researchers apply a series of tests, plots and subgroup analyses to assess the heterogeneity and robustness of the results. The latter step, along with the exhaustive and critical inclusion of studies, is of utmost importance in order to obtain unbiased meta-analytic conclusions.

With the aim of introducing the reader to the logics of a standard meta-analysis, in this section we will use as an example a meta-analysis of global gray matter volumes in patients with obsessive-compulsive disorder (OCD) (see Table 1). The included studies correspond to seven publications reporting global gray matter volume, which were included in a published meta-analysis of voxel-based morphometry studies in OCD [3].

Weighting of the studies

In order to summarize these seven studies, a simple meta-analysis could consist of calculating the mean difference in global gray matter volume between patients and controls as reported in the original studies [4]. Thus, we could summarize Table 1 by saying that the mean global gray matter volume is 8.4 mL inferior in patients than in healthy controls-this number is just the arithmetic mean of the differences shown in the table.

The use of the arithmetic mean, however, may be too simplistic, because the different studies should have different weights. For example, the number of patients in study 4 is four times larger than the number of patients in study 1. Clearly, we cannot give the same weight to both studies and should give more weight to study 4. Probably, we should give it about four times more weight, as it includes four times as many patients.

Including all the studies in Table 1 and weighting the mean difference by the sample sizes of the studies, we would conclude now that the mean global gray matter

volume is 8.8 mL inferior in patients than in controls. Note that when we previously calculated the mean difference as the simple arithmetic mean, we were indeed assuming that all the studies had the same sample size. This erroneous assumption had only a minor effect here (we thought that the difference was about 5% smaller than what we think now), but it could have important effects in other meta-analyses, especially if studies with smaller sample sizes inexplicably find more differences than studies with larger sample sizes-we will introduce how to detect this kind of bias later.

Unfortunately, weighting the calculations only by sample size would still be too simplistic, because the weight of a study should also include its precision. For example, study 1 included fewer patients than study 4, but its volume estimates seem much more precise, as its sample variance is approximately the half than that in study 4 (see Patients + controls column in Table 1). We do not know the reason for this higher precision (maybe the sample was more homogenous; maybe the technical procedures were cleaner; maybe it was just chance); however, we must take this precision into account by weighting by the inverse of the variance of the difference-which also includes the sample size.

Including all the studies in Table 1 and weighting by the inverse of the variance of the difference, we would conclude that the mean global gray matter volume is 8.9 mL inferior in patients than in controls (z-value = -1.55, $P = 0.121$). When previously we did not weight by sample variance we were assuming that all the studies had the same variance, though in this case this assumption was acceptable because the variance of the studies is rather homogeneous.

However, as explained in the next section, weighting the calculations only by the inverse of the variance of the difference may still be too simplistic.

Heterogeneity in the studies

Healthy individuals have different global gray matter volumes, that is, some have larger brains, some have thicker cortices, and so on. When conducting an analysis with original data, we are usually able to explain or

Table 1 Global gray matter volumes reported in seven studies on obsessive-compulsive disorder

	Reference	Patients		Controls		Patients + controls		Difference		Effect size	
		Number	Volume ± SD	Number	Volume ± SD	N	Variance	Estimate	Variance	Estimate	Variance
Study 1	[46]	18	773 ± 56	18	822 ± 56	36	3,114	-49	346	-0.854	0.122
Study 2	[47]	55	685 ± 74	50	708 ± 72	105	5,323	-23	203	-0.313	0.039
Study 3	[48]	25	850 ± 83	25	834 ± 71	50	5,997	+16	480	0.196	0.080
Study 4	[49]	72	739 ± 82	72	763 ± 78	144	6,404	-24	178	-0.298	0.028
Study 5	[50]	37	776 ± 69	26	747 ± 68	63	4,680	+29	307	0.418	0.067
Study 6	[51]	19	827 ± 44	15	836 ± 63	34	3,041	-9	363	-0.179	0.120
Study 7	[52]	71	740 ± 66	71	738 ± 63	142	4,119	+2	116	0.035	0.028

All volumes are in milliliters. SD: standard deviation.

model a part of this variability, but there is also a part of this variability that remains unexplained. This residual error may be due to unobserved variables, etiological heterogeneity within particular diagnoses, poor model fitting, or maybe just pure chance. This individual-based within-study variability cause the sample means to be variable, so that different studies obtain different results.

However, within-study variability is not the only source of the between-study variability or heterogeneity. Given the relatively small amount of robust findings in neuroimaging, it would be highly desirable that all researchers conducted their studies using the exact same inclusion criteria and methods so that all between-study variability was only related to the within-study variability. However, the fact is that clinical and methodological differences between studies are often substantial.

On the one hand, patients included in the individual studies may have been sampled from clinically different populations; for example, one study of major depressive disorder may include outpatients with mild reactive depressive episodes while another study may be focused on inpatients suffering from severe endogenous depressions with melancholic symptoms. Similarly, patients in different studies may be receiving different treatments, or be in different phases of the disorder (for example, having a first episode or having a history of multiple episodes).

On the other hand, researchers may have been investigated similar but still different aspects of a disorder; for example, one study may have described the blood oxygen level-dependent (BOLD) brain response to a task involving a high memory load, while another study may be interest in the BOLD response to a task related to decision-making. Or even if studying the same particular cognitive function, each study may employ a particular statistical package, and its large set of associated assumptions.

Finally, there may be a relevant part of the between-study heterogeneity which can be neither related to the within-study variability, nor explained by clinical or methodological differences between studies. This is called residual heterogeneity.

It is highly recommended to study the between-study variability or heterogeneity in any meta-analysis. For example, if the main analysis detects differences between patients and controls, it may be of interest to explore whether these differences depend on the severity of the disorder, or if they are related to special subtypes of the disorder. These questions may be assessed with meta-regressions. But even if the meta-analysis does not aim to explore the modulating effects of clinical variables on the main outcomes, heterogeneity should still be taken into account.

Indeed, there is agreement on always including the residual heterogeneity in the weighting of the calculations [5-8]. Meta-analyses conducted this way are said to follow random-effects models, in opposition to the fixed-effects models that we saw in the previous point, which did not include heterogeneity. In the example of Table 1 the use of a random-effects model would lead us to conclude that the mean global gray matter volume is 9.0 mL inferior in patients than in controls (z-value = -0.98, P = 0.328; see Figure 1, left). Note the increase of P-value in the random-effects model (from 0.121 to 0.328), thus better controlling the false positive rate.

Other complementary analyses

The above meta-analysis of global gray matter volumes in OCD was only aimed to help interpret the findings of a regional voxel-based meta-analysis, for which no other tests beyond a correctly weighted random-effects model would probably be required. However, if global gray matter volumes were the main outcome of a meta-analysis, some complementary plots and tests would be recommended to help the reader assess the reliability and robustness of the findings [9].

On the one hand, the meta-regressions described above may be useful for assessing if the findings are predominantly (or only) present in one group of patients, for example, in those with more severe forms of OCD. In this regard, specific meta-analyses of subgroups of patients may further confirm these hypotheses or, also important, may state that the abnormalities are present in all subgroups of patients, increasing the robustness of the findings. Similarly, sensitivity analyses consisting of repeating the meta-analysis many times, each time with a different combination of studies, may be useful to assess whether the findings are driven by one or few studies. Finally, funnel plots (see Figure 1, right) may be useful for appraising whether studies with small samples report more statistically significant findings than studies with larger samples. This is typical of subjects with publication bias, where studies with small samples are only published if their results match a priori hypotheses.

It is important to note that these kinds of tests and graphical aids are necessary but do not provide conclusive information, and should only be interpreted in the context of the field under investigation. A symmetrical funnel plot, for example, is not an amulet against publication bias, especially in some types of meta-analysis. ROI-based studies, for instance, may be more prone to be affected by publication biases, as the authors may decide which brain regions are reported and which are not. Conversely, an asymmetrical funnel plot would not necessarily invalidate a meta-analysis if publication bias appears unlikely. This may be the case of voxel-based studies, where the whole brain is included in the analysis.

Use of effect sizes

Most meta-analyses do not use the raw volume differences as we exemplified in the previous points, but rather, they use standardized volume differences, that is,

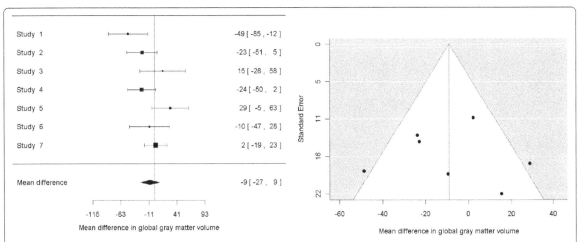

Figure 1 Forest (left) and funnel (right) plots of the mean differences in global gray matter volume between patients with obsessive-compulsive disorder and healthy controls (using a random-effects model). On the funnel plot, the included studies appear to be symmetrically distributed on either side of the mean difference, suggesting no publication bias towards positive or negative studies.

effect sizes [10]. Briefly, a raw difference is the difference in milliliters between patients' and controls' global gray matter volume, while a standardized difference is the difference is standard deviations-usually corrected for small sample size bias.

This subtle difference has a series of consequences. First, the unit of measure (milliliters, in this case) is lost, which makes the interpretation of the findings less straightforward but indeed more comparable with other measures, for example, an effect size of d = 0.5 is considered 'medium' independently of whether it refers to a difference in gray matter volume, in BOLD response or in a questionnaire score. Using the data from Table 1, the effect size of the difference in global gray matter volume between patients and controls is d = -0.122 (z-value = -0.93, P = 0.354; Figure 2), which is below the conventional range of 'small' effect (0.2 to 0.3) [11]. Second, a study reporting a larger difference may be found to have a smaller effect size, or vice versa, depending on the sample variance. For instance in Table 1, the raw difference is slightly larger in study 4 than in study 3, whilst the effect size is slightly larger in study 3 than in study 4. Third, and very important, effect size can be directly derived from many statistics like a *t*-value or a *P*-value, which are much more often reported than sample statistics; that is, we can often know the effect size but not the raw difference. This advantage usually allows a much more exhaustive inclusion of studies, thus clearly justifying the use of effect sizes in many meta-analyses.

Meta-analyses based on regions of interest
A ROI is a part of the brain that the authors of the study wish to investigate, usually based on *a priori*

hypotheses. ROI-based studies usually select a set of few ROIs and manually delimitate them on the raw images. Researchers then analyze the volume of these ROIs, their mean BOLD response to a stimulus, their positron emission tomography ligand volume of distribution, or any other measure of interest.

Region of interest-based meta-analyses
A typical ROI-based meta-analysis can be viewed as a set of different meta-analyses, each of them applied to a different ROI. These meta-analyses can usually be optimally conducted with all appropriate weightings and complementary analyses, as seen for example in the meta-analysis of regional brain volumes in OCD conducted by Rotge *et al.* [12], in which the analyses are based on effect sizes and random-effects models and complemented with explicit assessments of the heterogeneity, several sensitivity analyses, funnel plots and meta-regressions. Unfortunately, each original study included in this meta-analysis only investigated a small set of brain regions, causing the meta-analyses to include only a very small number of studies for each brain region. Indeed, only three or four studies could be included for highly relevant regions such as the putamen or the anterior cingulate cortex, both of which were found as abnormal in subsequent voxel-based meta-analyses [3,13]. Other brain regions could not be meta-analyzed because they had been investigated by too few or no studies. Needless to say, this would not be the case for those ROI studies reporting whole brain results in online supplements or similar, but this is seldom the case.

Moreover, it must be noted that some brain regions are more frequently studied than others, which causes the statistical power to differ depending on the brain

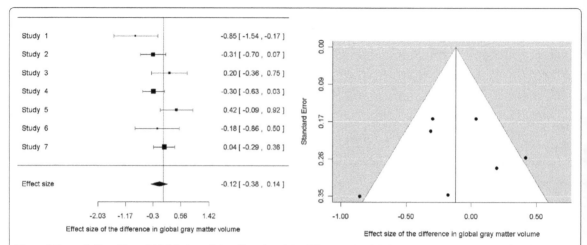

Figure 2 Forest (left) and funnel (right) plots of the effect size of the differences in global gray matter volume between patients with obsessive-compulsive disorder and healthy controls (using a random-effects model). On the funnel plot, the included studies appear to be symmetrically distributed on either side of the mean effect size, suggesting no publication bias towards positive or negative studies.

region under study. In the example, while data from five studies or more were available for the orbitofrontal cortex, the thalamus and the caudate nuclei, some brain regions could not be meta-analyzed at all.

Ultimately, the authors of the original studies have a set of *a priori* hypotheses which influence their decision to investigate differences in a given brain region at the expense of other regions. These decisions determine the number of studies investigating that brain region, and thus the statistical power to detect that brain region as significantly different between patients and controls in a ROI-based meta-analysis. Publication bias is also a problem as studies failing to report statistically significant differences on hypothesized ROIs may be less likely to ever be become publicly available. A recent analysis of more than 450 ROI-based neuroimaging studies in psychiatry illustrates this point well [14]. The author demonstrated that the number of studies reporting significant results was nearly the double than expected, suggesting strong publication biases in the ROI literature.

Another consideration is the heterogeneous definition or the boundaries of the ROIs, which may differ from one study to the other [12]. However, this variability might have a relatively small impact on effect sizes, as boundary definitions are the same for the patients and controls included in a study. Furthermore, the spatial error may probably be counteracted by the higher anatomical accuracy achieved by the manual delimitation of the ROIs in the original studies [15,16].

Label-based reviews

Some authors have used a simplified type of ROI-based meta-analysis, consisting of just counting how many times a particular ROI is detected as significantly abnormal in

patients versus healthy controls. This procedure has been called label-based review [17]. For example, in their functional neuroimaging meta-analysis of the brain's response to emotional tasks, Phan *et al.* [18] represented each activation peak as a dot in an atlas of the brain. They then divided the brain into 20 ROIs and counted how many studies had one or more activation peak in each ROI.

A fictitious example of such approach is shown in Figure 3A. Here, the studies would have reported that the patients with mood or anxiety disorders have increases of gray matter volume in the basal ganglia, extending to the anterior part of the right insula, as well as decreases of gray matter volume in the anterior cingulate and insular cortices. The authors of a label-based review would have first plotted the peaks of the clusters of significant increase (red) or decrease (blue) of gray matter volume in a brain template. Then, they would divide the brain into several regions, for example, anterior cingulate gyrus, left and right inferior frontal gyri, insulas, superior temporal gyri, caudate nuclei, putamen nuclei, and so on. Finally, they would have counted how many peaks lay within each of these regions.

This method may be useful when other approaches are not feasible, for example when not enough information is available for conducting a ROI-based or a voxel-based meta-analysis. Its simplicity, however, may conceal a series of important drawbacks which must be taken into account. First, no weighting of the studies is performed, which means that all studies are assumed to have the same sample size and precision. This is a strong and unrealistic assumption which may be violated in most meta-analysis. Fortunately, sample size information is always available, and so label-based meta-analyses should

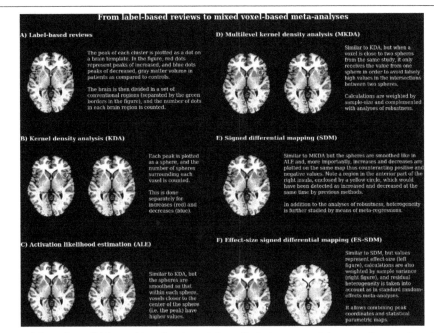

Figure 3 Summary of the main available voxel-based meta-analytic methods. Increases and decreases of gray matter volume are fictitious and have been manually plotted over a MRICroN template to illustrate the main features of the different methods.

at least be weighted by sample size. Second, the findings of the studies are binarized (significant versus not-significant), leading to a loss of information on the magnitude of the raw differences or on the effect sizes. Third, it is not clear whether studies reporting opposite findings in a particular ROI (for example, volume decrease in some studies and volume increase in others) are adequately dealt with. Finally, they may be also affected by the particular issues of ROI-based meta-analyses described above.

Voxel-based meta-analyses

Scanner three-dimensional images are composed of thousands of tiny cubes (or rectangular cuboids) called voxels, in the same way that digital photographs are composed of thousands of tiny squares called pixels. Voxel-based methods consist of conducting the meta-analytic calculations separately in each voxel of the brain, thus freeing the meta-analysis from aprioristic anatomical definitions. There are different types of voxel-based meta-analyses, including image-based, coordinate-based and mixed image- and coordinate-based meta-analyses.

Image-based meta-analyses

An image-based meta-analysis should be understood as a voxel-based version of the standard meta-analysis, that is, it consists of thousands of standard meta-analyses, each of them applied to a different voxel [2,19]. The data of each study is retrieved from its statistical parametric

maps (the three-dimensional images resulting from the comparison between patients and controls), and thus include the whole brain. This technique shares some limitations with any voxel-based analysis, mainly relating to the massive number of statistical tests (that is, one test for each voxel). The correction of multiple comparisons is an unsolved issue, with current methods being either too liberal or too conservative [19]. For this reason, thresholds based on uncorrected *P*-values and cluster-size are usually preferred [1,19,20]. Also, such massive-scale testing prevents a careful visual inspection of the analyses (for example, to describe relevant non-significant trends).

However, the biggest drawback of image-based meta-analyses is that the statistical parametric maps of the original studies are seldom available, therefore seriously limiting the inclusion of studies.

Coordinate-based meta-analyses

Given the poor availability of statistical parametric maps, early meta-analyses of voxel-based studies consisted of label-based (rather than image-based) reviews, as discussed earlier. These methods quickly evolved to coordinate-based meta-analyses, which in their simplest form consisted of counting, for each voxel, how many activation peaks had been reported within its surroundings [21]. In the fictitious example, the dots of the label-based review (Figure 3A) would be replaced with spheres (Figure 3B, C), and the brain would not be divided into conventional regions but rather the number of spheres surrounding each voxel would be counted, thus obtaining a count for each voxel. It must be noted that calculations in activation likelihood estimation (ALE) [22] are not exactly based on counting the number of spheres but on computing the probability of a union, though in practice, the latter behaves like the former.

The use of voxels rather than conventional divisions of the brain improved the anatomical localization of the findings. However, the first available methods, namely ALE and kernel density analysis (KDA) [21], had some additional issues which enlarged the list of drawbacks of label-based reviews. Specifically, they only counted the total number of peaks, independently of whether they came from the same or different studies, and thus the analysis could not be weighted by sample size and a single study reporting many peaks in close proximity could drive the findings of the whole analysis.

These drawbacks led to the creation of a second generation of coordinate-based meta-analytic methods, mainly evolved versions of KDA, such as multilevel KDA [23] and parametric voxel-based meta-analysis [24]; evolved versions of ALE [25,26]; and signed differential mapping (SDM) [3,27-30] (Figure 3D, E), which overcame these limitations by separating the peaks of each study. Moreover, some of these new methods weighted the studies by their sample size and included a series of complementary analyses to assess the reliability and robustness of the findings. One of the methods, SDM, also addressed between-study heterogeneity by reconstructing positive and negative maps in the same image, thus counteracting the effects of studies reporting findings in opposite directions [31] and incorporating meta-regression methods. Finally, SDM included templates for white matter [32], allowing multimodal meta-analyses which were not possible with previous methods [33]. However, these methods still did not employ the standard statistical methods of the ROI-based meta-analyses, for example, they did not weight by the precision of each study.

Several of these methods have recently been applied to mood and anxiety disorders. One such was a meta-analysis of studies investigating bipolar disorder [34] using SDM, which found patients to have gray matter reductions in the left medial frontal and/or anterior cingulate cortex (MF/ACC) and bilateral anterior insula, with complementary analyses showing findings in the left ACC and right insula to be robust, and left MF/ACC volume to be higher in samples where patients were being treated with lithium. An SDM meta-analysis of studies investigating major depressive disorder also found patients to have gray matter reductions in the MF/ACC [35], and complementary analyses showed this finding to be robust and more severe in multiple-episode samples. Recent SDM meta-analyses of studies investigating anxiety disorders have also found patients to have gray matter reduction in the MF/ACC [13], along with abnormalities in the basal ganglia. Specifically, patients with OCD were found to have increased gray matter volume in the bilateral putamen and caudate nuclei [3], with complementary analyses showing findings in the MF/ACC and left basal ganglia to be robust, and bilateral increases of basal ganglia volume to be higher in samples including patients with higher symptom severity. Conversely, patients with anxiety disorders other than OCD were found to have decreased gray matter volume in the left putamen nucleus [13].

An example of the use of these methods in functional neuroimaging is the recent study by Delvecchio *et al.* [36], which meta-analyzed the functional brain response to emotional faces using ALE. They found that both patients with bipolar disorder and patients with unipolar depression displayed limbic hyperactivations. However, only patients with bipolar disorder showed a set of hypoactivations in the prefrontal cortex and hyperactivations in the thalamus and basal ganglia. Conversely, only patients with major depressive disorder showed hypoactivations in the sensorimotor cortices. Another example from the anxiety disorders literature is a multilevel KDA meta-analysis, which found that patients showed hyperactivations in the amygdala and insula [37]. Interestingly, these hyperactivations were more observed in phobias, whilst patients with post-traumatic stress disorder displayed a hypoactivation of the MF/ACC. Finally, an ALE meta-analysis of functional differences in patients with OCD detected that symptom provocation was possibly associated with activation of the orbitofrontal cortex, prefrontal cortex, anterior cingulate cortex, precuneus, premotor cortex, superior temporal gyrus, basal ganglia, hippocampus and uncus [38].

These methods may also be applied to functional connectivity studies [39,40]. Laird *et al.*, for instance, studied the default mode network by first creating ALE maps, and then deriving meta-analytic co-activation maps [40]. With this approach, they could identify an affective subnetwork component. This approach is promising, given the increasing interest in functional connectivity studies in various mood and anxiety disorders.

Mixed image- and coordinate-based meta-analyses

Recently, effect size SDM (ES-SDM) was designed to allow the combination of studies from which images (statistical parametric maps) are available with studies from which only peak coordinates are reported, thus allowing a more exhaustive inclusion of studies, as well as more accurate estimations [19].

This is achieved by first using peak coordinates and their statistical values to recreate the statistical parametric maps, and then conducting an image-based meta-analysis. Thus, this method has some statistical advantages as compared to previous coordinate-based methods, namely the use of standard statistical methods (for example, weighting the calculations by both sample size and study precision, use of effect sizes, inclusion and assessment of residual heterogeneity, and so on).

In a meta-analysis of the BOLD response to emotional facial stimuli [19], the sensitivity to detect real activations (that is, the number of actually activated voxels appearing as significant in the meta-analysis, divided by the total number of actually activated voxels) was similar between ES-SDM (55%) and SDM (51%) when only using peak coordinates. However, the inclusion of the statistical parametric maps led to a gradual and substantial increase of the sensitivity of ES-SDM (73% when the statistical parametric map of one study was included, 87% when the statistical parametric maps of two studies were included, 93% when the statistical parametric maps of three studies were included, and so on). Therefore, given the potential of this new method, we would encourage authors to make their statistical parametric maps widely available to the community on their laboratory websites or via other means.

Online databases

In parallel with the development of new meta-analytical methods, several freely-available website-based databases of neuroimaging data have been made available. These online databases may be classified in three groups, namely: sets of original data (for example, the raw scanner images from several samples of individuals); summary statistics from the studies included in one meta-analysis (for example, the mean ± standard deviation ROI volumes); and sets of summary statistics of virtually all published studies.

The online sets of original data are composed of the raw and/or pre-processed brain images, along with the demographic and clinical characteristics of each of the many anonymous participants. These databases may be used by researchers to conduct their studies, thus being a useful resource for highly accurate data analyses. It must be noted, however, that analyses derived from these datasets should not be strictly considered meta-analyses, as they do not necessarily exhaustively include all available data. Examples of these datasets are BRAINNet (http://www.brainnet.net), the fMRI Data Center (http://www.fmridc.org) and OpenfMRI (http://www.openfmri.org).

Online databases containing the summary statistics from the studies included in particular meta-analyses represent a more interactive (and often complete) alternative to the traditional 'supplementary materials' that accompany published meta-analyses. Importantly, these online data may be used by other researchers to conduct updated or secondary analyses. Examples of this type of

databases are the Bipolar Disorder Neuroimaging Database (http://www.bipolardatabase.org) and the Major Depressive Disorder Neuroimaging Database (http://www.depressiondatabase.org) by Kempton and colleagues [41,42], as well as the series of peak-coordinate databases from SDM meta-analyses (http://www.sdmproject.com/database).

Finally, many sets of summary statistics of virtually all published neuroimaging studies exist, allowing a rapid retrieval of specific data in order to facilitate the meta-analytic process. The developers of BrainMap (http://www.brainmap.org), for instance, have been building and updating an impressive database of neuroimaging findings since 1987 [43]. Other available databases are the AMAT toolbox (http://www.antoniahamilton.com/amat.html), the Brede Database (http://neuro.imm.dtu.dk/services/brededatabase) [44], the Internet Brain Volume Database (http://www.cma.mgh.harvard.edu/ibvd) and the Surface Management System Database (http://sumsdb.wustl.edu/sums/index.jsp).

Another recent and promising online development called NeuroSynth (http://www.neurosynth.org) [45] deserves mentioning. NeuroSynth contains a set of summary statistics together with online functions aimed to conduct real-time meta-analyses online. Unfortunately, extraction of coordinates from publications is not manually verified, which may bias the results towards those regions that the authors of the original articles wanted to emphasize in the tables of the manuscripts. However, when the researcher's goal is to obtain a very fast and preliminary meta-analysis of the literature, NeuroSynth may be one of the first options.

Conclusions

In this paper we have reviewed the main types of meta-analytic methods available for neuroimaging studies, using examples from the mood and anxiety disorder literature to illustrate these methods.

ROI- and voxel-based methods each have advantages and disadvantages, which are summarized in Table 2. Specifically, ROI-based meta-analyses use optimal statistical methods, but they usually have a limited and likely biased inclusion of studies [14]. Conversely, voxel-based meta-analyses usually have a more exhaustive and unbiased inclusion of studies, but their statistical methods are less accurate. There are also relevant differences between the different available voxel-based meta-analytic methods. Fortunately, the field is rapidly evolving to develop more accurate and robust methods.

Although voxel-based meta-analyses minimize the effects of selectively reporting certain ROI, they are not totally immune to publication biases, as negative results may still be less likely to be published (what is known as the file drawer problem). Authors of the original

Table 2 Comparison of the main meta-analytic methods for neuroimaging studies comparing patients and controls

	ROI-based meta-analyses	Voxel-based meta-analyses			
		KDA/old ALE	Multilevel KDA/new ALE	SDM	ES-SDM
Selection of studies					
Exhaustive inclusion of studies	Limited, as information for a given brain region is present in few or no studies	Probable, as far as the included studies investigate the whole brain and not only some ROIs (in which case should be discarded)			More probable, because statistical parametric maps can also be included
Unbiased inclusion of studies	Limited, as information is only available for regions hypothesized a priori; ignoring the rest of the brain	Probable, as far as the included studies do not use different statistical thresholds for different parts of the brain (this is a strict inclusion criterion in SDM and ES-SDM)			
Statistical analyses					
Weighting of the studies	Complete (sample size and study precision)	None	Partial (only sample size)		Complete (sample size and study precision)
Control of the heterogeneity	Residual heterogeneity is correctly included in the analyses	Residual heterogeneity is not controlled, and increases and decreases are not counteracted, potentially leading to voxels being detected as increased and decreased at the same time		Residual heterogeneity is not included in the weightings, but increases and decreases are counteracted	Residual heterogeneity is correctly included in the weightings
Study of the heterogeneity	Possible, by means of meta-regressions and subgroup analyses	Limited to subgroup analyses		Possible, by means of meta-regressions and subgroup analyses	
Correction for multiple comparisons	Possible	Not possible, questionable or limited to conventional voxel-thresholded cluster-based methods			
Description of the effect sizes	Possible	Not possible		Possible though limited to pseudo-effect sizes based on the proportion of studies reporting significant findings	Possible
Description of relevant non-significant trends	Possible, as the number of ROIs is manageable	Not possible, or limited to the visual inspection of liberally thresholded maps, as the number of voxels is too massive for a more accurate individual inspection			

Please see text for further details. ALE: activation likelihood estimation; ES: effect size; KDA: kernel density analysis; ROI: region of interest; SDM: signed differential mapping.

papers are strongly encouraged to publish their results even if they perceive them as being disappointing or they do not find differences between patients and controls.

Finally, we suggest that in any meta-analysis of neuroimaging data, independently of the chosen method, authors should aim to: only include studies which explored the whole brain; ensure that the same threshold throughout the whole brain was used within each included study; and explore the robustness of the findings with several complementary analyses, for example, sensitivity analyses, quantification of the ROI- or voxel-based between-study heterogeneity [19], funnel plots of the values extracted from the meta-analytic clusters or their peaks, and so on, just like in any standard meta-analysis.

Author details
[1]Institute of Psychiatry, King's College London, De Crespigny Park, London, UK. [2]Research Unit, FIDMAG-CIBERSAM, Sant Boi de Llobregat, Barcelona, Spain.

Authors' contributions
All authors drafted, read and approved the final manuscript.

Competing interests
The authors declare that they have no competing interests.

References
1. Wager TD, Lindquist M, Kaplan L: **Meta-analysis of functional neuroimaging data: current and future directions.** *Soc Cogn Affect Neurosci* 2007, **2**:150-158.
2. Lazar NA, Luna B, Sweeney JA, Eddy WF: **Combining brains: a survey of methods for statistical pooling of information.** *Neuroimage* 2002, **16**:538-550.
3. Radua J, Mataix-Cols D: **Voxel-wise meta-analysis of grey matter changes in obsessive-compulsive disorder.** *Br J Psychiatry* 2009, **195**:391-400.
4. Mulrow CD, Oxman AD: *Cochrane Collaboration Handbook* Oxford: Cochrane Collaboration; 1996.
5. DerSimonian R, Laird N: **Meta-analysis in clinical trials.** *Control Clin Trials* 1986, **7**(3):177-188.
6. Viechtbauer W: **Bias and efficiency of meta-analytic variance estimators in the random-effects model.** *J Educ Behav Stat* 2005, **30**:261-293.
7. Fleiss JL, Gross AJ: **Meta-analysis in epidemiology, with special reference to studies of the association between exposure to environmental tobacco smoke and lung cancer: a critique.** *J Clin Epidemiol* 1991, **44**:127-139.
8. Ades AE, Higgins JPT: **The interpretation of random-effects meta-analysis in decision models.** *Med Decis Making* 2005, **25**:646-654.
9. Elvik R: **Evaluating the statistical conclusion validity of weighted mean results in meta-analysis by analysing funnel graph diagrams.** *Accid Anal Prev* 1998, **30**(2):255-266.
10. Hedges LV, Olkin I: *Statistical Methods for Meta-Analysis* Orlando, FL: Academic Press; 1985.
11. Cohen J: *Statistical Power Analysis for the Behavioral Sciences* Hillsdale, NJ: Lawrence Erlbaum Associates; 1988.
12. Rotge JY, Guehl D, Dilharreguy B, Tignol J, Bioulac B, Allard M, Burbaud P, Aouizerate B: **Meta-analysis of brain volume changes in obsessive-compulsive disorder.** *Biol Psychiatry* 2009, **65**(1):75-83.
13. Radua J, van den Heuvel OA, Surguladze S, Mataix-Cols D: **Meta-analytical comparison of voxel-based morphometry studies in obsessive-compulsive disorder vs other anxiety disorders.** *Arch Gen Psychiatry* 2010, **67**(7):701-711.

14. Ioannidis JPA: **Excess significance bias in the literature on brain volume abnormalities.** *Arch Gen Psychiatry* 2011, **68**(8):773-780.
15. Uchida RR, Del-Ben CM, Araujo D, Busatto-Filho G, Duran FL, Crippa JA, Graeff FG: **Correlation between voxel based morphometry and manual volumetry in magnetic resonance images of the human brain.** *An Acad Bras Cienc* 2008, **80**(1):149-156.
16. Bergouignan L, Chupin M, Czechowska Y, Kinkingnehun S, Lemogne C, Le Bastard G, Lepage M, Garnero L, Colliot O, Fossati P: **Can voxel based morphometry, manual segmentation and automated segmentation equally detect hippocampal volume differences in acute depression?** *Neuroimage* 2009, **45**(1):29-37.
17. Laird AR, McMillan KM, Lancaster JL, Kochunov P, Turkeltaub PE, Pardo JV, Fox PT: **A comparison of label-based review and ALE meta-analysis in the Stroop task.** *Hum Brain Mapp* 2005, **25**(1):6-21.
18. Phan KL, Wager T, Taylor SF, Liberzon I: **Functional neuroanatomy of emotion: a meta-analysis of emotion activation studies in PET and fMRI.** *Neuroimage* 2002, **16**(2):331-348.
19. Radua J, Mataix-Cols D, Phillips ML, El-Hage W, Kronhaus DM, Cardoner N, Surguladze S: **A new meta-analytic method for neuroimaging studies that combines reported peak coordinates and statistical parametric maps.** *Eur Psychiatry* 2011.
20. Eickhoff SB, Bzdok D, Laird AR, Kurth F, Fox PT: **Activation likelihood estimation meta-analysis revisited.** *Neuroimage* 2012, **59**(32):2349-2361.
21. Wager TD, Phan KL, Liberzon I, Taylor SF: **Valence, gender, and lateralization of functional brain anatomy in emotion: a meta-analysis of findings from neuroimaging.** *Neuroimage* 2003, **19**(3):513-531.
22. Turkeltaub PE, Eden GF, Jones KM, Zeffiro TA: **Meta-analysis of the functional neuroanatomy of single-word reading: method and validation.** *Neuroimage* 2002, **16**(3 Pt 1):765-780.
23. Wager TD, Barrett LF, Bliss-Moreau E, Lindquist K, Duncan S, Kober H, Joseph J, Davidson M, Mize J: **The neuroimaging of emotion.** In *The Handbook of Emotion*. Edited by: Lewis M, Haviland-Jones JM, Barrett LF. New York: Guilford Press; 2008:.
24. Costafreda SG, David AS, Brammer MJ: **A parametric approach to voxel-based meta-analysis.** *Neuroimage* 2009, **46**(1):115-122.
25. Ellison-Wright I, Ellison-Wright Z, Bullmore E: **Structural brain change in Attention Deficit Hyperactivity Disorder identified by meta-analysis.** *BMC Psychiatry* 2008, **8**:51.
26. Eickhoff SB, Laird AR, Grefkes C, Wang LE, Zilles K, Fox PT: **Coordinate-based activation likelihood estimation meta-analysis of neuroimaging data: a random-effects approach based on empirical estimates of spatial uncertainty.** *Hum Brain Mapp* 2009, **30**(9):2907-2926.
27. Nakao T, Radua J, Rubia K, Mataix-Cols D: **Gray matter volume abnormalities in ADHD: voxel-based meta-analysis exploring the effects of age and stimulant medication.** *Am J Psychiatry* 2011, **168**(11):1154-1163.
28. Via E, Radua J, Cardoner N, Happe F, Mataix-Cols D: **Meta-analysis of gray matter abnormalities in Autism Spectrum Disorder.** *Arch Gen Psychiatry* 2011, **68**:409-418.
29. Fusar-Poli P, Radua J, McGuire P, Borgwardt S: **Neuroanatomical maps of psychosis onset: voxel-wise meta-analysis of antipsychotic-naive VBM studies.** *Schizophr Bull* 2011.
30. Palaniyappan L, Balain V, Radua J, Liddle PF: **Structural correlates of auditory hallucinations in schizophrenia: a meta-analysis.** *Schizophr Res* 2012.
31. Radua J, Mataix-Cols D: **Heterogeneity of coordinate-based meta-analyses of neuroimaging data: an example from studies in OCD-Authors' reply.** *Br J Psychiatry* 2010, **197**(1):77.
32. Radua J, Via E, Catani M, Mataix-Cols D: **Voxel-based meta-analysis of regional white matter volume differences in Autism Spectrum Disorder vs. healthy controls.** *Psychol Med* 2010, **41**:1539-1550.
33. Bora E, Fornito A, Radua J, Walterfang M, Seal M, Wood SJ, Yucel M, Velakoulis D, Pantelis C: **Neuroanatomical abnormalities in schizophrenia: a multimodal voxelwise meta-analysis and meta-regression analysis.** *Schizophr Res* 2011, **127**(1-3):46-57.
34. Bora E, Fornito A, Yucel M, Pantelis C: **Voxelwise meta-analysis of gray matter abnormalities in bipolar disorder.** *Biol Psychiatry* 2010, **67**(11):1097-1105.
35. Bora E, Fornito A, Pantelis C, Yucel M: **Gray matter abnormalities in Major Depressive Disorder: a meta-analysis of voxel based morphometry studies.** *J Affect Disord* 2011.

36. Delvecchio G, Fossati P, Boyer P, Brambilla P, Falkai P, Gruber O, Hietala J, Lawrie SM, Martinot JL, McIntosh AM, Meisenzahl E, Frangou S: Common and distinct neural correlates of emotional processing in Bipolar Disorder and Major Depressive Disorder: a voxel-based meta-analysis of functional magnetic resonance imaging studies. *Eur Neuropsychopharmacol* 2011, **22(2)**:100-113.

37. Etkin A, Wager TD: Functional neuroimaging of anxiety: a meta-analysis of emotional processing in PTSD, social anxiety disorder, and specific phobia. *Am J Psychiatry* 2007, **164(10)**:1476-1488.

38. Rotge JY, Guehl D, Dilharreguy B, Cuny E, Tignol J, Bioulac B, Allard M, Burbaud P, Aouizerate B: Provocation of obsessive-compulsive symptoms: a quantitative voxel-based meta-analysis of functional neuroimaging studies. *J Psychiatry Neurosci* 2008, **33(5)**:405-412.

39. Neumann J, Fox PT, Turner R, Lohmann G: Learning partially directed functional networks from meta-analysis imaging data. *Neuroimage* 2010, **49(2)**:1372-1384.

40. Laird AR, Eickhoff SB, Li K, Robin DA, Glahn DC, Fox PT: Investigating the functional heterogeneity of the default mode network using coordinate-based meta-analytic modeling. *J Neurosci* 2009, **29(46)**:14496-14505.

41. Kempton MJ, Geddes JR, Ettinger U, Williams SC, Grasby PM: Meta-analysis, database, and meta-regression of 98 structural imaging studies in bipolar disorder. *Arch Gen Psychiatry* 2008, **65(9)**:1017-1032.

42. Kempton MJ, Salvador Z, Munafo MR, Geddes JR, Simmons A, Frangou S, Williams SC: Structural neuroimaging studies in major depressive disorder. Meta-analysis and comparison with bipolar disorder. *Arch Gen Psychiatry* 2011, **68(7)**:675-690.

43. Laird AR, Lancaster JL, Fox PT: BrainMap: the social evolution of a functional neuroimaging database. *Neuroinformatics* 2005, **3**:65-78.

44. Nielsen FA, Hansen LK, Balslev D: Mining for associations between text and brain activation in a functional neuroimaging database. *Neuroinformatics* 2004, **2(4)**:369-380.

45. Yarkoni T, Poldrack RA, Nichols TE, Van Essen DC, Wager TD: Large-scale automated synthesis of human functional neuroimaging data. *Nat Methods* 2011, **8(8)**:665-670.

46. Carmona S, Bassas N, Rovira M, Gispert JD, Soliva JC, Prado M, Tomas J, Bulbena A, Vilarroya O: Pediatric OCD structural brain deficits in conflict monitoring circuits: a voxel-based morphometry study. *Neurosci Lett* 2007, **421(3)**:218-223.

47. van den Heuvel OA, Remijnse PL, Mataix-Cols D, Vrenken H, Groenewegen HJ, Uylings HB, van Balkom AJ, Veltman DJ: The major symptom dimensions of obsessive-compulsive disorder are mediated by partially distinct neural systems. *Brain* 2009, **132(Pt 4)**:853-868.

48. Kim JJ, Lee MC, Kim J, Kim IY, Kim SI, Han MH, Chang KH, Kwon JS: Grey matter abnormalities in obsessive-compulsive disorder: statistical parametric mapping of segmented magnetic resonance images. *Br J Psychiatry* 2001, **179**:330-334.

49. Pujol J, Soriano-Mas C, Alonso P, Cardoner N, Menchon JM, Deus J, Vallejo J: Mapping structural brain alterations in obsessive-compulsive disorder. *Arch Gen Psychiatry* 2004, **61(7)**:720-730.

50. Szeszko PR, Christian C, Macmaster F, Lencz T, Mirza Y, Taormina SP, Easter P, Rose M, Michalopoulou GA, Rosenberg DR: Gray matter structural alterations in psychotropic drug-naive pediatric obsessive-compulsive disorder: an optimized voxel-based morphometry study. *Am J Psychiatry* 2008, **165(10)**:1299-1307.

51. Valente AA Jr, Miguel EC, Castro CC, Amaro E Jr, Duran FL, Buchpiguel CA, Chitnis X, McGuire PK, Busatto GF: Regional gray matter abnormalities in obsessive-compulsive disorder: a voxel-based morphometry study. *Biol Psychiatry* 2005, **58(6)**:479-487.

52. Yoo SY, Roh MS, Choi JS, Kang DH, Ha TH, Lee JM, Kim IY, Kim SI, Kwon JS: Voxel-based morphometry study of gray matter abnormalities in obsessive-compulsive disorder. *J Korean Med Sci* 2008, **23(1)**:24-30.

4

Epigenetic modifications associated with suicide and common mood and anxiety disorders

Abdulrahman M El-Sayed[1,2*], Michelle R Haloossim[3], Sandro Galea[4] and Karestan C Koenen[5]

Abstract

Epigenetic modifications are those reversible, mitotically heritable alterations in genomic expression that occur independent of changes in gene sequence. Epigenetic studies have the potential to improve our understanding of the etiology of mood and anxiety disorders and suicide by bridging the gap in knowledge between the exogenous environmental exposures and pathophysiology that produce common mood and anxiety disorders and suicide. We systematically reviewed the English-language peer-reviewed literature about epigenetic regulation in these disorders between 2001–2011, summarizing and synthesizing this literature with respect to directions for future work. Twenty-one articles met our inclusion criteria. Twelve studies were concerned with epigenetic changes among suicide completers; other studies considered epigenetic regulation in depression, post-traumatic stress disorder, and panic disorder. Several studies focused on epigenetic regulation of amine, glucocorticoid, and serotonin metabolism in the production of common mood and anxiety disorders and suicide. The literature is nascent and has yet to reach consensus about the roles of particular epigenetic modifications in the etiology of these outcomes. Future studies require larger sample sizes and measurements of environmental exposures antecedent to epigenetic modification. Further work is also needed to clarify the link between epigenetic modifications in the brain and peripheral tissues and to establish 'gold standard' epigenetic assays.

Keywords: Epigenetics, Mood disorders, Anxiety disorders, Suicide, Depression, PTSD, Histone modification, Methylation

Introduction

Nearly 50% of adults in the United States have experienced a mood or anxiety disorder at some point in their lives. Mood and anxiety disorders are among the most debilitating diseases worldwide—the World Health Organization's latest Global Burden of Disease report ranked depression among the top three most prevalent causes of disability globally, accounting for the highest single proportion of years lived with disability around the world [1,2]. Panic disorder, as well as self-inflicted injury, which is often precipitated by depression, were also high on the WHO list [2]. Mood, anxiety disorders and self-inflicted injury are also profoundly expensive, imposing high direct and indirect costs on individuals, industry, and health systems, alike [3].

The search for causes of common mood and anxiety disorders and suicide has spanned at least a century of research in a wide range of disciplines. However, a gap remains between studies focused on exogenous environmental determinants such as negative life events [4] or neighborhood social context [5,6] and studies focused on genetic determinants and biological correlates such as abnormalities in brain circuitry [7]. The recent growth in interest in epigenetic studies in human populations has been fueled, in part, by the potential of epigenetics to bridge this divide [8].

Epigenetic modifications are those reversible, mitotically heritable alterations in genomic expression that occur independent of changes in gene sequence [9]. Rather they occur via methylation of DNA or alterations to chromatin structure that either impede or facilitate access to the

* Correspondence: ame2145@columbia.edu
[1]Department of Epidemiology, Mailman School of Public Health, Columbia University, 722 W. 168th Street, R521, New York, NY 10032, USA
[2]College of Physicians and Surgeons, Columbia University, New York, NY, USA
Full list of author information is available at the end of the article

DNA by transcription factors and associated complexes [9]. Epigenetic modification of expression has been demonstrated to mediate the interplay between environmental stimuli and physiologic—and pathophysiologic— change throughout the life course [10]. Early research has been promising [11], demonstrating epigenetic involvement in the pathophysiology of depression [12], anxiety disorders [13], and suicide [14]. However, a central challenge to understanding the role of epigenetic modifications in psychopathology is limited access to brain tissue in extant studies, where inference has been limited to assessments of epigenetic modification of peripheral tissue samples which may not be related to pathophysiologic processes underlying psychopathology.

Given the growing interest in behavioral epigenetics it appears to be the appropriate time to take stock, and to synthesize the peer-reviewed literature about epigenetic modification in the etiology of common mood and anxiety disorder and suicide. In reviewing the existing literature, we aimed to summarize the state of the science, identify methodological challenges, and offer potential solutions to address these challenges.

Methods

We systematically reviewed the literature about epigenetic factors in the etiology of mood and anxiety disorders and suicide. We restricted our search to English-language, peer-reviewed articles. Our review encompassed the literature published between January 1st, 2001 and December 1st, 2011—we limited our review to the years following the sequencing of the human genome to reflect current thinking about the genetics of psychopathology. The literature reviewed here was identified via the MEDLINE and PSYCHINFO databases.

Our original search yielded 1273 articles, 600 of which were judged to consider epigenetic factors in the etiology of mood and anxiety disorders and/or suicide after screening by title. Another 368 were discarded after screening by abstract because they did not consider epigenetic mechanisms or disease outcomes of interest. Of the remaining 232, articles were included in the review if they fulfilled the following criteria:

- Included original data about a n > 1 sample of human subjects
- Used DSM-III, DSM-IV, or ICD-10 criteria to classify participants as having common mood or anxiety disorders (including and limited to PTSD, GAD, Phobias, Panic Disorder, or Depression) OR used coroners' reports to classify cause of death by self-inflicted injury
- Objectively assessed epigenetic mechanisms relating to the etiology of mood and anxiety disorders or suicide

After reading the complete manuscripts, 211 were excluded because they did not meet our criteria, above. This left 21 articles from the original search considered in this review. Reference lists from these articles were searched, and yielded no further articles which fulfilled the inclusion criteria, yielding a final total of 21 articles reviewed here. Figure 1 shows a flow diagram of our search strategy.

Because of the diversity of outcomes in which we were interested, the genetic pathways considered in the extant literature, and the methods used to both assess for epigenetic mechanisms and statistically analyze the findings, a meta-analysis of the results would not have been appropriate or feasible. For each of the 21 papers, we extracted the following information: the outcome of interest; sample population; proportion male; proportion White; number of cases and controls; loci considered; tissues sampled; laboratory techniques used; statistical analyses employed; and summary of the findings.

Results

Table 1 includes a detailed review of each of the studies included in our review. The majority (12) of the studies included in the literature considered epigenetic modification in the etiology of suicide [14-25]. Five studies considered epigenetic factors and mood disorders (all five were concerned with depression) [12,26-29], and the remaining four studies considered epigenetic factors in the etiology of anxiety disorders (three considered PTSD and one considered panic disorder) [13,30-32].

All of the studies concerned with epigenetic factors in suicide assessed gene expression and methylation profiles in the post-mortem brains of suicide completers relative to non-suicide controls [14-25], although one study also included adjuvant data about methylation profiles in peripheral leukocytes [17]. Among studies regarding epigenetic factors in the etiology of depression, one study assessed methylation and expression profiles in the post-mortem brain [27], another assessed methylation and expression of tissue in buccal cells [28], and the remaining three assessed methylation and expression profiles in peripheral blood [12,26,29]. All four studies about epigenetic mechanisms in anxiety disorders assessed methylation and expression in whole blood [13,30-32].

Epigenetic modifications in the etiology of suicide

There were twelve studies concerned with epigenetic mechanisms in the etiology of suicide [14-25]. Three studies assessed epigenetic mechanisms involved in the expression of Brain Derived Neurotrophic Factor (BDNF) and its receptor, Tropomyosin-Related Kinase B (TrkB). In a study of post-mortem brain tissue from 10 suicide completers and 10 controls matched on age, gender, post-mortem interval and brain pH, Ernst and

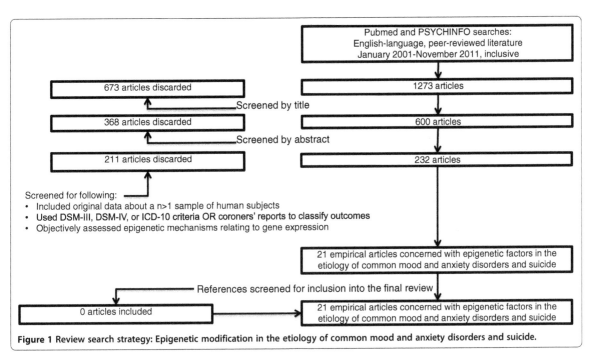

Figure 1 Review search strategy: Epigenetic modification in the etiology of common mood and anxiety disorders and suicide.

colleagues [18] found significantly higher methylation of the TrkB.T1 promoter in the frontal cortices of suicide completers relative to controls, and that methylation frequency at sites 2 and 5 of the promoter were associated with lower TrkB.T1 expression. By contrast, Keller and colleagues [22] demonstrated that no significant differences in TrkB.T1 methylation in Wernecke's areas of suicide completers relative to non-suicide controls. However, in a 2010 study from the same sample, the group demonstrated that suicide completers had higher rates of methylation at BDNF promoter IV than non-suicide controls, and that BDNF promoter IV methylation was predictive of lower BDNF mRNA expression in cases relative to controls [21].

Several studies considered epigenetic modification of genes involved in amine metabolism in the brain. Three studies using data from the Quebec Suicide Brain Bank and non-suicide controls from the same area considered the role of histone methylation at different locations in the etiology of suicide with conflicting results. The first found no association between H3K4me3 methylation at either spermine synthase (SMS) or spermine oxidase (SMOX) and suicide [25]. In addition, there was no association between methylation at either site and risk of suicide [25]. Another found higher H3K4me3 methylation levels, a marker of more open chromatin, at the antizyme 1 (OAZ1) promoter [23]. H3K4me3 methylation was correlated with higher expression of OAZ1 and arginase II (ARG2). A third study by the same group also concerned

with epigenetic modification of genes involved in amine metabolism found that spermidine/spermine N^1-acetyltransferase (SAT1) methylation was not associated with suicide. Similarly, there was no association between H3K27me3 methylation and suicide. A fourth study using post-mortem brain samples of 20 suicide cases and 20 non-suicide controls from the Geneva Institute for Forensic Medicine considered methylation of the spermine/spermidine N^1-acetyltransferase (SSAT) gene promoter in the ventral prefrontal cortex in the etiology of suicide and found no association between methylation and suicide.

One study was concerned with epigenetic modifications of genes involved in 5-HT metabolism. De Luca and colleagues studied both the post-mortem brains of suicide completers as well as peripheral blood methylation expression profiles of suicide attempters to assess the role of epigenetic modification of the 5-HT2A C102 in the etiology of suicide [17]. Comparing 10 suicide completers to non-suicide controls matched on genotype, age at death, and previous psychiatric diagnoses, they found no difference in methylation at C102 in the dorsolateral pre-frontal cortex [17]. They also compared methylation profiles at this location in the leukocytes of both suicide attempters and non-suicide controls all of whom had a history of bipolar disorder or schizophrenia. While there were no differences in methylation among bipolar patients, suicide attempters with schizophrenia had significantly higher methylation levels at the C102 location [17].

Poulter and colleagues used post-mortem brain samples from several brain regions from 10 suicide completers and 10 non-suicide controls in Budapest to assess the role of DNA methyltransferase (DNMT) expression and subsequent GABA$_A$ promoter hypermethylation [15]. They found differential DNMT expression in the frontopolar cortices, dorsal vagal complexes, and hippocampi of suicide completers relative to controls, and no difference in the amygdala. Moreover, DNMT-3B upregulation predicted hypermethylation of CpG islands 2 and 4 in the GABA$_A$ promoter [15].

One study considered the role of epigenetic regulation of the neuron-specific glucocorticoid receptor (NR3C1) in suicide etiology among those with a history of childhood abuse [19]. McGowan and colleagues found that in the hippocampi of post-mortem brain tissue among patients matched on age, gender and post-mortem interval, suicide completers with a history of child abuse had higher rates of CpG methylation and lower expression of NR3C1 mRNA than non-abused suicide completers [19]. There were no differences between non-abused suicide completers and non-suicide controls [19]. Another study by the same group also considered the role of epigenetic modification in the etiology of suicide among those abused during childhood [14]. They found more heavy methylation of the rRNA promoter in the hippocampi of suicide completers relative to non-suicide controls [14]. There was, however, no difference in methylation of the rRNA promoter in the cerebellum of suicide completers relative to controls [14].

A final study considered the etiology of suicide among depressive patients. Klempan and colleagues assessed differences in methylation and expression of the oligodendrocyte-specific RNA binding protein (QKI) in suicide completers with a history of major depression relative to age-matched non-suicide controls [20]. Although they found that suicide completers had significantly lower mRNA levels of QKI in 11 cortical regions as well as in the amygdala, there were no significant differences in methylation levels between suicide completers and non-suicide controls [20].

Epigenetic modifications in the etiology of mood disorders

There were five studies concerned with the role of epigenetic modification in the etiology of mood disorders—all five were concerned specifically with depression [12,26-29]. Two studies were concerned with epigenetic influences in genes involved in 5-HT metabolism and depression with mixed results [26,28]. In a study of participants in the Iowa Adoption Study, Philibert and colleagues assessed the relationship between methylation at the 5-HT transporter (SLC6A4) in lymphoblasts and both history of and current major depression—they found no association between SLC6A4 methylation or mRNA expression and either outcome [26]. Another study assessed the relation between 5-HT transporter promoter methylation in buccal cells and depression in a nested cohort from the Victorian Adolescent Health Study in Victoria, Australia. While 5-HT transporter promoter methylation did not predict depression on its own, there was a significant interaction between methylation and the short "s-type" allele in predicting depression.

A study by Alt and colleagues assessed the relationship between glucocorticoid receptor (GR) promoter methylation in several regions of the post-mortem brains of depressed patients relative to non-depressed controls from the Dutch Brain Bank matched on age, sex, brain weight, post-mortem delay, and pH of the cerebrospinal fluid [27]. There were no differences in GR mRNA expression levels by disease status nor in methylation patterns in any of the brain regions sampled (amygdala, hippocampus, inferior postulate gyrus, cingulate gyrus, and nucleus accumbens) [27].

In a study of a Japanese sample of depressed patients and non-depressed controls recruited from four academic medical centers, Fuchikami and colleagues assessed the relation between BDNF promoter methylation in white blood cells and depression [29]. They found that BDNF promoter methylation at CpG site 1 was associated with depression, although there was no association between CpG methylation at site 4 and the outcome [29].

A final study considered "functional annotation clusters" (FACs) of epigenetic modifications in the whole blood of a community-based sample in Detroit, MI [12]. The authors found that cases had fewer uniquely unmethylated and methylated genes than controls, and that methylation predicted lower gene expression. FACs associated with multicellular organismal development, lipoprotein activity, and hydrolase activity were uniquely unmethylated, while those associated with protease activity, metabolic processes, and cell development were uniquely methylated among depressed subjects [12]. In controls, FACs involved in brain development, tryptophan metabolism, and neuromuscular processes were uniquely unmethylated, while those involved in signaling, lipocalin, and tissue development were uniquely methylated [12].

Epigenetic modifications in the etiology of anxiety disorders

There were four studies that considered epigenetic mechanisms in the etiology of anxiety disorders [13,30-32]. Three studies were concerned with the etiology of post-traumatic stress disorder (PTSD) [30-32] and one was concerned with panic disorder [13].

With respect to PTSD, none of the three studies considered epigenetic modification of one specific gene pathway. Rather each considered non-specific sets of

Table 1 *Studies about epigenetic modifications involved in the etiology of common mood and anxiety disorders and suicide, January 2010-November 2011

Author (Year)	Outcome	Sample	% Male	% White	N Cases	N Controls
Suicide						
Poulter et al., 2008 [15]	Completed suicide	Department of Forensic Medicine, Semmelweis University Medical School, Budapest	50% in methylation analyses	100%	10 for methylation analysis	10 for methylation analysis
McGowan et al., 2008 [14]	Completed suicide following child abuse	Quebec Suicide Brain Bank matched on age, gender, and post-mortem interval; 5 cases and 1 control used for RNA expression analyses, separate 13 cases and 11 controls used for other analyses	100%	100%	18	12
Guipponi et al., 2008 [16]	Completed suicide	Geneva, Switzerland Institute for Forensic Medicine	55% cases; 50% controls	N/I	20	20
De Luca et al., 2009 [17]	Completed suicide	Stanley Medical Research Institute array collection; suicide and non-suicide controls matched on genotype, diagnosis, age at death, and sex	40% cases; 60% controls	N/I	10	10
	Suicide attempt	48 schizophrenics (24 suicide attempts and 24 non-attempters) pooled from Toronto Schizophrenia, and SMR populations	67% cases; 75% controls	N/I	24	24
	Suicide attempt	57 bipolar subjects (29 suicide attempts and 28 non-attempters) pooled from Toronto Bipolar and SMR populations	34.4% cases; 35.7% controls	N/I	29	28
Ernst et al., 2009 [18]	Completed suicide	Quebec Suicide Brain Bank (28 suicide completers and 11 controls); matched on age, postmortem interval, and pH. Epigenetic analyses performed on 10 subjects with low TrKB expression and 10 matched controls.	100%	100%	10 (of 28 possible)	10 (of 11 possible)
McGowan et al., 2009 [19]	Completed suicide following child abuse	Quebec Suicide Brain Bank matched on age, gender, and post-mortem interval	100%	100%	24 (12 with history of child abuse; 12 without such a history)	12
Klempan et al., 2009 [20]	Completed suicide among depressive patients	Quebec Suicide Brain Bank matched on age	100%	100%	16 (4 included in methylation analysis)	13 (4 included in methylation analysis)
Keller et al., 2010 [22]	Completed suicide	Biological Bank of the Institut za Varovanje Zdravja, Ljubljana (Slovenia)	48% cases; 48% controls	100%	44	33
Fiori et al., 2010 [25]	Completed suicide	Quebec Suicide Brain Bank as well as a Quebecois sample of healthy controls	100%	100%	10 (of 40 possible)	10 (of 56 possible)
Fiori et al., 2011a [24]	Completed suicide	Quebec Suicide Brain Bank as well as a Quebecois sample of healthy controls	100%	100%	10	10
Fiori et al., 2011b [23]	Completed suicide	Quebec Suicide Brain Bank as well as a Quebecois sample of healthy controls; suicide completers selected on over-expression of AMD1, ARG2, OAZ1, and OAZ2	100%	100%	34	34

Table 1 *Studies about epigenetic modifications involved in the etiology of common mood and anxiety disorders and suicide, January 2010-November 2011 (Continued)

Study	Disorder	Sample				
Keller et al., 2011 [21]	Completed suicide	Biological Bank of the Institut za Varovanje Zdravja, Ljubljana (Slovenia)	61% cases; 52% controls	N/I	18	18
Mood Disorders						
Philibert et al., 2008 [26]	Major depression	Iowa Adoption Study participants	50%	93%	68 (history of MD); 17 (current MD)	124 (no history of MD); 175 (no current MD)
Alt et al., 2009 [27]	Major Depressive Disorder	Dutch Brain Bank; Matched on age, sex, brain weight, post-mortem delay and pH of CSF	67% cases; 50% controls	N/I	6	6
Olsson et al., 2010 [28]	Depression	Nested cohort from the Victorian Adolescent Health Cohort Study, a population-representative sample of 2032 young Australians in Victoria	55%	96%	25	125
Fuchikami et al., 2011 [29]	Major depression	Japanese sample of DSM-IV criteria depressed patients and health controls from four academic medical centers	N/I	N/I	20	18
Uddin et al., 2011 [12]	Lifetime Depression	Detroit Neighborhood Health Survey, a multiethnic representative survey of low-income neighborhoods in Detroit, MI	40%	14%	33	67
Anxiety Disorders						
Elser et al., 2006 [13]	Panic disorder	N/I	N/I	N/I	24	N/I
Uddin et al., 2010 [30]	Post-traumatic stress disorder	Detroit Neighborhood Health Survey, a multiethnic representative survey of low-income neighborhoods in Detroit, MI	40%	14%	27	77
Uddin et al., 2011 [31]	Post-traumatic stress disorder	Detroit Neighborhood Health Survey, a multiethnic representative survey of low-income neighborhoods in Detroit, MI	40%	14%	27	77
Smith et al., 2011 [32]	Lifetime post-traumatic stress disorder	Cohort of African-American participants recruited at clinical waiting rooms in a low-income, urban context	63% of cases; 60% of controls	0%	51 (25 with childhood trauma)	53 (21 with childhood trauma)

Table 1 *Studies about epigenetic modifications involved in the etiology of common mood and anxiety disorders and suicide, January 2010-November 2011 (Continued)

Suicide

Author (Year)	Gene (s)/loci	Tissue	Assay	Statistical analysis	Summary
Poulter et al., 2008 [15]	DNMT mRNA expression in the frontopolar cortex, hippocampus, amygdala, and dorsal vagal complex; GABAa promoter	post-mortem brain	qPCR; Methylation Mapping; Western Blot	ANOVA and t-tests with Bonferroni corrections; chi-square tests	DNMT-1 was downregulated, and DNMT-3B was upregulated among suicide completers relative to controls in the frontopolar cortex. There was no association between DNMT expression and suicide in the amygdala. In the hippocampus, DNMT-1 and 3B were downregulated in suicide completers relative to controls. DNMT-3B was elevated in the hypothalamus and the dorsal vagal complex. CG2 and 4 were hypermethylated in suicide completers relative to controls in the GABAa alpha1 subunit, and this was associated with DNMT-3b upregulation.
McGowan et al., 2008 [14]	rRNA promotor in the hippocampus and cerebellum	post-mortem brain	RT-PCR; methylation mapping; nearest neighbor quantification	factorial ANOVA, Bonferroni corrections; linear regression for site-specific differences	rRNA promotor was more heavily methylated in the hippocampus of suicide subjects than of controls. 21 of 26 sites had higher methylation frequency in suicide subjects relative to controls in the hippocampus. These differences were not observed in the cerebellum.
Guipponi et al., 2008 [16]	SSAT promotor in ventral prefrontal cortex	post-mortem brain	Pyrosequencing	ANOVA and t-tests	There was no association between promotor methylation and suicide.
De Luca et al., 2009 [17]	5-HT2A C102 allele in the dorsolateral pre-frontal cortex	post-mortem brain	HpaII treatment followed by TaqMan Assay Q-PCR	independent t-tests	No significant difference in methylation levels of C102 were found in Brain-tissue between suicide completers and controls.
	5-HT2A C102 allele in the white blood cells	leukocytes	HpaII treatment followed by TaqMan Assay Q-PCR	independent t-tests, corrected by Bonferroni	Suicide attempters had significantly higher methylation of 102 C in peripheral leukocytes relative to controls.
	5-HT2A C102 allele in the white blood cells	leukocytes	HpaII treatment followed by TaqMan Assay Q-PCR	independent t-tests, corrected by Bonferroni	There was no significant difference in methylation of 102 C in the peripheral leukocytes of suicide attempters and controls.
Ernst et al, 2009 [18]	TrKB.T1 promoter region in the frontal cortex	post-mortem brain	Methylation mapping; Q-PCR and Western blot analysis; HG-U133 plus 2 microarray chip	t-test on mean methylation at two CpG dinucleotides	There was a significant difference in TrKB.T1 expression among suicide completers and non-completers. In suicide completers, downregulation was correlated with methylation frequency at sites 2 and 5 in the TrKB.T1 promotor.
McGowan et al, 2009 [19]	NR3C1 neuron-specific glucocorticoid receptor promotor in the hippocampus	post-mortem brain	RT-PCR; methylation mapping	factorial ANOVA, Bonferroni corrections	There was decreased glucocorticoid receptor mRNA and increased cytosine methylation in abused suicide completers as compared to non-abused completers. There were no differences between non-abused completers and non-completers.

Table 1 *Studies about epigenetic modifications involved in the etiology of common mood and anxiety disorders and suicide, January 2010-November 2011 (Continued)

Klempan et al., 2009 [20]	QKI promotor in the orbitofrontal cortex	post-mortem brain	HG-U133 A/B microarray; methylation mapping; TaqMan gene expression assays	t-test	Suicide completers had significantly lower mRNA levels of QKI in 11 cortical regions and in the amygdala. However, there were no significant differences in methylation levels at the QKI promotor by suicide status.
Keller et al., 2010 [22]	Overall methylation in Wernicke's area; BDNF promotor region methylation in Wernicke's area	post-mortem brain	Pyrosequencing; MassARRAY; bisulfite genomic sequencing	ANOVA and ANCOVA adjusted for sex and age	BDNF promotor IV methylation was significantly higher in suicide completers relative to controls. Higher BDNF methylation was associated with lower BDNF transcript IV. There was no difference in genome-wide methylation levels between suicide completers and controls. In suicide completers with high methylation levels, there were lower BDNF mRNA levels.
Fiori et al., 2010 [25]	SMS and SMOX promotor region in the BA 8/9, as well as histone methylation of H3K27me3	post-mortem brain	Methylation mapping and chromatin immunoprecipitation	t-test with correction for multiple testing	There were no associations between methylation at any locus and suicide. Histone H3k27me3 methylation was not associated with suicide.
Fiori et al., 2011a [24]	SAT1 promotor in the prefrontal cortex; histone methylation of H3K27me3	post-mortem brain	Methylation mapping and chromatin immunoprecipitation	t-test	CpG methylation at the SAT1 promotor was not associated with suicide, although it did predict decreased SAT1 expression. Histone H3k27me3 methylation was not associated with suicide completion.
Fiori et al., 2011b [23]	Histone H3Kme3 in the inferior frontal gyrus	post-mortem brain	Chromatin immunoprecipitation	t-test and pearson correlation	Suicide completers had significantly higher H3Kme3 levels at OAZ1. H3Kme3 was positively correlated with expression of ARG2 and OAZ1.
Keller et al., 2011 [21]	BDNF receptor (TrkB) in Wernicke's area; BDNF promotor in Wernicke's area	post-mortem brain	MassArray	t-tests	There were no significant differences in TrkB promotor methylation between suicide completers and controls. BDNF promotor IV methylation was significantly higher in suicide completers relative to controls.
Mood Disorders					
Philibert et al., 2008 [26]	5HTT promotor SLC6A4	lymphoblast	RT-PCR; MassArray quantitative methylation	ANOVA and linear regression with Bonferroni corrections	There was no relationship between methylation and mRNA expression overall. There was no relationship between SLC6A4 expression and life history of MD or current MD.
Alt et al., 2009 [27]	Glucocorticoid receptor promotor region (1 J, 1E, 1B, 1 F) of amygdala, hippocampus, inferior postulate gyrus, cingulate gyrus, nucleus accumbens	post-mortem brain	QIAamp DNA Mni kit (Qiagen); pyrosequencing	Mann–Whitney U-test, corrected by Bonferroni	GR transcript levels were homogenous by disease status. Exon 1 F expression was reduced among MDD patients relative to controls. There were no significant differences in methylation patterns between groups between different brain regions.
Olsson et al., 2010 [28]	5HTT promotor	buccal cells	MassArrray	logistic regression, Bonferroni corrections	Buccal cell 5HTT methylation and depression were not associated either over the entire promotor or in subregions identified by PCA. However, there was a joint effect of 5HTT methylation and the s-allele variant on risk for depression.
	BDNF promotor		MassArray		

Table 1 *Studies about epigenetic modifications involved in the etiology of common mood and anxiety disorders and suicide, January 2010-November 2011 (*Continued*)

Study	Gene	Tissue	Platform	Analysis	Results
Fuchikami et al., 2011 [29]		white blood cells		2-dimensional hierarchical clustering and t-tests	Mean methylation rates of CpG 1 but not 4 at the BDNF promotor was associated with depression.
Uddin et al., 2011 [12]	non-specific	whole blood	HumanMethylation 27 beadchip; pyrosequencing of two loci	McNemar's chi-squared tests for overall methylation; Functional annotation clustering analyzed via Wilcoxon test, alpha < 0.01	Cases had fewer uniquely unmethylated and methylated genes than controls. Methylated genes were associated with lower gene expression. FACs associated with multicellular organismal development, lipoprotein activity, and hydrolase activity were uniquely unmethylated, while those associated with protease activity, metabolic processes, and cell development were uniquely methylated in cases. In controls, FACs associated with brain development, tryptophan metabolism, and neuormuscular processes were uniquely unmethylated, while those involved in signaling, lipocalin, and tissue development were uniquely methylated.
Anxiety Disorders					
Elser et al., 2006 [13]	NET promotor and exon 9	white blood cells	CpGenome DNA modification it and ABI Prism 7700 Sequence Detection System; chromatin immunoprecipitation	t-test on mean methylation in promotor region	There was a significant difference in NET promotor methylation among patients with panic disorder relative to healthy controls. Promotor regions were also enriched with the MeCP2 co-repressor complex.
Uddin et al., 2010 [30]	non-specific	whole blood	HumanMethylation 27 beadchip	McNemar's chi-squared tests for overall methylation; Functional annotation clustering analyzed via Wilcoxon test, alpha < 0.01	There was no difference in overall methylation level among PTSD cases relative to controls, however the number of uniquely methylated genes did differ by disease status. Uniquely unmethylated genes in PTSD cases were associated immune system involvement, including TLR1, TLR3 (innate immune system), IL8, LTA, and KLRG-1 (adaptive immune system).
Uddin et al., 2011 [31]	33 genes previously described in the literature as associated with PTSD	whole blood	HumanMethylation 27 beadchip	Logistic regression to assess the relation between site-specific methylation and lifetime traumatic events adjusted for race, smoking, gender, age, socioeconomic status, peripheral cell count, and medication	Only MAN2C1 methylation interacted with number of potentially traumatic events to significantly predict lifetime PTSD. Increases in both factors were associated with increased lifetime PTSD risk.
Smith et al., 2011 [32]	non-specific	whole blood	HumanMethylation 27 beadchip	linear mixed model adjusted for age, sex, and chip effects, with adjustment for multiple testing using the false discovery rate method	Lifetime PTSD was associated with increased methylation overall. Lifetime PTSD was associated with increased methylation in TPR, ANXA2, CLEC9A, ACP15, and TLR8 compared to controls. CPG site methylation at BDNF and CXCL1 were associated with lifetime PTSD. There was no association between methylation at NR3C1 and SLC6A4 and PTSD.

*N/I; not indicated.

pathways. A study by Smith and colleagues of a cohort of African-American participants recruited at clinical waiting rooms in a low income context used linear mixed models adjusted for age, sex, and assay effects, found that increased methylation in white blood cells was associated with lifetime PTSD [32]. Moreover, those with lifetime PTSD had increased methylation at several sites, including translocated promoter region (TPR), annexin 2 (ANXA2), c-type lectin-like receptor 9A (CLEC9A), testicular acid phosphatase 5 (ACPT5) and toll-like receptor 8 (TLR8). Methylation at specific CpG islands in BDNF and chemokine ligand 1 (CXCL1) were also associated with lifetime PTSD [32]. Another study by Uddin and colleagues considered unique methylation and unmethylation by FAC [30] in white blood cells of a community-based sample in Detroit, MI. There was no difference in overall methylation levels among PTSD cases relative to controls, however the number of uniquely methylated genes did differ among cases and controls [30]. Uniquely unmethylated genes in PTSD cases were associated immune system involvement, including toll-like receptor 1 (TLR1), toll-like receptor 3 (TLR3) (innate immune system), interleukin 8 (IL8), lymphotoxin alpha (LTA), and killer cell lectin-like receptor G1 (KLRG-1) (adaptive immune system) [30]. Another study among the same population demonstrated effect modification of the relationship between the number of reported potentially traumatic events and the degree of mannosidase 2 C1 (MAN2C1) methylation, such that among those with increased methylation at MAN2C1 a larger number of potentially traumatic events was more strongly related to PTSD risk [31].

A fourth study was concerned with the role of epigenetic modification of the promoter as well as exon 9 of the neuroepithelial cell transforming (NET) gene promotor and exon 9 in the etiology of panic disorder [13]. Using peripheral blood, the authors demonstrated a significant difference in NET promotor methylation relative to healthy controls. Moreover, they noted an enrichment of the MeCP2 co-repressor complex at the promoter regions of NET among cases relative to controls [13].

Discussion

We systematically reviewed the peer-reviewed literature about the role of epigenetic modification in the etiology of common mood and anxiety disorders and suicide. Twenty-one papers were published between 2001, the publication of the human genome project, and 2011. The majority (12) of studies we found were concerned with evidence of epigenetic changes in the post-mortem brains of suicide completers, with other studies considering epigenetic factors in the etiology of depression, PTSD, and panic disorder. A plurality focused on epigenetic regulation of genes involved in amine,

glucocorticoid, and serotonin metabolism in the production of common mood and anxiety disorders and suicide; studies also considered epigenetic modification of a diverse array of other genes.

Given the small number of studies, drawing substantive conclusions about how epigenetic modifications in specific genes may be operating in the etiology of the diseases in question is not possible at this stage. Our review occasions a synthesis of methodological limitations of the extant literature and recommendations on how investigators may best approach this area in future studies.

Five methodological limitations to this literature emerge from our review. The first is that studies in this area have suffered from small sample sizes, the consequences of which include lack of power and increased false discovery rates. Second, existing studies have been limited to assessing epigenetic modification in the postmortem brain or the peripheral blood following disease diagnosis, and drawing inference from either tissue type is problematic. Third, studies have used different techniques to assess epigenetic modifications that may produce heterogeneous results. Fourth, few studies have assessed environmental antecedents to epigenetic modifications in extant studies. Fifth, there appears to be little consensus regarding genome-wide vs. candidate-gene approaches.

The first methodological limitation to this literature is the use of small sample sizes in most studies, a ubiquitous problem in molecular epidemiology [33]. Of the studies we reviewed, only one included more than fifty cases (e.g., subjects with the outcome). Compounding small sample sizes in studies overall, many of the studies we reviewed limited epigenetic analysis to a subset of the total study population. Small sample sizes limit study power, therefore increasing the likelihood of type II error (e.g., the proportion of false negative findings) [33]. More dangerously, underpowered studies also increase the "false discovery rate" or the number of significant findings that fall into type I error (e.g., the proportion of false positive findings), as demonstrated in Equation 1 [34-36].

$$FDR = \frac{\alpha(1 - prior)}{\alpha(1 - prior) + power * prior} \tag{1}$$

^ "prior" indicates the proportion of tested hypotheses that are actually correct.

In this equation, the false discovery rate (FDR) is inversely proportional to power (1-beta), such that low power also yields high FDR, driving up Type I error. Therefore, given the small sample sizes employed in the majority of studies we reviewed, it is likely that the findings suffer from high proportions of both type I and type II error.

A second limitation is the use post-mortem brain or peripheral cell tissues for epigenetic analyses. Seven of the 21 studies we reviewed analyzed epigenetic modification in peripheral blood cells, and one study analyzed epigenetic modification in buccal mucosa. Although all human cells carry the full endowment of genetic material, cells modify gene expression to efficiently carry out their diverse functions as they specialize, silencing some genes while activating others in line with their physiologic responsibilities. Epigenetic modification is the physiologic process by which genes are silenced or primed for expression [37,38]. The pathophysiology of mood-anxiety disorders and suicide is localized to the brain and it remains therefore unclear how gene expression in peripheral tissues correlates with physiologically meaningful gene expression in the brain. However, even epigenetic studies using post-mortem brain tissue have challenges. Three of the 21 studies we reviewed analyzed post-mortem brain tissue. While these studies assessed epigenetic changes in the appropriate organ, assessing post-mortem brain tissue carries its own challenges. This is problematic with respect to temporality between exposure and outcome, because post-mortem brains, by definition, can only be harvested after death, and therefore epigenetic modification can only be ascertained after the occurrence of the outcome. Moreover, death often involves acidosis, which may contribute to the instability of genetic material [39-41], increasing the likelihood of misclassifying epigenetic modification and increasing the chances of spurious findings. Therefore, much more work is needed to help us understand the physiologic significance of both peripheral tissue and brain methylation patterns.

A third limitation to the literature is that published studies used different laboratory techniques to measure the degree of epigenetic modification. With respect to DNA methylation alone, there are a number of gene-specific assays currently in use, including bisulfite reaction based DNA sequencing methods, which include bisulfite genomic sequencing PCR [42] and/or methylation specific PCR [43]; genome-wide screens, such as CpG island microarrays [44] and Restriction Landmark Genomic Scanning for Methylation (RLGS-M) techniques [45]; and methylated DNA immunoprecipitation (MeDIP) [46]. There are few studies that have compared the sensitivity and specificity of each method, although a recent study compared two bisulfite sequence-based assays (which are very similar) head-to-head and found as much as an 18% difference in identification of methylated CpG islands in biological replicates of human embryonic stem cells [47]. To our knowledge, there are no "gold standard" assays for most epigenetic markers. Therefore, differential use of assays may present a source

of misclassification bias in studies, which would ultimately increase the rate of type II error rate in the extant literature.

Fourth, studies in our review largely failed to assess the environmental exposures thought to produce epigenetic change to begin with. Only three out of 21 of the studies reviewed here included any assessment of a common environmental stressor with respect to epigenetic modifications and their relationship with common mood and anxiety disorders and suicide [14,19,20]. This is an important limitation, as there is ample data demonstrating the importance of environmental stressors in the etiology of these disorders [48]. Without assessing common environmental stressors antecedent to epigenetic modifications, our studies fail to adequately test dominant hypotheses about the mediating role of epigenetic changes between environments and outcomes in common mood and anxiety disorders and suicide.

The fifth limitation is the lack of consensus regarding genome-wide vs. candidate-gene approaches in epigenetic studies. Three of the studies we reviewed used genome-wide approaches [12,30,32], while the remaining 18 studies assessed for epigenetic modifications of candidate genes. Both approaches have limitations. With respect to genome-wide studies, the analyses (and findings) are often unfocused. Unlike in genome-wide association studies, there is no agreed upon method for analysis and synthesis of data or for adjustment for multiple comparisons in genome-wide epigenetic studies. In particular, appropriate adjustment for multiple comparisons can be problematic, increasing the proportion of false-positive findings [49]. Candidate-gene approaches benefit from being hypothesis-driven, and therefore more amenable to thoughtful, model-based study designs. However, candidate-gene approaches face their own limitations. Candidate-gene studies are more likely to yield overall negative results, as these studies test only one hypothesis, as compared to genome-wide studies which test more global hypotheses about the role of epigenetic modification *anywhere* in the genome influencing risk for outcomes of interest. As candidate-gene approaches are more likely to yield negative overall findings, there is a high probability of publication bias, whereby the literature about candidate-gene epigenetic modification is likely to be highly enriched for positive findings [35].

Limitations of the review

The reader should be aware of several limitations when considering the findings of our systematic review. First, we limited our review to the published peer-reviewed literature. Therefore, it is plausible that our selection of studies may have been subject to a publication bias, affecting the veracity of our inferences. Second, we organized studies by outcome. This organizational scheme may have also, in part, shaped the inferences drawn here. However, because we limited our inferences largely to methodological critiques of the literature, it is unlikely that either limitation would have had a substantial influence on our interpretation of our findings. Third, our review was limited to only the English-language literature published in journals indexed in two databases. It is plausible that we may have missed literature about epigenetics in relation to common mood and anxiety disorders and suicide published in other languages or in journals that were not indexed in MEDLINE or PSYCHINFO. However, this is less likely, as a detailed search of the citations of included studies yielded no further studies for inclusion in the review.

Conclusions

Research into the epigenetic mechanisms that may underlie common mood and anxiety disorders and suicide has the potential to unite the heretofore disparate bodies of work that have characterized the pathophysiology of these disorders and their population causes, respectively. However, at this nascent stage in the development of this literature, there are several methodological challenges, discussed above, that have yet to be addressed. With respect to these challenges moving forward, studies about the role of epigenetic regulation in the etiology of common mood and anxiety disorders can improve in the following ways.

As sufficient power and small sizes have dogged extant studies in this area, future studies require larger sample sizes, maximizing power and minimizing the false discovery rate. Furthermore, systematic comparisons of assays used to assess epigenetic modifications are needed as is consensus around what constitute 'gold standard' laboratory techniques for assessing epigenetic modification. Another challenge to this literature is the validity of using epigenetic data from peripheral blood, epithelial tissue, or post-mortem brain specimens. However, given the obvious limitations to sampling brain tissue in representative populations of living subjects, sampling these tissues may, in the long-term, remain the best available option. Future work associating epigenetic modifications with changes in gene expression and correlating epigenetic modifications in peripheral tissues with brain function may offer one way to address these limitations. Moreover, work in neuroscience to characterize the relationship between real-time brain imaging studies and epigenetic modification in brain regions sampled among patients undergoing neurosurgery, when living-patient brain samples can be collected, could yield imaging markers of epigenetic regulation in the brain. These approaches represent a handful of the many lines of inquiry that could improve our capacity to assess epigenetic modification in the brain. Future studies in this area would also do well to measure epigenetic modification in relation to its environmental antecedents so as to better assess dominant

hypotheses about the mediation of the relationship between environmental exposures and common mood and anxiety disorders and suicide by epigenetic modification.

Lastly, both genome-wide and candidate gene approaches have their role in epigenetic analyses. Genome-wide approaches may be more appropriate for exploratory analyses [50]. However, candidate gene approaches may be better suited for hypothesis-testing regarding the roles of individual genes or sets of genes hypothesized to function in a particular way in disease etiology. It is important that investigators in this area are attuned to the particular strengths and weakness of each approach so that each is used appropriately in studies about the role of epigenetics in the etiology of common mood and anxiety disorders and suicide.

Competing interests
The authors declare that they have no competing interests.

Authors' contributions
AME extracted data from studies and drafted the manuscript. MRH carried out the literature search and edited the manuscript for intellectual content. SG edited the manuscript for intellectual content. KCK conceived the review, specified review inclusion and exclusion criteria, and edited the manuscript for intellectual content. All authors have read and approve the final version.

Acknowledgments
AME was funded by the Columbia University Medical Scientist Training Program. KCK was funded by NIH grants MH078928, DA022720, and 5P51RR000165. Funding bodies had no role in the design, interpretation, or presentation of findings.

Author details
[1]Department of Epidemiology, Mailman School of Public Health, Columbia University, 722 W. 168th Street, R521, New York, NY 10032, USA. [2]College of Physicians and Surgeons, Columbia University, New York, NY, USA. [3]Department of Sociomedical Sciences, Mailman School of Public Health, Columbia University, 722 W. 168th Street, New York, NY 10032, USA. [4]Department of Epidemiology, Mailman School of Public Health, Columbia University, 722 W. 168th Street, 1508, New York, NY 10032, USA. [5]Department of Epidemiology, Mailman School of Public Health, Columbia University, 722 W. 168th Street, R720G, New York, NY 10032, USA.

References
1. Hyman S, Chisholm D, Kessler R, Patel V, Whiteford H: **Mental Disorders**. In *Disease control priorities in developing countries*. 2 editionth edition. Edited by Jamison DT, Breman JG, Measham AR, *et al*. Geneva: World Health Organization; 2006.
2. Mathers CD, Stein C, Fat DM: *Global Burden of Disease: 2004 Update*. Geneva: World Health Organization; 2008.
3. Luppa M, Heinrich S, Angermeyer MC, König H, Riedel-Heller SG: **Cost-of-illness studies of depression: A systematic review**. *J Affect Disord* 2007, **98**(1–2):29–43.
4. Risch N, Herrell R, Lehner T, Liang KY, Eaves L, Hoh J, Griem A, Kovacs M, Ott J, Merikangas KR: **Interaction between the serotonin transporter gene (5-HTTLPR), stressful life events, and risk of depression: a meta-analysis**. *JAMA* 2009, **301**(23):2462–2471.
5. Beard JR, Cerda M, Blaney S, Ahern J, Vlahov D, Galea S: **Neighborhood characteristics and change in depressive symptoms among older residents of New York City**. *Am J Public Health* 2009, **99**(7):1308–1314.
6. Galea S, Ahern J, Nandi A, Tracy M, Beard J, Vlahov D: **Urban neighborhood poverty and the incidence of depression in a population-based cohort study**. *Ann Epidemiol* 2007, **17**(3):171–179.

7. Liu Y, Blackwood DH, Caesar S, de Geus EJ, Farmer A, Ferreira MA, Ferrier IN, Fraser C, Gordon-Smith K, Green EK, Grozeva D, Gurling HM, Hamshere ML, Heutink P, Holmans PA, Hoogendijk WJ, Hottenga JJ, Jones L, Jones IR, Kirov G, Lin D, McGuffin P, Moskvina V, Nolen WA, Perlis RH, Posthuma D, Scolnick EM, Smit AB, Smit JH, Smoller JW, St Clair D, van Dyck R, Verhage M, Willemsen G, Young AH, Zandbelt T, Boomsma DI, Craddock N, O'Donovan MC, Owen MJ, Penninx BW, Purcell S, Sklar P, Sullivan PF: Wellcome Trust Case–control Consortium: Meta-analysis of genome-wide association data of bipolar disorder and major depressive disorder. Mol Psychiatry 2011, 16(1):2–4.

8. Galea S, Uddin M, Koenen K: The urban environment and mental disorders: Epigenetic links. Epigenetics 2011, 6(4):400–404.

9. Henikoff S, Matzke MA: Exploring and explaining epigenetic effects. Trends Genet 1997, 13(8):293–295.

10. Jirtle RL, Skinner MK: Environmental epigenomics and disease susceptibility. Nat Rev Genet 2007, 8(4):253–262.

11. Tsankova N, Renthal W, Kumar A, Nestler EJ: Epigenetic regulation in psychiatric disorders. Nat Rev Neurosci 2007, 8(5):355–367.

12. Uddin M, Koenen KC, Aiello AE, Wildman DE, de los Santos R, Galea S: Epigenetic and inflammatory marker profiles associated with depression in a community-based epidemiologic sample. Psychol Med 2011, 41(05):997–1007.

13. Esler M, Alvarenga M, Pier C, Richards J, El-Osta A, Barton D, Haikerwal D, Kaye D, Schlaich M, Guo L, Jennings G, Socratous F, Lambert G: The neuronal noradrenaline transporter, anxiety and cardiovascular disease. J Psychopharmacol 2006, 20(4 suppl):60–66.

14. McGowan PO, Sasaki A, Huang TC, Unterberger A, Suderman M, Ernst C, Meaney MJ, Turecki G, Szyf M: Promoter-wide hypermethylation of the ribosomal RNA gene promoter in the suicide brain. PLoS One 2008, 3(5):e2085.

15. Poulter MO, Du L, Weaver ICG, Palkovits M, Faludi G, Merali Z, Szyf M, Anisman H: GABAA Receptor Promoter Hypermethylation in Suicide Brain: Implications for the Involvement of Epigenetic Processes. Biol Psychiatry 2008, 64(8):645–652.

16. Guipponi M, Deutsch S, Kohler K, Perroud N, Le Gal F, Vessaz M, Laforge T, Petit B, Jollant F, Guillaume S, Baud P, Courtet P, La Harpe R, Malafosse A: Genetic and epigenetic analysis of SSAT gene dysregulation in suicidal behavior. Am J Med Genet B Neuropsychiatr Genet 2009, 150B(6):799–807.

17. Luca VD, Viggiano E, Dhoot R, Kennedy JL, Wong AHC: Methylation and QTDT analysis of the 5-HT2A receptor 102 C allele: Analysis of suicidality in major psychosis. J Psychiatr Res 2009, 43(5):532–537.

18. Ernst CC, Deleva V, Deng X, Sequeira A, Pomarenski A, Klempan T, Ernst N, Quirion R, Gratton A, Szyf M, Turecki G: Alternative Splicing, Methylation State, and Expression Profile of Tropomyosin-Related Kinase B in the Frontal Cortex of Suicide Completers. Arch Gen Psychiatry 2009, 66(1):22–32.

19. McGowan PPO: Epigenetic regulation of the glucocorticoid receptor in human brain associates with childhood abuse. Nat Neurosci 2009, 12(3):342–348.

20. Klempan TA, Ernst C, Deleva V, Labonte B, Turecki G: Characterization of QKI Gene Expression, Genetics, and Epigenetics in Suicide Victims with Major Depressive Disorder. Biol Psychiatry 2009, 66(9):824–831.

21. Keller S, Sarchiapone M, Zarrilli F, Videtic A, Ferraro A, Carli V, Sacchetti S, Lembo F, Angiolillo A, Jovanovic N, Pisanti F, Tomaiuolo R, Monticelli A, Balazic J, Roy A, Marusic A, Cocozza S, Fusco A, Bruni CB, Castaldo G, Chiariotti L: Increased BDNF Promoter Methylation in the Wernicke Area of Suicide Subjects. Arch Gen Psychiatry 2010, 67(3):258–267.

22. Keller S, Sarchiapone M, Zarrilli F, Tomaiuolo R, Carli V, Angrisano T, Videtic A, Amato F, Pero R, di Giannantonio M, Iosue M, Lembo F, Castaldo G, Chiariotti L: TrkB gene expression and DNA methylation state in Wernicke area does not associate with suicidal behavior. J Affect Disord 2011, 135(1–3):400–404.

23. Fiori LM, Gross JA, Turecki G: Effects of histone modifications on increased expression of polyamine biosynthetic genes in suicide. Int J Neuropsychopharmacol 2011, 19:1–6.

24. Fiori LM, Turecki G: Epigenetic regulation of spermidine/spermine N1-acetyltransferase (SAT1) in Suicide. J Psychiatr Res 2011, 45(9):1229–1235.

25. Fiori LM, Turecki G: Genetic and epigenetic influences on expression of spermine synthase and spermine oxidase in suicide completers. Int J Neuropsychopharmacol 2010, 13(6):725–736.

26. Philibert RA, Sandhu H, Hollenbeck N, Gunter T, Adams W, Madan A: The relationship of 5HTT (SLC6A4) methylation and genotype on mRNA expression and liability to major depression and alcohol dependence in subjects from the Iowa Adoption Studies. Am J Med Genet B Neuropsychiatr Genet 2008, 147B(5):543–549.

27. Alt SR, Turner JD, Klok MD, Meijer OC, Lakke EAJF, DeRijk RH, Muller CP: Differential expression of glucocorticoid receptor transcripts in major depressive disorder is not epigenetically programmed. Psychoneuroendocrinology 2010, 35(4):544–556.

28. Olsson CA, Foley DL, Parkinson-Bates M, Byrnes G, McKenzie M, Patton GC, Morley R, Anney RJL, Craig JM, Saffery R: Prospects for epigenetic research within cohort studies of psychological disorder: A pilot investigation of a peripheral cell marker of epigenetic risk for depression. Biol Psychol 2010, 83(2):159–165.

29. Fuchikami M, Morinobu S, Segawa M, Okamoto Y, Yamawaki S, Ozaki N, Inoue T, Kusumi I, Koyama T, Tsuchiyama K, Terao T: DNA Methylation Profiles of the Brain-Derived Neurotrophic Factor (BDNF) Gene as a Potent Diagnostic Biomarker in Major Depression. PLoS One 2011, 6(8):e23881.

30. Uddin M, Aiello AE, Wildman DE, Koenen KC, Pawelec G, de los Santos R, Goldmann E, Galea S: Epigenetic and immune function profiles associated with posttraumatic stress disorder. Proc Natl Acad Sci 2010, 107(20):9470–9475.

31. Uddin M, Galea S, Aiello AE, Wildman DE, de los Santos R, Koenen KC: Gene expression and methylation signatures of MAN2C1 are associated with PTSD. Dis Markers 2011, 30(2):111–121.

32. Smith AK, Conneely KN, Kilaru V, Mercer KB, Weiss TE, Bradley B, Tang Y, Gillespie CF, Cubells JF, Ressler KJ: Differential immune system DNA methylation and cytokine regulation in post-traumatic stress disorder. Am J Med Genet B Neuropsychiatr Genet 2011, 156(6):700–708.

33. Burton PR, Hansell AL, Fortier I, Manolio TA, Khoury MJ, Little J, Elliott P: Size matters: just how big is BIG?: Quantifying realistic sample size requirements for human genome epidemiology. Int J Epidemiol 2009, 38(1):263–273.

34. Benjamini Y, Hochberg Y: Controlling the false discovery rate: a practical and powerful approach to multiple testing. J R Statist Soc B 1995, 57(1):289–300.

35. Duncan LE, Keller MC: A Critical Review of the First 10 Years of Candidate Gene-by-Environment Interaction Research in Psychiatry. Am J Psychiatry 2011, 168(10):1041–1049.

36. Wacholder S, Chanock S, Garcia-Closas M, El Ghormli, Rothman N: Assessing the Probability That a Positive Report is False: An Approach for Molecular Epidemiology Studies. J Natl Cancer Inst 2004, 96(6):434–442.

37. Spencer VA, Davie JR: Role of covalent modifications of histones in regulating gene expression. Gene 1999, 240(1):1–12.

38. Berger SL: The complex language of chromatin regulation during transcription. Nature 2007, 447(7143):407–412.

39. Vawter MP, Tomita H, Meng F, Bostad B, Li J, Evans S, Choudary P, Atz M, Shao L, Neal C, Walsh DM, Burmeister M, Speed T, Myers R, Jones EG, Watson SJ, Akil H, Bunney WE: Mitochondrial-related gene expression changes are sensitive to agonal-pH state: implications for brain disorders. Mol Psychiatry 2006, 11(7):663–679.

40. Tomita H, Vawter MP, Walsh DM, Evans SJ, Choudary PV, Li J, Overman KM, Atz ME, Myers RM, Jones EG, Watson SJ, Akil H, Bunney WE Jr: Effect of agonal and postmortem factors on gene expression profile: quality control in microarray analyses of postmortem human brain. Biol Psychiatry 2004, 55(4):346–352.

41. Ernst C, McGowan PO, Deleva V, Meaney MJ, Szyf M, Turecki G: The effects of pH on DNA methylation state: In vitro and post-mortem brain studies. J Neurosci Methods 2008, 174(1):123–125.

42. Darst RP, Pardo CE, Ai L, Brown KD, Kladde MP: Bisulfite Sequencing of DNA, In Current Protocols in Molecular Biology. John Wiley & Sons, Inc: Ausubel FM, Brent R, Kingston RE, Moore DD, Seidman JG, Smith JA, Struhl K. Hoboken; 2001.

43. Herman JG, Graff JR, Myöhänen S, Nelkin BD, Baylin SB: Methylation-specific PCR: a novel PCR assay for methylation status of CpG islands. Proc Natl Acad Sci 1996, 93(18):9821–9826.

44. Yan PS, Chen C, Shi H, Rahmatpanah F, Wei SH, Huang TH: Applications of CpG Island Microarrays for High-Throughput Analysis of DNA Methylation. J Nutr 2002, 132(8):2430S–2434S.

45. Akama TO, Okazaki Y, Ito M, Okuizumi H, Konno H, Muramatsu M, Plass C, Held WA, Hayashizaki Y: Restriction Landmark Genomic Scanning (RLGS-M)-based Genome-wide Scanning of Mouse Liver Tumors for Alterations in DNA Methylation Status. Cancer Res 1997, 57(15):3294–3299.

46. Mohn F, Weber M, Schubeler D, Roloff TC: **Methylated DNA Immunoprecipitation (MeDIP).** *Methods Mol Biol* 2009, **507**(part iii):55–64.

47. Harris RA, Want T, Coarfa C, Nagarajan RP, Hong C, Downey SL, Johnson BE, Fouse SD, Delaney A, Zhao Y, Olshen A, Ballinger T, Zhou X, Forsberg KJ, Gu J, Echipare L, O'Green H, Lister R, Pelizzola M, Xi Y, Epstein CB, Bernstein BE, Hawkins RD, Ren B, Chung WY, Gu H, Bock C, Gnirke A, Zhang MQ, Haussler D, Ecker JR, Li W, Farnham PJ, Waterland RA, Meissner A, Marra A, Hirst M, Milosavljevic A, Costello JF: **Comparison of sequencing-based methods to profile DNA methylation and identification of monoallelic epigenetic modifications.** *Nat Biotechnol* 2010, **28**(10):1097–1105.

48. Kim D: **Blues from the neighborhood? Neighborhood characteristics and depression.** *Epidemiol Rev* 2008, **30**(1):101–17.

49. Johnson RC, Nelson GW, Troyer JL, Lautenberger JA, Kessing BD, Winkler BD, Winkler CA, O'Brien SJ: **Accounting for multiple comparisons in a genome-wide association study (GWAS).** *BMC Genomics* 2010, **11**(1):724.

50. Hirschhorn JN, Daly MJ: **Genome-wide association studies for common diseases and complex traits.** *Nat Rev Genet* 2005, **6**(2):95–108.

5

Contextual modulation of medial prefrontal cortex to neutral faces in anxious adolescents

Tara S Peris[1][*][†] and Adriana Galván[2,3][†]

Abstract

Background: Although interpretation biases are well documented among youth with anxiety disorders, understanding of their neural correlates is limited. In particular, there has been little study of how anxious youth neurobiologically represent changing contextual cues that may trigger anxiety. This study examined neural responses during a task in which participants viewed neutral faces paired with experimentally manipulated contextual stimuli.

Methods: Participants (16 youth with a primary anxiety disorder diagnosis and 15 age- and gender-matched controls) passively viewed neutral faces that were paired with either neutral descriptive vignettes or with vignettes that were potentially anxiety provoking (for example, those that involved performance/social evaluation).

Results: The two groups were differentiated by their medial prefrontal cortex (mPFC) responses, such that context modulated mPFC activation in anxious youth while non-anxious youth demonstrated no such differentiation. Counter to expectations, the performance/evaluation frames were not associated with amygdala reactivity for either group.

Conclusions: The present investigation is among the first to identify how context modulates mPFC responding to neutral stimuli among anxious youth. It takes an important step toward understanding the neurobiological correlates underlying interpretation biases of neutral stimuli in this population.

Keywords: Anxiety disorders, Adolescence, FMRI

Background

Anxiety disorders occur frequently in children and adolescents [1] affecting up to 25% of the youth population [2-4]. Characterized by marked distress and functional impairment in the short-term, anxiety disorders can derail the normal developmental trajectory and place youth at risk for a host of poor outcomes over the long term. Indeed, when left untreated, youth with these conditions are at risk for diminished school performance [5], compromised family functioning [6], and increased rates of psychiatric disorder in adulthood [7]. These risks constitute a significant public health burden, and they underscore the importance of continued efforts to understand the etiology and course of youth anxiety.

Information-processing models provide one strategy for understanding how anxiety emerges and is maintained over time. These models emphasize biases in how youth attend to, process, and interpret potentially threatening information as central to anxiety, and they have received considerable empirical support [8,9]. Research using traditional descriptive and experimental paradigms has found that anxious youth are apt to interpret neutral or ambiguous information as threatening [8-10]. These cognitive biases are thought to fuel the distress and avoidance behavior that characterize anxiety disorders, and they are viewed as potential explanatory mechanisms for understanding their etiology [10,11]. However, the neural correlates of biased interpretations of neutral stimuli in these youth remain relatively sparse. In particular, the neural locus that transforms neutral information as 'threatening' in anxious youth remains unknown. A candidate brain region that may underlie this phenomenon is the medial prefrontal cortex (mPFC). The mPFC has garnered substantial interest in the adolescent literature because of its role in self-concept and mentalizing [12-14], its engagement in social and emotional processes [15,16], and its protracted development

* Correspondence: tperis@mednet.ucla.edu
[†]Equal contributors
[1]Division of Child and Adolescent Psychiatry, UCLA Semel Institute for Neuroscience and Human Behavior, 760 Westwood Plaza, Room 67-439, Los Angeles, CA 90095, USA
Full list of author information is available at the end of the article

throughout childhood and adolescence [17]. There is also some evidence that the ventromedial PFC is associated with trait anxiety [18] and that the ventrolateral PFC in anxious youth is hyper-responsive to fear states when viewing emotional faces [19]. Medial regions of the PFC exhibit increased activation in anxious versus non-anxious youth in response to emotional faces [20] and during viewing of others' opinions [21]. In particular, the ventromedial PFC has been implicated in evaluative functions associated with affective processing [22] while dorsal regions of the medial PFC have been linked to appraisal of emotions [23]. These converging studies suggest that activation in mPFC is significantly implicated in anxiety.

There is to our knowledge little study of how anxious youth respond to changing contextual cues that may trigger anxiety. Research suggests that neural responses to threat are sensitive to subtle differences in context [24]. In particular, in a study examining amygdala-PFC linkages in response to surprised faces, Kim et al. [24] presented non-anxious adults with surprised faces that were preceded by vignettes that provided either a positive or negative context (for example, he just found/lost $500 dollars). They found that faces preceded by negative contextual frames were associated with increased amygdala and ventrolateral PFC activation relative to those preceded by positive frames while comparisons involving positive *versus* negative frames produced greater activation within the ventromedial PFC [24].

Based on studies suggesting heightened mPFC activation in anxious youth [18,20,21], the present investigation evaluated neurodevelopmental features of mPFC response during contextual modulation of neutral faces in anxious and non-anxious youth. These faces were paired with both descriptively neutral vignettes ('He is watching a presentation') and those that were potentially anxiety-provoking ('He is about to give a presentation'). We hypothesized that: (1) the mPFC and amygdala would discriminate neutral faces based on context; and (2) that this response would be greater for anxious youth compared to healthy controls.

Method
Participants
Thirty-two adolescents participated (Table 1). Participants in the anxious group (ANX; n=16; mean age, 13.05 years; 6 girls), were required to meet Diagnostic and Statistical Manual of Mental Disorders-Fourth Edition (DSM-IV) [25] criteria for a current primary diagnosis of separation anxiety, social phobia, or GAD. Co-morbidity among these diagnoses was permitted; however, participants were excluded from participation if they met criteria for any other DSM-IV diagnosis (for example, major depressive disorder). All youth in the ANX arm were

Table 1 Demographic characteristics

	Anxious group	Healthy control group
	M (SD)	M (SD)
n	16 (6 girls)	15 (5 girls)
Age	13.05 (2.87)	13.69 (2.28)
IQ	110.35 (13.39)	100.46 (14.77)
MASC[a]		
Total score	58.81 (9.53)[b]	47.53 (10.38)[b]
Harm avoidance	59.87 (8.00)[b]	52.00 (12.38)[b]
Social anxiety	58.50 (10.83)[b]	49.53 (8.16)[b]
Physical symptoms	48.68 (9.22)	42.61 (7.95)

[a]Multidimensional anxiety scale for children.
[b]Significant group differences P <0.05.

treatment-seeking, and they were excluded if they had a prior history of cognitive behavior therapy or pharmacotherapy. The healthy controls (HC) (n=15; mean age, 13.69 years; 5 girls) did not meet criteria for any current or lifetime DSM-IV diagnosis. Adolescents in both conditions were excluded if they were currently taking psychotropic medication, had a positive pregnancy test, endorsed current drug or alcohol abuse, or met criteria for MRI restrictions. One HC participant was excluded for excess motion.

Procedure
Prior to conducting the study, written informed consent was obtained from the parents of participants, and written assent was obtained from the participants. This study was conducted approved by the UCLA Institutional Review Board (#11-002606). Participants were recruited via advertisements and flyers and direct calls from families to a pediatric anxiety specialty program at a large, academic medical center. Interested families completed an initial telephone screening to assess preliminary eligibility. They were then invited to the laboratory for two separate visits. At the first visit, participants provided written informed consent/assent and were diagnosed using the Anxiety Disorders Interview Schedule-4th edition, [26], a widely-used semi-structured clinical interview for diagnosing pediatric anxiety [24], by a licensed clinical psychologist. They also completed the Wecshler Abbreviated Scale of Intelligence [27] as a measure of IQ. Participants were also acclimated to the scanner environment with a mock scanner. At visit two, participants received a brain scan. Prior to the scan, participants were given verbal and written instructions about the task. To ensure that the youngest children understood the instructions, they were read to all participants by an experimenter. After completion of the experiment participants were given monetary compensation.

fMRI task

Participants performed a modified version of a task [24], in which a face was preceded by a vignette that was intended to modulate contextual interpretation of the face. On each trial, presentation of a neutral face (1 s) was preceded by a vignette (5 s) that described either a socially neutral situation (for example, 'She is listening to an important presentation') or the same situation with a potentially anxiety-provoking component (for example, 'She is about to give an important presentation') (Figure 1). To maintain attention, they were asked to press one button if the face was male and a different button if the face was female. There were two runs (n=36 trials/run; 6 min 18 s), and 12 vignette-face pairs presented per run. There were two versions of the task. In Version A, faces 1 to 6 were always paired with an anxiety-provoking vignette and faces 7 to 12 were always paired with a neutral vignette. In Version B, the opposite pairing was presented. Vignette-face pairs were never presented more than once per run. Versions A and B were counterbalanced across participants. Eprime software [28] was used to generate stimuli and to collect responses. Stimuli were visualized through MRI-compatible goggles.

After the task, participants were presented with each of the faces and vignettes and asked to rate how anxious/nervous they felt on a Likert scale based on the following: 'Imagine being in the situation described or recall a situation in which you witnessed someone else in that situation and indicate how anxious/nervous the face/vignette made you feel'. During scanning, participants responded by pressing either of two buttons on a button-response box with the pointer and middle fingers of their right hand. During the rating component of the scan, they used all four buttons of the response box.

Stimuli and apparatus

The neutral face stimuli were taken from the NimStim Set of Facial Expressions [29]. This stimuli set is available in the public domain and was developed using actors of various genders and races who were asked to portray a range of facial expressions (for example, fearful, happy, sad, neutral) [29]. Male and female faces were counterbalanced with vignette pairing to ensure that half of each of the anxiety-provoking and neutral vignettes were paired with female faces.

The following criteria were used to generate the vignettes used in this study: (1) vignettes described common, everyday situations (for example, school, softball field, interaction with another person); (2) anxiety-provoking conditions included potential evaluation by peers, colleagues, or superiors or the potential for personal evaluation of performance; and (3) neutral conditions were as similar to anxiety-provoking conditions as possible but involved more passive observation of the target situation (that is, watching a presentation *versus* giving a presentation). Sentences in the two conditions were openly pilot tested on an initial case series of youth.

Measures
Anxiety disorders interview schedule-fourth edition (ADIS-IV)
The ADIS-IV [30] is a semi-structured diagnostic interview that assesses the major DSM-IV anxiety, mood, and externalizing disorders [30]. The instrument also assigns clinical severity ratings (CSRs) following an 8-point scale (0= not at all, 8= very, very much) for each diagnosis; scores of four or higher indicate a clinically significant anxiety disorder. The ADIS-IV has well-documented psychometric properties including sound reliability, and

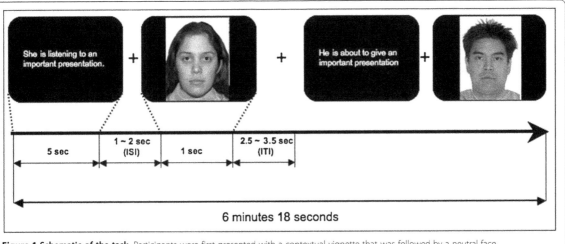

Figure 1 Schematic of the task. Participants were first presented with a contextual vignette that was followed by a neutral face.

it is widely considered the gold standard instrument for assessing anxiety [30]. Within the present study, anxious youth were required to meet criteria for at least one current anxiety disorder diagnosis (CSR ≥4); youth who received sub-threshold ratings for anxiety (that is, a CSR ≤3) or who had a history of anxiety but did not currently meet criteria for a DSM-IV anxiety disorder diagnosis were excluded from participating in either arm of the study.

Multidimensional anxiety scale for children (MASC)

All participants completed the MASC [31], a widely used and psychometrically sound measure that assesses anxiety symptoms [2]. ANX participants had significantly higher MASC total scores compared to HC (F (1,30) = 9.25), P <0.005). On the subscales, the ANX had significantly higher scores *versus* HC for harm avoidance (F (1,30) =4.28), P=0.04) and social anxiety (F (1,30) = 6.07), P=0.02); there was a trend for physical symptoms (F (1,30)=3.5), P=0.07; Table 1).

MRI data acquisition

Imaging data were collected on a 3 T Siemens Trio MRI scanner. For each run, 182 functional T2*-weighted echoplanar images (EPI) were acquired (slice thickness, 4 mm; 34 slices; TR, 2 s; TE, 30 ms; flip angle, 90°; matrix, 64 × 64; field of view (FOV), 200 mm; voxel size, 3 × 3 × 4 mm^3]. Four volumes, collected at the beginning of each run to allow for T1 equilibrium effects, were discarded. A T2-weighted, matched-bandwidth (MBW) and high-resolution, anatomical scan and magnetization-prepared rapid-acquisition gradient echo (MPRAGE) scan were acquired for each subject for registration (TR, 2.3 s; TE, 2.1 ms; FOV, 256 mm; matrix, 192 × 192; sagittal plane; slice thickness, 1 mm; 160 slices).

After the scan, participants completed a rating scale about the scanning procedure ranging from 1 ('the scanner was not scary at all') to 4 ('the scanner was very scary. I could not wait to get out'). There were no group differences on this scale (F (1,30)=1.9, P>0.5) and ratings in both the AG (M=1.82, SD=.72) and the HC (M=1.53, SD=.66) groups were low.

Image preprocessing and registration

Imaging data were analyzed using the FSL 4.1.6 toolbox. Images were realigned to compensate for small head movements. All data reported are from scans that exhibited ≤2 mm in movement. There were no group differences in motion (AG: M=.12 mm; HC: M=.30 mm). The data were smoothed using a 5-mm FWHM Gaussian kernel, and filtered in the temporal domain using a non-linear high-pass filter (66-s cutoff). EPI images were first registered to the MBW scan, then to the

MPRAGE scan, and finally into standard MNI space (MNI152, T1 2 mm) for group analyses.

The following events were modeled: neutral vignette, anxiety-provoking vignette, neutral face, and anxiety-provoking face. Events were modeled at the time of the stimulus presentation with 5 s and 1 s duration for vignettes and faces, respectively. Temporal derivatives were included as covariates of no interest to improve statistical sensitivity. Null events were not explicitly modeled and therefore constituted an implicit baseline.

As we were most interested in how social context modulates interpretations of a neutral social stimulus, we focused on analyses of face presentation but not vignette presentation. Only neutral faces were presented in this study but half were paired with a neutral vignette and half were paired with an anxiety-provoking vignette. For each participant, the following four contrasts were computed: (1) neutral-paired face - baseline; (2) anxiety-paired face - baseline; (3) neutral-paired face - anxiety-paired face; and (4) anxiety-paired face - neutral-paired face. Statistical modeling was first performed separately for each imaging run. Regressors of interest were created by convolving a *delta* function representing trial onset times with a canonical (double-gamma) hemodynamic response function. The six movement parameters that were obtained during realignment showed that rotation and translation movement within each subject and session was <2 mm in all participants; nonetheless, the movement parameters were modeled as regressors of no interest at the first level. A second-level, fixed effects analysis combined runs for each participant. A 2 (group) × 2 (vignette) × 2 (choice) repeated measures Analysis of Variance (ANOVA) was conducted at the group level using the FMRIB Local Analysis of Mixed Effects (FLAME1) module in FSL [31-33]. Z (Gaussianised T) statistic images were thresholded using clusters determined by Z >2.3 and a (whole-brain corrected) cluster significance threshold of P <0.05 using Gaussian Random Fields theory [34]. Tests were corrected for family-wise errors (FWE).

To examine correlations between behavioral measures and neural activity, variables of interest were modeled as explanatory variables at the third-level. For regression analyses, the outlier rejection tool in FSL (automatic outlier de-weighting) was used. This tool automatically detects outlier data points (for each voxel, each subject's data are considered with respect to the other subjects to determine if it is an outlier) [35]. Outliers are then automatically de-weighted in the multi-subject statistics. Anatomical localization within each cluster was obtained by searching within maximum likelihood regions from the FSL Harvard-Oxford probabilistic atlas. All fMRI data shown were cluster-corrected for multiple comparison at z=2.3, P <0.05. For visualization purposes, percent MR signal change for regions that showed significant correlations with behavioral variables of interest were extracted and plotted against the behavioral measures.

Results
Behavioral results
A 2 (group) × 2 (vignette) × 2 (choice) repeated measures analysis of variance (ANOVA) was conducted to examine post-scan ratings of the vignettes. There was a significant main effect of vignette type on ratings F (1,30) =8.54, P=0.007 ($M_{anxiety-provoking}$=1.57 (range, 0–6.5); $M_{neutral}$=0.81 (range, 0–2.3)) such that the anxiety-provoking vignettes elicited greater feelings of anxiety. There were no significant effects of group or interactions. There were no significant effects of reaction time, as determined by ANOVA. After the task, participants were presented with the neutral faces and asked to provide a rating of how anxiety-provoking they were (1=not anxiety-provoking, 4=very anxiety-provoking); there was a trend towards a group difference [F(1,30)=3.02, P=0.06] with the anxious group (M=2.04) rating the faces as more anxiety-provoking than the control group (M=1.65).

fMRI results
A repeated measures ANOVA revealed a main effect of group and interaction on activation in the mPFC (x=−6,

x=52, z=−2) (z=4.34) (Figure 2A). The anxious group showed significantly greater activation to faces paired with anxiety-provoking vignettes (M=.13) relative to the control group (M=−0.12) [t(31)=4.65, P=0.03] and relative to faces paired with neutral vignettes (M=0.02) [t(31)= 2.89, P <0.05]; the control group significantly differed from baseline in both conditions (P <0.05) (Figure 2B). Greater activation in mPFC was significantly correlated with ratings of the anxiety-provoking vignettes in the anxious group (r=0.56, P=0.03) but not in the control group (r=0.01, ns). mPFC activation was not correlated with neutral ratings for either group (anxious group: r=0.33, ns; control group: r=0.04, ns).

Discussion
This study is among the first to examine how anxious youth and their non-anxious counterparts differ in their neural responses to neutral stimuli framed by different contextual cues. As predicted, the two groups were differentiated by their mPFC responses, with anxious youth showing significantly greater activation to faces paired with anxiety-provoking vignettes than control youth and minimal activation to faces paired with neutral vignettes. The control group showed no difference in activation to the two conditions. Counter to expectations, the

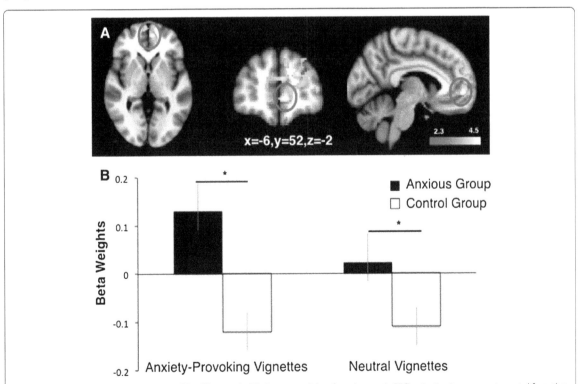

Figure 2 Neural activation in anxious and healthy youth. (A) Greater medial prefrontal cortex (mPFC) activation in response to neutral faces that had been paired with anxiety-provoking *versus* neutral contexts. **(B)** Parameter estimates from the mPFC (circled in **A**) illustrate greater activation in anxious *versus* control participants.

performance/evaluation frames were not associated with amygdala reactivity for either group. We speculate that perhaps this null finding was due to the fact that the participant was an observer of the anxiety-provoking event so it was not a direct threat to them.

Efforts to understand the etiology and course of youth anxiety disorders have long emphasized the role of interpretation biases in eliciting and maintaining anxiety [9,36]. These biases include the tendency to interpret neutral stimuli as dangerous, and are thought to fuel the distorted thinking and avoidance behavior that characterize anxiety disorders. This study builds on existing work to highlight the role of the mPFC in contributing to interpretation biases for anxious youth. When viewing the same neutral faces paired with different contextual cues, anxious adolescents exhibited heightened mPFC responding to the frames that involved performance and/or evaluation, a pattern that was distinct from their non-anxious counterparts.

These findings parallel earlier work with healthy adults demonstrating that neural responses to threat are sensitive to changes in context and that these changes may modulate patterns of neural responding [24]. The role of the mPFC is of particular interest given prior research implicating it in mentalizing tasks (that is, those that require the subject to infer what another person is feeling [37]) and anxiety [19-21]. In the present investigation, anxious youth may have been more sensitive to the feelings that they associated with the performance/evaluation frames and inferred those feelings as present for the individuals depicted on the stimuli.

Interestingly, we did not find the expected group differences in amygdala reactivity. Given its established role as a threat sensor in anxious youth (see Pine et al. [38] for review), it is possible that the task involved in this study was not viewed by subjects as threatening. Indeed, the stimuli presented in this study involved neutral faces that were not designed to be evocative. Certainly, the absence of findings among healthy controls is in keeping with earlier work demonstrating that comparison subjects do not show amygdala activity when passively viewing fearful faces [39].

The present results should be interpreted in light of several study limitations. First, the sample employed in this study was small and further replication is needed. Second, anxious youth were identified based on the presence of a primary anxiety disorder and were excluded if any other co-morbid conditions were present. While this bolsters confidence that the present findings are specific to youth with anxiety disorders, the vast majority of children and adolescents with anxiety disorders present with more than one mental health condition, which may limit generalization of these findings. Finally, while our focus was on adolescents, for purposes of this

pilot work, adolescence was defined broadly and the sample included a broad age range.

Conclusions

These limitations notwithstanding, the present investigation is among the first to demonstrate that context modulates mPFC responding to neutral stimuli among anxious youth. It takes an important step toward understanding how these youth make sense of neutral stimuli and the conditions under which they might elicit heightened patterns of activation. Future research is needed to examine more definitively the role of the mPFC in adolescent anxiety and the extent to which it may serve as a biomarker for illness. In addition, research aimed at understanding the mechanisms by which current anxiety disorder treatments serve to neutralize this pattern of responding is needed.

Competing interests
The authors declared that they have no competing interests.

Authors' contributions
Both authors contributed equally to this investigation. TP and AG conceived of the study, and participated in its design and coordination and helped to draft the manuscript. TP conducted all diagnostic assessments; AG oversaw all imaging procedures. Both authors read and approved the final manuscript.

Acknowledgments
We gratefully acknowledge assistance with data collection from Kristine McGlennen and Monica Wu. This research was supported by a NARSAD Young Investigator Award (Peris) and funding from NIMH (K23 MH085058; PI: Peris), NSF (BCS 0963750; PI: Galván) and UCLA institutional funds to AG.

Author details
[1]Division of Child and Adolescent Psychiatry, UCLA Semel Institute for Neuroscience and Human Behavior, 760 Westwood Plaza, Room 67-439, Los Angeles, CA 90095, USA. [2]Department of Psychology, University of California, Los Angeles, USA. [3]Brain Research Institute, University of California, Los Angeles, USA.

References
1. Cartwright-Hatton S, McNicol K, Doubleday E: Anxiety in a neglected population: prevalence of anxiety disorders in pre-adolescent children. Clin Psych Review 2006, 26:817–833.
2. Costello EJ, Mustillo S, Erkanli A, Keeler G, Angold A: Prevalence and development of psychiatric disorders in childhood and adolescence. Arch Gen Psychiatry 2003, 60:837–844.
3. Ford T, Goodman R, Meltzer H: The British child and adolescent mental health survey 1999: the prevalence of DSM-IV disorders. J Am Acad Child Adolesc Psychiatr 2003, 42:1203–1211.
4. Kashani JH, Orvaschel H: A community study of anxiety in children and adolescents. Am J Psychiatry 1990, 147:313–318.
5. Last CG, Hansen C, Franco N: Cognitive behavioral treatment of school phobia. J Am Acad Child Adolesc Psychiatry 1998, 37:404–411.
6. Keeton CP, Ginsburg GS, Drake KL, Sakolsky D, Kendall PC, Birmaher B, Albano AM, March JS, Rynn M, Piacentini J, Walkup JT: Benefits of child-focused anxiety treatments for parents and family functioning. Depress Anxiety 2013. epub ahead of print.
7. Aschenbrand SG, Kendall PC, Webb A, Safford SM, Flannery-Schroeder E: Is childhood separation anxiety disorder a predictor of adult panic disorder and agoraphobia? A seven-year longitudinal study. J Am Acad Child Adolesc Psychiatr 2003, 42:1478–1485.

8. Taghavi MR, Moradi AR, Neshat-Doost HT, William Y, Tim D: **Interpretation of ambiguous emotional information in clinically anxious children and adolescents.** *Cognit Emot* 2000, **14**:809–822.

9. Vasey MW, MacLeod C: **Information-processing factors in childhood anxiety: A review and developmental perspective.** In *The Developmental Psychopathology of Anxiety.* Edited by Vasey MW, MacLeod C. New York: Oxford University Press; 2001:253–277.

10. Clark DM, McManus F: **Information processing in social phobia.** *Biol Psychiatry* 2002, **51**:92–100.

11. MacLeod C, Rutherford E, Campbell L, Ebsworthy G, Holker L: **Selective attention and emotional vulnerability: assessing the causal basis of their association through the experimental manipulation of attentional bias.** *J Abnorm Psychol* 2002, **111**:107–123.

12. Somerville LH, Jones RM, Ruberry EJ, Dyke JP, Glover G, Casey BJ: **Medial prefrontal cortex and the emergence of self-conscious emotion in adolescence.** *Psychol Sci* 2013, **24**:1554–1562.

13. Sebastian CB, Burnett S, Blakemore SJ: **The development of self-concept during adolescence.** *Trends Cogn Sci* 2008, **12**:441–446.

14. Pfeifer JH, Lieberman MD, Dapretto M: **"I know you are, but what am I?!": Neural bases of self and social knowledge retrieval in children and adults.** *J Cogn Neurosci* 2007, **19**:1323–1337.

15. Amodio DM, Frith CD: **Meeting of minds: the medial frontal cortex and social cognition.** *Nat Rev Neurosci* 2006, **7**:268–277.

16. Roy M, Shohamy D, Wager T: **Ventromedial prefrontal-subcortical systems and the generation of affective meaning.** *Trends Cogn Sci* 2012, **16**:147–156.

17. Shaw P, Kabani NJ, Lerch JP, Eckstrand K, Lenroot R, Gogtay N, Greenstein D, Clasen L, Evans A, Rapoport JL, Giedd JN, Wise SP: **Neurodevelopmental trajectories of the human cerebral cortex.** *J Neurosci* 2008, **28**:3586–3594.

18. Hare TA, Tottenham N, Galvan A, Voss HU, Glover GH, Casey BJ: **Biological substrates of emotional reactivity and regulation in adolescence during an emotional go-nogo task.** *Biol Psychiatry* 2008, **63**:927–934.

19. McClure EB, Monk CS, Nelson EE, Parrish JM, Adler A, Blair RJ, Fromm S, Charney DS, Leibenluft E, Ernst M, Pine DS: **Abnormal attention modulation of fear circuit function in pediatric generalized anxiety disorder.** *Arch Gen Psychiatry* 2007, **64**(1):97–106.

20. Labuschagne I, Phan KL, Wood A, Angstadt M, Chua P, Heinrichs M, Stout JC, Nathan PJ: **Medial frontal hyperactivity to sad faces in generalized social anxiety disorder and modulation by oxytocin.** *Int J Psychopharm* 2011, **14**:1–14.

21. Blair KS, Geraci M, Otero M, Majestic C, Odenheimer S, Jacobs M, Blair RJ, Pine DS: **Atypical modulation of medial prefrontal cortex to self-referential comments in generalized social phobia.** *Psychiatry Res* 2011, **193**:38–45.

22. Grabenhorst F, Rolls ET: **Value, pleasure, and choice in the ventral prefrontal cortex.** *Trends Cogn Sci* 2011, **15**:56–67.

23. Etkin A: **Functional neuroanatomy of anxiety: a neural circuit perspective.** *Curr Top Behav Neurosci* 2010, **2**:251–277.

24. Kim H, Somerville LH, Johnstone T, Polis S, Alexander AL, Shin LM, Whalen PJ: **Contextual modulation of amygdala responsivity to surprised faces.** *J Cogn Neurosci* 2004, **16**:1730–1745.

25. American Psychiatric Association: *Diagnostic and Statistical Manual of Mental Disorders.* 4th edition. Washington, DC: American Psychiatric Association; 1994.

26. Silverman W, Albano A: *Anxiety Disorders Interview Schedule for DSM-IV: Parent Version.* San Antonio, TX: Graywing; 1996.

27. Wechsler D: *Wechsler Abbreviated Scale of Intelligence™ (WASI™).* New York, (NY); 1999.

28. Pittsburgh, PA: Psychology Software Tools Inc.

29. Tottenham N, Tanaka JW, Leon AC, McCarry T, Nurse M, Hare TA, Marcus DJ, Westerlund A, Casey BJ, Nelson C: **The NimStim set of facial expressions: judgments from untrained research participants.** *Psychiatry Res* 2009, **168**:242–249.

30. Silverman W, Saavedra L, Pina A: **Test-retest reliability of anxiety symptoms and diagnoses with the anxiety disorders interview schedule for DSM-IV: children and parent versions.** *J Am Acad Child Adolesc Psychiatry* 2001, **40**:937–944.

31. March JS, Parker JDA, Sullivan K, Stallings P, Conners CK: **The Multidimensional Anxiety Scale for Children (MASC): factor structure, reliability, and validity.** *J Am Acad Child Adolesc Psychiatr* 1997, **36**:554–565.

32. Poline J-B, Worsley KJ, Evans A, Friston K: **Combining spatial extent and peak intensity to test for activations in functional imaging.** *Neuroimage* 1997, **5**:83–96.

33. Beckmann C, Jenkinson M, Smith S: **General multilevel linear modeling for group analysis in fMRI.** *Neuroimage* 2003, **20**:1052–1063.

34. Woolrich MW, Behrens TE, Beckmann CF, Jenkinson M, Smith SM: **Multilevel linear modeling for fMRI group analysis using Bayesian inference.** *Neuroimage* 2004, **21**:1748–1761.

35. Woolrich M: **Robust group analysis using outlier inference.** *Neuroimage* 2008, **41**:286–301.

36. Kendall PC: **Anxiety disorders in youth.** In *Child and Adolescent Therapy: Cognitive Behavioral Procedures.* 4th edition. Edited by Kendall PC. New York: Guilford Press; 2012:143–190.

37. Sebastian CL, Fontaine NM, Bird G, Blakemore SJ, Brito SA, McCrory EJ, Viding E: **Neural processing associated with cognitive and affective Theory of Mind in adolescents and adults.** *Soc Cogn Affect Neurosci* 2012, **7**:53–63.

38. Pine D: **Research review: a neuroscience framework for pediatric anxiety disorders.** *J Child Psychol Psychiatry* 2007, **48**:631–648.

39. Thomas KM, Drevets WC, Dahl RE, Ryan ND, Birmaher B, Eccard CH, Axelson D, Whalen PJ, Casey BJ: **Amygdala response to fearful faces in anxious and depressed children.** *Arch Gen Psychiatry* 2001, **58**:1057–1063.

Facial emotion processing in major depression: a systematic review of neuroimaging findings

Anja Stuhrmann[1], Thomas Suslow[1,2] and Udo Dannlowski[1*]

Abstract

Background: Cognitive models of depression suggest that major depression is characterized by biased facial emotion processing, making facial stimuli particularly valuable for neuroimaging research on the neurobiological correlates of depression. The present review provides an overview of functional neuroimaging studies on abnormal facial emotion processing in major depression. Our main objective was to describe neurobiological differences between depressed patients with major depressive disorder (MDD) and healthy controls (HCs) regarding brain responsiveness to facial expressions and, furthermore, to delineate altered neural activation patterns associated with mood-congruent processing bias and to integrate these data with recent functional connectivity results. We further discuss methodological aspects potentially explaining the heterogeneity of results.

Methods: A Medline search was performed up to August 2011 in order to identify studies on emotional face processing in acutely depressed patients compared with HCs. A total of 25 studies using functional magnetic resonance imaging were reviewed.

Results: The analysis of neural activation data showed abnormalities in MDD patients in a common face processing network, pointing to mood-congruent processing bias (hyperactivation to negative and hypoactivation to positive stimuli) particularly in the amygdala, insula, parahippocampal gyrus, fusiform face area, and putamen. Furthermore, abnormal activation patterns were repeatedly found in parts of the cingulate gyrus and the orbitofrontal cortex, which are extended by investigations implementing functional connectivity analysis. However, despite several converging findings, some inconsistencies are observed, particularly in prefrontal areas, probably caused by heterogeneities in paradigms and patient samples.

Conclusions: Further studies in remitted patients and high-risk samples are required to discern whether the described abnormalities represent state or trait characteristics of depression.

Keywords: Facial emotion processing, fMRI, neuroimaging, depression, emotion, amygdala, anterior cingulate, orbitofrontal cortex, functional connectivity

Background

Major depression ranks among the most debilitating diseases worldwide and is estimated to produce the second largest disease burden by the year 2020 [1]. Despite an increasing amount of empirical studies investigating abnormalities in affective processing in unipolar depression, understanding the neurobiological underpinnings is still a major research goal and is essential for novel treatment developments. In a large body of behavioral studies, depression has been characterized by mood congruent emotion processing biases in different aspects of cognition [2-5]. Apparently, these cognitive biases have been reported to be particularly prominent for emotional faces. Depressed patients seem to be less sensitive in the identification of emotional faces and, in addition, a negative response bias was found: they tend to interpret neutral faces as sad and happy faces as neutral (for review see [6,7]).

While negative faces seem to be processed more rapidly and deeply, processing of positive facial expressions appears to be impaired [8-10]. Furthermore, behavioral biases towards sad faces seem to persist even after

* Correspondence: Udo.Dannlowski@ukmuenster.de
[1]University of Münster, Department of Psychiatry, Albert-Schweitzer-Campus 1, Building, A9, 48149 Münster, Germany
Full list of author information is available at the end of the article

recovery from depression [11], increasing the risk for future depressive episodes [12]. Interestingly, rapid, automatic stages of emotion processing are also affected in depression, as suggested by studies employing subliminal presentation conditions [13,14]. Figure 1 presents the main emotion processing stages as supposed by Phillips *et al.* [15], extended about separate pathways for stimulus presentation with or without conscious awareness.

Faces are a very important component of daily human visual communication. Since the processing of facial expressions is a fundamental step in social functioning, guiding adequate social interaction [16], biased processing of emotional faces in depression could be a strong determinant of the frequently observed interpersonal problems, including social withdrawal, feelings of interpersonal rejection and restriction of non-verbal expressiveness [17].

Brain imaging techniques, such as functional magnetic resonance imaging (fMRI), have already made substantial contributions to the understanding of how faces and facial expressions are processed in humans [18-21].

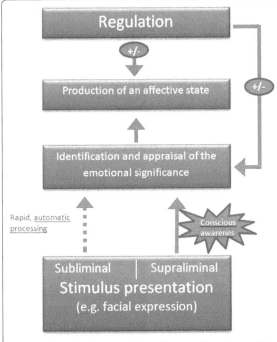

Figure 1 Emotional perception and processing stages. After stimulus presentation (subliminal or supraliminal) the central emotion perception and processing stages are: (1) the identification and appraisal of stimulus significance, taking place with or without conscious awareness; (2) the generation of an affective state, expression of emotion and behavioral response; and (3) up or down regulation (circles with positive/negative signs) of the affective state and identification process. Modified from Phillips *et al.* [15].

According to neurobiological models of emotional face processing, successful encoding of emotional expressions depends on multiple interactions between complimentary systems: a neural core system for the visual analysis of faces consists of the bilateral inferior occipital gyrus, the lateral fusiform gyrus and the superior temporal sulcus. Changeable and invariant aspects of the face representation have distinct representations in this system. A second, extended system supports the processing of facial information such as meaning and significance. It is composed of additional brain areas generally involved in representing and producing emotions. Major components include the amygdala, insula, orbitofrontal areas and somatosensory cortex [22]. Notably, most if not all of these areas have already been implicated in the etiology of major depression (see [23-25] for reviews). Thus, presenting facial emotional stimuli is a valid and reliable approach in order to activate brain areas crucial for emotion processing in general and crucial for the pathophysiology of depression specifically [18]. Unsurprisingly, emotional faces have been frequently employed in neuroimaging studies in depressed patients, contributing to the refinement of neurobiological models of depression [24-26]. Put simply, these models postulate increased activity in brain regions essential for emotional identification and production (that is, amygdala, orbitofrontal cortex (OFC), striatum) and decreased neural activity within regions important for emotion regulation such as the dorsolateral prefrontal cortex (DLPFC) and anterior cingulate cortex (ACC).

However, currently available data on emotional face processing in depression are far from being consistent. The heterogeneity of study samples (for example, state of illness, medication status and so on), imaging paradigms (for example, implicit or explicit processing paradigms, stimulus material, baseline condition), and analysis strategies (for example, activation or connectivity analyses) is reflected in apparently heterogeneous and partly conflicting findings at first sight. Given the importance of emotional face processing in major depression, the goal of the present review is to provide a comprehensive overview of neuroimaging studies investigating facial emotion processing in acutely depressed patients compared with healthy controls. Particular effort was made to delineate altered neural activation patterns associated with mood-congruent processing bias and to integrate these findings with functional connectivity results.

First, we describe in detail the results of all available fMRI studies comparing facial emotion-related brain activation in patients with major depressive disorder (MDD) and healthy control (HC) subjects. In addition to whole brain and region of interest (ROI) data, recent functional connectivity data will also be considered.

Finally, the summarized results will be discussed in the context of current models of depression and their possible role for 'trait' or 'state' aspects of depression.

Methods

To identify relevant functional neuroimaging studies focusing on emotional face processing in major depression, a database search of journal articles via Medline, Embase and Scopus was conducted from the year 2000 to August 2011. We used combinations of the keywords 'fMRI', 'functional magnetic resonance', 'depression', 'MDD', 'face', 'facial expression', and 'emotion'. All studies were limited to English language publications. We further examined the reference lists of review articles on MDD and all studies identified for inclusion to check for potentially useful studies not identified by computerized literature search.

Studies were included if they: (1) were fMRI studies, (2) statistically compared a group of adult patients with MDD to a group of healthy volunteers (3) utilized facial emotion expressions as stimuli (4) conducted a whole brain analysis, ROI analysis or functional connectivity analysis (5) reported results in acute depression (during current episode). Thus, we did not consider results reported in remitted patients. We did not include fMRI studies simply correlating imaging data with clinical features without any comparison to HCs.

Variables of interest extracted from the studies were differences in neural activations during facial emotion processing in MDD patients compared to HCs. Therefore, we extracted the neuroimaging data of between-group comparisons regarding experimental conditions reflected by 'emotion vs baseline' contrasts (for example, MDD > HC, HC > MDD).

Results

The literature search yielded a total of 25 studies meeting the inclusion criteria (see Table 1). A total of 20 studies reported between-group results in terms of whole brain and/or ROI data, whereas only 1 study found no differences between MDD patients and the healthy control group at a pretreatment baseline [27]. Functional connectivity data were reported by six studies. One study reported both whole-brain and FC results [28].

Neurobiological differences in 'activation' by emotional faces

Abnormal limbic activity

Amygdala Of the 20 included fMRI studies, 10 reported significant differences in amygdala responsiveness in MDD patients compared to HCs during exposure to facial emotions. Two recent studies by Victor *et al.* [29] and Suslow *et al.* [30], both using subliminal stimuli presentation, reported a similar differential response

pattern of higher amygdala response to sad facial stimuli and decreased responses to happy facial stimuli in MDD patients compared to HCs. Related to negative stimuli, supporting findings were reported earlier by Surguladze *et al.* [31] and Fu *et al.* [32,33]; both groups observed amygdala hyperactivation to overtly presented sad facial expressions. In addition, increased amygdala activation to fearful facial expressions was reported by Sheline *et al.* [34]. The result of amygdala hyper-responsiveness to sad/fearful faces (combined contrast) was again supported by Peluso *et al.* [35] and recently for fearful/angry faces (combined contrast) by Zhong *et al.* [36]. Two results contradicting this pattern should also be mentioned: first, decreased amygdala activation in response to fearful faces in MDD patients compared to HCs in a study investigating bipolar patients as a second control group [37] and second, increased activation to happy facial stimuli [34]. Finally, Matthews *et al.* [28] described in a comparatively young patient sample with early depression onset hyperactivation of the amygdala in MDD patients versus HCs in a combined contrast including fear, angry and happy faces.

In summary, half of the 20 relevant studies report increased amygdala activation in response to emotional faces in MDD patients compared to HCs. Across the aforementioned studies, results indicate predominantly hyper-responsiveness to negative facial expressions, in particular to sadness. Available data on subliminal happy facial processing further suggests hyporesponsiveness of the amygdala in MDD patients.

Hippocampus Although several activations observed in parts of the amygdala extended to (para)hippocampal regions [33,37], only one activation peak has been observed directly in the hippocampus [38]. The observed result showed decreased hippocampus activity to sad facial expressions in MDD patients.

Insula, parahippocampal gyrus/thalamus So far, only one study by Surguladze *et al.* [39] investigated responses to faces displaying different degrees of disgust in MDD patients vs HCs. The authors observed greater activation in the left insula in depressed patients compared to HCs. Apart from altered processing of disgust in MDD patients, additional altered activation to other emotional faces has been reported in the insula: Suslow *et al.* [30] demonstrated higher insula and parahippocampal gyrus (PHG) activation to sad faces and decreased activation to happy faces. This was supported by the results of earlier studies indicating the same direction of insula and PHG responsiveness to sad and happy stimuli, respectively. Zhong *et al.* [36] observed increased insula activation to fearful/angry (combined contrast) faces in a young sample of MDD patients. Additionally, thalamic hyper-responsiveness to sad facial stimuli has been reported by Fu *et al.* [32].

Table 1 Description of fMRI studies on facial emotion processing, comparing a group of major depressive disorder (MDD) patients to healthy controls (HCs)

Author/year	Reference	Participants	Patient mean age (SD)	Patient (a) mean duration of illness in months; (b) mean episodes	Medication	Emotions	Paradigm and stimulus type	Stimulus duration	Analysis approach
Whole brain and/or ROI data:									
Almeida et al. 2010	[62]	15 MDD, 15 HC, (15 BDD), (15 BDDr)	32.74 (9.87)	(a) 13.67 ± 9.87; (b) not reported	Yes	Fear, sad, happy	Facial expression processing paradigm. Ekman faces. Morphed 50% and 100% intensity. Explicit task: label emotion.	2 s	ROI
Frodl et al. 2009	[43]	12 MDD, 12 HC	43.3 (11.2)	Not reported	Yes	Sad, angry	Emotion face-matching task. Ekman faces. Explicit task: match emotion. Implicit task: match gender. Control task: match shapes.	5.3 s	Whole brain, ROIs
Frodl et al. 2011	[27]	24 MDD, 15 HC	38.9 (10.4)	(a) 56.0 ± 63.4; (b) 1.6 ± 0.7	No	Sad, angry	Emotion face-matching task. Faces from Gur and colleagues. Explicit task: match the emotion. Implicit task: match the gender. Control task: match shapes.	5.3 s	Whole brain
Fu et al. 2004; Fu et al. 2007	[32,63]	19 MDD, 19 HC	43.2 (8.8)	Not reported	No	Sad, happy	Facial expression processing paradigm. Ekman faces. Morphed to express low, medium and high intensities. Implicit task: indicate the sex of the face.	3 s	Whole brain
Fu et al. 2008	[33]	16 MDD, 16 HC	40.0 (9.4)	(a) not reported; (b) 0.63	No	Sad	Facial expression processing paradigm. Ekman faces. Morphed to express low, medium and high intensities. Implicit task: indicate the sex of the face.	3 s	Whole brain
Gotlib et al. 2005	[45]	18 MDD, 18 HC	35.2	Not reported	Yes	Sad, happy, neutral	Facial expression processing paradigm. Ekman faces. Implicit task: indicate the sex of the face.	3 s	Whole brain
Keedwell et al. 2005	[42]	12 MDD, 12 HC	43 (9.8)	Not reported	Yes	Sad, happy, neutral	Mood provocation paradigm. Individual autobiographical memory prompts played prior to the presentation of mood congruent facial expressions. Ekman faces. Task: oral subjective rating of mood.	2 s	Whole brain
Lawrence et al. 2004	[37]	9 MDD, 11 HC, (12 BDD)	41[a] (11)	(a) 96 ± 60; (b) not reported	Yes	Sad, fear, happy, neutral	Facial expression processing paradigm. Ekman faces. Morphed 50% and 100% intensity. Implicit task: indicate the sex of the face.	2 s	Whole brain, ROIs
Lee et al. 2008	[38]	21 MDD, 15 HC	46.8 (9.1)	(a) 14.8 ± 3.3; (b) 1.9 ± 0.8	Yes	Sad, angry, neutral	Face viewing paradigm. Data set of Korean faces. Task: evaluative ratings (arousal, valence).	1.5 s	ROIs
Matthews et al. 2008	[28]	15 MDD, 16 HC	24.5 (5.5)	(a) not reported; (b) 4.46	No	Angry, fear, happy	Emotion face-matching task. Emotional faces. Task: match faces.	5 s	ROI

Table 1 Description of fMRI studies on facial emotion processing, comparing a group of major depressive disorder (MDD) patients to healthy controls (HCs) *(Continued)*

Study	Ref	Sample	Age		Med free	Emotions	Task	Timing	Region
Peluso et al. 2009	[35]	14 MDD, 15 HC	37.9 (14)	Not reported	No	Angry, fear	Emotion face-matching task. Ekman faces. Explicit task: match emotion. Implicit task: match faces. Control task: match shapes.	5 s	Whole brain, ROI
Scheuerecker et al. 2010	[41]	13 MDD, 15 HC	37.9 (10.1)	(a) 52.3 ± 71.5; (b) 1.45 ± 0.68	No	Sad, angry	Emotion face-matching task. Faces from Gur and colleagues. Explicit task: match the emotion. Implicit task: match the gender. Control task: match shapes.		Whole brain
Sheline et al. 2001	[34]	11 MDD, 11 HC	40.3	Not reported	No	Fear, happy, neutral	Subliminal emotion paradigm. Masked Ekman faces. Task: indicate the sex of the face.	Prime: 40 ms; mask: 160 ms	ROI
Surguladze et al. 2010	[39]	9 MDD, 9 HC	42.8 (7.2)	(a) 96 ± 61.2; (b) not reported	Yes	Disgust, fear, neutral	Facial expression processing paradigm. Ekman faces. Morphed 50% and 100% intensity. Implicit task: indicate the sex of the face + offline facial affect recognition task.	2 s	Whole brain
Surguladze et al. 2005	[31]	16 MDD, 14 HC	42.3 (8.4)	(a) 90 ± 61.2; (b) not reported	Unknown	Sad, happy, neutral	Facial expression processing paradigm. Ekman faces. Morphed 50% and 100% intensity. Implicit task: indicate the sex of the face.	2 s	Whole brain, ROIs
Suslow et al. 2010	[30]	30 MDD, 26 HC	38.8 (11.4)	(a) 72.2 ± 75.0; (b) 2.7 ± 2.0	Yes	Sad, happy, neutral	Subliminal emotion paradigm. Masked Ekman faces. Task: evaluative ratings of the neutral mask face (valence) + offline detection task.	Prime: 33 ms; mask: 467 ms	Whole brain, ROI
Townsend et al. 2010	[40]	15 MDD, 15 HC	46.6 (11.2)	(a) 176.4 ± 159.6; (b) 3 (median)	No	Sad, fearful	Emotion face-matching task. Ekman faces. Explicit task: match emotion. Control task: match shapes.		Whole brain, ROIs
Victor et al. 2010	[29]	22 MDD (16 MDDr), 25 HC	33.2 (5.0)	Not reported	No	Sad, happy, neutral	Subliminal emotion paradigm. NimStim set of facial expressions. Task: remember the neutral target face and respond to indicate whether this target face appears during the current trial.	Prime: 26 ms; mask: 107 ms	Whole brain, ROI
Zhong et al. 2011	[36]	29 MDD, 31 HC, (26 CV subjects)	20.45 (1.82)	Not reported	No	Fearful, angry	Emotion face-matching task. Standardized set of Chinese facial expressions. Implicit task: match faces. Control task: match shapes.	5 s	ROI, Whole brain
Functional connectivity studies:									
Almeida et al. 2009	[47]	16 MDD, 16 HC, (15 BDD)	32.3 (9.7)	(a) 13.4 ± 9.6; (b) not reported	Yes	Sad, happy, neutral	Facial expression processing paradigm. Ekman faces. Morphed 50% and 100% intensity. Explicit task: label emotion.	2 s	Dynamic causal modeling
Carballedo et al. 2011	[48]	15 MDD, 15 HC	39.87 (8.57)	Not reported	No	Sad, angry	Emotion face-matching task. Ekman faces. Explicit task: match emotion. Control task: match shapes.	5.25 s	Structural equation modeling

Table 1 Description of fMRI studies on facial emotion processing, comparing a group of major depressive disorder (MDD) patients to healthy controls (HCs) *(Continued)*

Chen *et al.* 2008	[49]	19 MDD, 19 HC	34.3 (8.6)	Not reported	No	Sad	Facial expression processing paradigm. Ekman faces. Morphed to express low, medium and high intensities. Implicit task: indicate the sex of the face.	3 s	Functional connectivity
Dannlowski *et al.* 2009	[50]	34 MDD, 31 HC	38.6 (12.2)	(a) 125.0 ± 125.5; (b) 4.7 ± 5.3	Yes	Sad, angry, happy, neutral	Passive face viewing paradigm. Ekman faces.	500 ms	Functional connectivity
Frodl *et al.* 2010	[51]	25 MDD, 15 HC	39.4 (10.4)	(a) 51.8 ± 63.9; (b) 1.52 ± 0.6	No	Sad, angry	Emotion face-matching task. Ekman faces. Explicit task: match emotion. Implicit task: match gender. Control task: match shapes.		Functional connectivity
Mathews *et al.* 2008	[28]	15 MDD, 16 HC	24.5 (5.5)	(a) not reported; (b) 4.46	No	Angry, fear, happy	Emotion face-matching task. Emotional faces. Task: match faces.	5 s	Functional connectivity

BDD, bipolar disorder; BDDr, bipolar disorder remitted; CV, cognitive vulnerability; MDDr, major depressive disorder remitted; ROI, region of interest

There is a clear trend for similar activation patterns between the insula, PHG area and amygdala, supporting the hypothesis of an emotion bias in limbic structures in MDD patients, with hyper-responsiveness to negative facial expressions and hyporesponsiveness to happy facial expressions. Nevertheless, one group detected decreased activity in the insula in a combined contrast of sad and fear [40] which differs from this pattern.

Striatum Aberrant activity in striatal structures also resembles the activation pattern observed in the amygdala and insula. Again, predominant putamen/caudate nucleus hyper-responsiveness to sad/angry facial expressions and rather hyporesponsiveness in response to happy facial expressions has been observed [32,33,37,41].

Abnormal frontal activity

Motor cortex and prefrontal cortex Initially, there is good agreement among the results reported for the motor cortex, a brain area that has been given little attention in emotion processing. Hyperactivated motor cortex (Brodmann's area (BA) 6, BA 4) during sad and angry facial processing in MDD patients compared to HCs was reported by four studies [32,33,41,42]. Findings in the lateral prefrontal cortex (PFC) are less consistent: comparing aberrant increased to decreased activation to sad and angry facial stimuli in DLPFC in MDD patients, we find both reported nearly equally often [30,36,37,42,43]. Similar inconsistencies were reported regarding neural responsiveness to happy facial stimuli in DLPFC and in more ventral, lateral PFC areas (see Table 2 for details). Even though altered neuronal responses in DLPFC are a prevalent finding in MDD patients, it is hardly possible to draw a final conclusion about a general hyper/hypoactivation of the DLPFC

during facial emotion processing in unipolar depression, underlining the variability in neuroimaging results. In OFC several independent studies detected decreased activation in inferior and medial OFC areas in response to either sad, fear or angry facial stimuli [37,38,42]. Furthermore, Surguladze *et al.* [39] reported hyperactivation to disgust in OFC in MDD patients.

Cingulate gyrus Aberrant activation in the posterior, mid and anterior cingulum in MDD patients compared to HCs has been almost solely reported to facial expressions of sadness.

Findings in posterior cingulate responsiveness are contradictory: Fu *et al.* [32] and Keedwell *et al.* [42] reported enhanced activity in the posterior cingulum, whereas in a later therapy study by Fu and colleagues [33] weakened activity in MDD patients compared to HCs in closely related areas emerged. In the middle cingulate gyrus, two independent studies point to rather enhanced neural responses to sad/angry facial stimuli in MDD patients compared to HCs [32,43]. Of particular concern in the pathophysiology of affective disorders is the role of the ACC [23,44]. Decreased responses to sad facial stimuli in MDD patients compared to HCs in dorsal parts of the ACC were reported by Lawrence *et al.* [37] and Fu *et al.* [33]. However, one study revealed a contradictory finding of rather increased responsiveness in dorsal ACC to sad facial expressions [32]. Interestingly, Gotlib *et al.* [45] reported two hyperactivated clusters in different subgenual parts of the ACC in the MDD group to sad and happy facial expressions, respectively. Figure 2 presents a summary of altered activation loci for facial emotion processing tasks within the posterior, middle and anterior cingulum in unipolar depression.

Table 2 Emotional face processing studies: between group fMRI findings (major depressive disorder (MDD) > healthy controls (HCs))

Brain region	BA	Sad > Baseline	Fear > Baseline	Angry > Baseline	Happy > Baseline	Disgust > Baseline	Author/year	Reference
Limbic lobe								
Amygdala		↑					Fu et al. 2004	[32]
Amygdala			↑	↑			Peluso et al. 2009	[35]
Amygdala			↑a		↑a		Sheline et al. 2001	[34]
Amygdala		↑			↓		Suslow et al. 2010	[30]
Amygdala		↑			↓		Victor et al. 2010	[29]
Amygdala			↑	↑			Zhong et al. 2011	[36]
Extended amygdala			↑	↑	↑		Matthews et al. 2008	[28]
Amygdala/hippocampus		↑					Fu et al. 2008	[33]
PHG/amygdala		↑b					Surguladze et al. 2005	[31]
Amygdala/hippocampus			↓				Lawrence et al. 2004	[37]
Hippocampus		↓					Lee et al. 2008	[38]
Extended limbic system								
Insula		↑					Fu et al. 2004	[32]
Insula	13				↓		Gotlib et al. 2005	[45]
Insula		↑					Keedwell et al. 2005	[42]
Insula						↑	Surguladze et al. 2010	[39]
Insula	13		↑	↑			Zhong et al. 2011	[36]
Insula		↓	↓				Townsend et al. 2010	[40]
Insula/PHG		↑			↓		Suslow et al. 2010	[30]
PHG		↑					Fu et al. 2008	[33]
PHG/globus pallidus/anterior thalamus			↓		↓		Lawrence et al. 2004	[37]
Thalamus		↑					Fu et al. 2004	[32]
Striatum								
Putamen		↑					Fu et al. 2008	[33]
Putamen		↑b			↓b		Surguladze et al. 2005	[31]
Putamen		↓	↓				Townsend et al. 2010	[40]
Putamen/globus pallidus		↑					Fu et al. 2004	[32]
Uncus/amygdala/caudate/putamen					↓		Lawrence et al. 2004	[37]
Caudate		↑					Fu et al. 2004	[32]
Caudate		↓					Lee et al. 2008	[38]
Caudate		↑		↑			Scheuerecker et al. 2010	[41]
Frontal lobe								
Motor cortex								
Premotor cortex	6	↑					Fu et al. 2004	[32]
Middle frontal gyrus	6	↑					Fu et al. 2008	[33]
SMA		↑		↑			Scheuerecker et al. 2010	[41]
Precentral gyrus	4	↑					Fu et al. 2004	[32]
Precentral gyrus	4	↑					Fu et al. 2008	[33]
Precentral gyrus	4				↑		Keedwell et al. 2005	[42]
Precentral gyrus	4,6				↓		Keedwell et al. 2005	[42]
Precentral gyrus		↑		↑			Scheuerecker et al. 2010	[41]
Postcentral gyrus	1, 2, 3	↑					Fu et al. 2004	[32]
Postcentral gyrus		↑		↑			Frodl et al. 2009	[43]
Postcentral gyrus	2	↑					Keedwell et al. 2005	[42]

Table 2 Emotional face processing studies: between group fMRI findings (major depressive disorder (MDD) > healthy controls (HCs)) *(Continued)*

Region	BA						Study	Ref
DLPFC								
DLPFC	44, 45, 9	↓	↓		↓		Lawrence *et al.* 2004	[37]
DLPFC	9	↑					Keedwell *et al.* 2005	[42]
Superior frontal gyrus		↑[a]		↑			Frodl *et al.* 2009	[43]
Superior frontal gyrus	8				↑		Gotlib *et al.* 2005	[45]
Superior frontal gyrus	8	↓					Fu *et al.* 2008	[33]
Superior frontal gyrus	8		↓	↓			Zhong *et al.* 2011	[36]
Middle frontal gyrus		↑[a]		↑			Frodl *et al.* 2009	[43]
Middle frontal gyrus		↑			↓		Suslow *et al.* 2010	[30]
Middle frontal gyrus	8	↓					Fu *et al.* 2008	[33]
Middle frontal gyrus	8	↓					Keedwell *et al.* 2005	[42]
VLPFC								
VLPFC	10, 47, 45, 46				↓		Lawrence *et al.* 2004	[37]
VLPFC	11				↑		Gotlib *et al.* 2005	[45]
VLPFC	10/47	↓					Keedwell *et al.* 2005	[42]
Middle frontal gyrus	10/47				↑		Keedwell *et al.* 2005	[42]
Middle frontal gyrus		↑		↑			Scheuerecker *et al.* 2010	[41]
Cingulum								
Anterior cingulum	32	↑					Fu *et al.* 2004	[32]
Anterior cingulum	24/32	↓					Fu *et al.* 2008	[33]
Anterior cingulum	25		↓	↓			Zhong *et al.* 2011	[36]
Sg anterior cingulum	25	↑					Gotlib *et al.* 2005	[45]
Sg anterior cingulum	24/32				↑[a]		Gotlib *et al.* 2005	[45]
Anterior cingulum	24	↓					Lawrence *et al.* 2004	[37]
Middle cingulum	23/24	↑					Fu *et al.* 2004	[32]
Middle cingulum	33/24, 32/24	↓					Fu *et al.* 2008	[33]
Middle cingulum		↑[a]		↑			Frodl *et al.* 2009	[43]
Middle cingulum	23				↑		Keedwell *et al.* 2005	[42]
Posterior cingulum	23/31, 29/31	↑					Fu *et al.* 2004	[32]
Posterior cingulum	31	↓					Fu *et al.* 2008	[33]
Posterior cingulum	31				↓		Fu *et al.* 2007	[63]
Posterior cingulum	31	↑					Keedwell *et al.* 2005	[42]
Medial PFC								
Inferior frontal gyrus	47	↑					Gotlib *et al.* 2005	[45]
Inferior frontal gyrus	47/45	↓					Gotlib *et al.* 2005	[45]
Inferior frontal gyrus	45	↑					Keedwell *et al.* 2005	[42]
Inferior frontal gyrus	47		↓	↓			Zhong *et al.* 2011	[36]
Medial PFC	10, 11, 47		↓				Lawrence *et al.* 2004	[37]
DMPFC	8				↑		Keedwell *et al.* 2005	[42]
VMPFC	10/32				↑		Keedwell *et al.* 2005	[42]
Orbitofrontal cortex								
Orbitofrontal cortex	47					↑	Surguladze *et al.* 2010	[39]
Orbitofrontal cortex	11	↓					Lawrence *et al.* 2004	[37]
Orbitofrontal cortex	11	↓					Keedwell *et al.* 2005	[42]
Orbitofrontal cortex		↓		↓			Lee *et al.* 2008	[38]

Table 2 Emotional face processing studies: between group fMRI findings (major depressive disorder (MDD) > healthy controls (HCs)) *(Continued)*

Orbitofrontal cortex		↓	↓	Lee *et al.* 2008	[38]
Temporal lobe					
Middle temporal gyrus	21	↓		Gotlib *et al.* 2005	[45]
Middle temporal gyrus	21/22		↓	Keedwell *et al.* 2005	[42]
Middle temporal gyrus	21		↑	Surguladze *et al.* 2010	[39]
Middle temporal gyrus		↑	↓	Suslow *et al.* 2010	[30]
Middle temporal gyrus/inferior temporal gyrus		↑	↓	Suslow *et al.* 2010	[30]
Middle temporal gyrus	21, 37	↓		Townsend *et al.* 2010	[40]
Inferior temporal gyrus	20		↓	Gotlib *et al.* 2005	[45]
Inferior temporal gyrus	37		↑	Surguladze *et al.* 2010	[39]
Inferior temporal gyrus	20	↓		Townsend *et al.* 2010	[40]
Superior temporal gyrus	42	↑		Fu *et al.* 2008	[33]
Superior temporal gyrus	42	↑		Keedwell *et al.* 2005	[42]
Fusiform gyrus	37	↓		Fu *et al.* 2008	[33]
Fusiform gyrus	20	↑		Keedwell *et al.* 2005	[42]
Fusiform gyrus	19	↑[b]	↓[b]	Surguladze *et al.* 2005	[31]
Fusiform gyrus		↑	↓	Suslow *et al.* 2010	[30]

The table includes whole brain and region of interest (ROI) results of the described studies in Table 1, section 'Whole Brain and ROI studies'. The table does not include results on other study aspects such as treatment response or connectivity analyses.

[a]Due to deactivations in controls.

[b]Linear trend for increasing intensities of sadness/happiness.

BA, Brodmann's area; DLPFC, dorsolateral prefrontal cortex; DMPFC, dorsomedial prefrontal cortex; PFC, prefrontal cortex; PHG, parahippocampal gyrus; SMA, supplementary motor area; Sg, subgenual; VLPFC, ventrolateral prefrontal cortex; VMPFC, ventromedial prefrontal cortex.

Abnormal temporal activity

Lateral: middle temporal gyrus (MTG: BA 21), inferior temporal gyrus (ITG: BA 20), superior temporal gyrus (STG: BA 22, 42) In MDD patients, several hyperactivations in MTG, ITG and STG in response to sad facial stimuli have been detected [30,33,42], contrary to two observed hypoactivated clusters. In addition, noticeable deactivation to happy facial expressions stimuli has been observed, too [40,45]. Specific to the emotion of disgust, Surguladze *et al.* [39] described increased activation in MTG and STG in MDD patients.

Medial: fusiform gyrus/fusiform face area (BA 37) Suslow *et al.* [30] and Surguladze *et al.* [31] both reported a pattern of increased activation to sad facial expression and decreased activation to happy facial expression in fusiform gyrus in MDD patients compared to HCs. One study supported this pattern [42], also observing increased activation to sad facial stimuli, whereas a deactivation in fusiform gyrus during sad facial processing has also been detected [33].

Differential effects of valence (positive versus negative facial emotions)

In limbic regions, the combined results of aberrant negative face processing in MDD patients revealed predominantly exaggerated responsiveness of the amygdala, PHG and insula (for details, see section above). In striatal regions, further increased responsiveness to negative stimuli has been detected in putamen and caudate nucleus [31-33,41]. By contrast, data on the processing of positive facial stimuli rather indicate decreased responsiveness in MDD patients compared to HCs in the amygdala, insula, PHG and putamen [29-31,37,45]. In frontal lobe structures a deviant neural response picture emerged: exaggerated responses to negative facial stimuli in MDD patients occurred particularly in the motor cortex [32,33,41,42] and in the middle and subgenual cingulum (see Figure 2), whereas rather decreased responsiveness was dominant in the OFC [37,38,42]. Concerning the processing of positive facial stimuli in frontal areas, increased as well as decreased activity has been observed in MDD patients (see Table 2). Thus, the present data suggest group × valence interactions particularly in areas involved in the generation of affective responses, indicating a neurobiological substrate of mood-congruent processing bias. However, unfortunately only a few studies explicitly investigated group × valence interactions in factorial designs. Brain areas showing group × valence interactions include the amygdala [29,30], insula, PHG [30], the fusiform gyrus [30,31] and putamen [31].

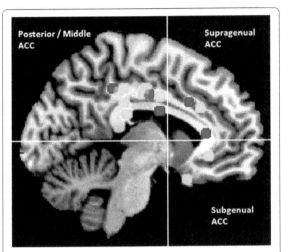

Figure 2 Increased and decreased cingulate activation in major depressive disorder (MDD) patients in emotional face processing studies. Paramedian slice of a Montreal Neurological Institute (MNI) template depicting abnormal cingulate activation during emotional face processing in major depressive disorder. Peak activation coordinates reported by primary authors in Talairach coordinates were converted into MNI space. Light blue: hyperactivation, dark blue: hypoactivation. ACC = anterior cingulate cortex.

Connectivity results

Connectivity analysis in functional neuroimaging can be subdivided into two general classes: functional connectivity (FC), which examines simple correlations between neural activity in two anatomically distinct brain areas; and effective connectivity (EC), which measures the directional influence that one neural system exerts over another [46]. The most influential models of depressive disorders assume that depressive symptoms might rather result from abnormal interactions between several brain regions than from differences in single (isolated) local brain function [7,23,25]. However, relatively few functional neuroimaging studies have investigated connectivity within these postulated networks. To date, six studies have examined neural connectivity in MDD patients compared to HCs during the processing of facial expressions [28,47-51]. One of the first studies by Chen et al. [49] in 19 unmedicated patients with MDD and 19 HCs used regression analysis between the amygdala and all other brain regions on neural activity to sad facial expressions. The authors found decreased FC of bilateral amygdala in depressed patients compared to matched HCs in the hippocampus, putamen, insula, PHG, inferior, middle, and superior temporal cortices, and inferior/middle frontal cortices before antidepressant treatment. Antidepressant treatment was associated with a significant increase in FC between the amygdala and right frontal cortex, supragenual ACC, striatum and

thalamus in MDD subjects. Matthews et al. [28] focused explicitly on differences in amygdala-cingulate FC during emotional face processing in 15 MDD patients and 16 HCs. The results indicate increased FC between the bilateral amygdala and subgenual ACC and decreased FC between the amygdala and supragenual ACC in MDD patients. Furthermore, greater depressive symptom severity was positively correlated with decreased coactivation of the supragenual cingulate in MDD subjects. Dannlowski et al. [50] calculated FC of the amygdala with prefrontal areas based on neural activity during passive viewing of negative emotional faces in a large sample of 34 MDD patients with relatively long illness history and 32 HC subjects. Depressed patients showed significantly reduced connectivity of the amygdala with the dorsal ACC and DLPFC. Taken together, all three FC studies show comparable results concerning abnormally reduced FC between the amygdala and dorsal/supragenual ACC regions in acute depression, while amygdala-subgenual ACC connectivity seems to be increased. Recently, Frodl et al. [51] selected the OFC instead of the amygdala as the 'seed region' for functional connectivity analysis. In 15 unmedicated MDD patients and 15 HC subjects, functional connectivity between the OFC and other brain regions was assessed during negative facial emotion processing. Results between patients and HCs demonstrate that the OFC coactivated less with the dorsal ACC, precuneus, and cerebellum and more with the right DLPFC, right inferior frontal operculum, and left motor areas in the patient group.

To the best of our knowledge, facial emotion processing in MDD patients has only twice been investigated with effective connectivity techniques. Almeida et al. [47] used dynamic causal modeling (DCM) to examine EC between the amygdala and medial OFC. Their data showed reduced left-sided top-down OFC-amygdala EC in the happy and sad facial processing paradigm in a sample of predominantly female depressed subjects compared to HCs. Recently, Carballedo et al. [48] used structural equation modeling (SEM) to calculate the differences in effective connectivity between 15 MDD patients and 15 HCs. The authors proposed an emotional model including the amygdala, OFC, ACC and PFC. Bilaterally, the path analysis revealed attenuated connectivity strengths from the amygdala to OFC during sad and angry facial processing in patients compared to controls. Additionally, for the right hemisphere, patients show lower connectivity from the amygdala to the ACC and from ACC to PFC, whereas controls show lower connectivity in the opposite direction, namely from ACC to the amygdala. One should note that both EC studies reviewed here found lower left-sided influences between the amygdala and OFC, although the study by

Almeida *et al.* [47] showed top-down alterations and the one by Carballedo *et al.* [48] bottom-up alterations.

In summary, functional connectivity between the amygdala and other brain areas shows (a) decreased amygdala coupling with other limbic regions (hippocampus, putamen, insula, PHG), temporal regions, and in particular with the supragenual/dorsal ACC and DLPFC, and (b) increased coupling with subgenual ACC. Of particular concern seems to be the role of the ACC, resembling results identified with conventional fMRI analysis. The longitudinal data by Chen *et al.* [49] provide first evidence that decreased FC coupling between the amygdala and supragenual ACC increases after pharmacological intervention.

Discussion

The present review aimed to summarize available empirical data regarding the neural correlates of abnormal emotional face processing in acute unipolar depression (during the current episode). Presenting differential facial expressions activates a common face-processing network in HCs and MDD patients, including primary visual pathways as well as further supporting brain areas crucial for emotion processing in general. The amygdala belongs to the latter group, the extended limbic system and specific frontal areas, namely the ACC, OFC and ventromedial prefrontal cortex (VMPFC). These regions are of particular interest for understanding the pathophysiology of unipolar depression. Our analysis indicates evidence of abnormal neural face processing in MDD patients, especially in the amygdala, the insula, PHG, ACC and OFC. Although neural alterations were reported in several other brain regions, the Discussion section focuses on these areas because they are (a) crucial for evaluating the neural mood-congruent face processing hypothesis, and (b) are core domains in an altered functional connectivity network in MDD patients during emotional face processing.

Neural mood-congruent face processing

Neural responses in MDD patients associated with mood-congruent processing patterns are most evident in the amygdala [29,30], insula and PHG [30], the fusiform gyrus [30,31] and putamen [31].

The amygdala plays a pivotal role in emotion processing and in the perception and processing of emotional salience in facial expressions (for reviews see [52-54]). Furthermore, the amygdala is a key region within the neurobiological framework of depressive disorder. Several authors have suggested that, for MDD, mood-congruent bias in behavioral measures is strongly linked to amygdala hyper-responsiveness to negative stimuli [2,55,56]. Findings of increased amygdala responsiveness to negative emotional faces are well in line with several

imaging studies employing other stimuli, including negative words [57,58], individualized self-referential sentences [59], or in expectation of negative pictures [60]. Furthermore, these findings are supported by studies in depressed adolescents [61].

However, not all fMRI studies have found evidence for altered amygdala activation in MDD. In detail, 10 of the 20 included studies reported differences in amygdala activation between MDD patients and HCs using face emotion processing tasks [28-37], while the other studies found no significant group effects [27,38-43,45,62,63]. Nevertheless, focusing on the observed differences in amygdala responsiveness, studies provide compelling support for amygdala mood-congruent processing in MDD patients. First, abnormal amygdala responsiveness has been shown to negative and positive facial expressions, corroborating amygdala function in processing salient stimuli, independent of stimuli valence [64]. Second, as hypothesized in mood congruent processing theories of depression, the majority of results show exaggerated amygdala response to sad stimuli, and in addition decreased amygdala response to happy facial stimuli, although replications with happy facial expressions are still rare. These results indicate that, in convergence with behavioral measures, neurobiological assessment can be a sensitive measure for mood-congruent biases in unipolar depression. Of note are two recent studies using subliminal presentation conditions pointing to mood congruency effects to negative and positive stimuli already at early, automatic processing stages [29,30].

In conclusion, the findings of our analysis support the assumption that amygdala hyperactivity is associated with negatively biased facial emotion processing implicated in the pathophysiology of major depression, although this became evident in only one-half of the reviewed studies. Studies investigating the question of whether abnormalities in amygdala responses to emotional faces demonstrated in acute depression represent a state marker of acute depressive episodes or vulnerability factors for depression are rare. In remitted patients, Neumeister *et al.* [65] demonstrated enhanced regional cerebral blood flow responses to sad facial expressions in the amygdala relative to HCs, but others have failed to replicate these findings in remitted patients [66,67]. In people at risk for depression, van der Veen *et al.* [68] and Monk *et al.* [69] reported greater abnormal amygdala activation to negative facial expression, but again inconsistent findings exist [70]. Interestingly, Zhong *et al.* [36] reported higher amygdala activation evident in both MDD subjects and a sample of healthy people with high cognitive vulnerability to depression compared to HCs. Increased left amygdala responsiveness was positively associated with CSQ scores (measures causal attributions, consequences and self-worth characteristics). In addition, Cremers et al. [71] reported that right amygdala-dorsomedial PFC connectivity for negative faces vs neutral faces was positively associated with neuroticism scores, a personality trait related to the development of affective disorders. Finally, a recent study by Dannlowski et al. [72] investigated long-term effects of childhood maltreatment with fMRI in psychologically healthy participants. The observed association between childhood maltreatment and amygdala responsiveness during emotional face processing resembles findings in depressed patients, suggesting that these functional changes might constitute a predisposition for developing affective disorders.

Hyperactivated amygdala to negative emotional faces in remitted patients and people at high risk for depression is indicative of trait vulnerability. This interpretation receives support from imaging genetics and twin studies, suggesting that amygdala responsiveness to emotional faces as well as amygdala prefrontal connectivity are under strong genetic influence [73-78].

Some methodological aspects explaining the heterogeneity of studies should be discussed here. With regard to presentation modus, all three studies using subliminal presentation of facial expressions reported differences in amygdala activation [29,30,34]. Victor et al. [29] even observed differences in amygdala activation specific to masked presentation of sad and happy faces, absent to unmasked stimuli, supporting the assumption that subliminal stimuli presentation maybe an advantage in identifying emotional-processing biases in MDD with focus on amygdala activation. It may be subliminal stimulus presentation prevents confounding with other cognitive processes prevalent in depression such as rumination on negative thoughts/preservation of attention to negative faces [34]. Comparing paradigms presenting facial stimuli supraliminally, only about half of the investigations implementing either face-matching paradigms or the 'face recognition task' observed amygdala differences. Scheuerecker et al. [41] suggested that participants probably used more visual and cognitive strategies to solve the face-matching task, causing ACC and PFC activation maybe inhibiting amygdala activation. Concerning task type (that is, explicit or implicit), an implicit task, requiring participants to focus on gender aspects of the face, seems to be sufficient to elicit amygdala activation [28,31-33,35,36]. As amygdala and frontal responsiveness depends on task complexity, face type and attention focus, future research should take into account such variations in designing facial processing paradigms.

Furthermore, medication status has an important impact on neural activation patterns: seven of the ten studies reporting altered amygdala activation were performed on unmedicated patients. This result is not surprising regarding the converging evidence, that amygdala is a key region for antidepressant effects, reducing abnormal amygdala responsiveness to negatively valenced faces in MDD patients (for a recent meta-analysis see [79]). Other possible influencing factors may be methodological aspects such as experimental design (for example, event-related vs block design) or the selection of different baseline conditions (for example, neutral faces or a no-face condition) as well as clinical and non-diagnostic variables such as age, comorbidity, treatment history and number of prior episodes (for details see Table 1). Furthermore, difficulties in detecting altered amygdala responsiveness in MDD patients may be caused by a 'ceiling' effect. As noted by Townsend et al. [40], several PET studies have shown increased resting blood flow in the amygdala in MDD patients [80-84], making it difficult to detect group differences in activation tasks if amygdala baseline activation was already increased.

Aside from the amygdala, several other subcortical brain structures show activation patterns supporting mood-congruent processing in depressed patients. Insula hyperactivation to sad facial stimuli is a prominent result, and furthermore two independent studies observed hypoactivation to happy facial stimuli (see Table 2). Apart from having a pivotal role in the processing of disgust [39] the insula has strong functional connections to the amygdala [85]. Insula projections to inferior parietal cortex and the amygdala are involved in identifying/representing motivational salient information, social cues and the expression of conditioned responses: particularly on implicit processing pathways [86,87]. Furthermore, activity in the putamen and caudate nucleus also resembles mood-congruent activation patterns in MDD patients, although contributions to the processing of facial expressions are still under debate [87]. In visual face areas, fusiform gyrus responsiveness also indicates mood-congruent processing in terms of increased activation to sad facial expressions and decreased activation to happy faces. In addition to encoding face traits and facial identity [20], recent studies revealed that fusiform regions are also sensitive to facial emotional expression (for a review see [88]). The authors suggest that the modulation by emotional effects can be explained by direct connections between visual cortex and the amygdala, facilitating direct feedback signals from the amygdala [89] to visual processing areas.

In summary, neuronal correlates of mood-congruent facial affect processing in MDD patients are most prominent in limbic and subcortical regions, compromising the amygdala, insula and putamen/caudate nucleus. In a larger context these regions are hypothesized to be part of an extended emotional face processing system [20] and furthermore constitute a ventral stream in emotion-cognition processing, appraising emotional behavior and producing affective states, altered in unipolar depression [25]. As described, these alterations may even influence visual processing areas such as the fusiform face gyrus. Studies in remitted patients and in people at risk for depression provide the first indications that enhanced limbic neural responses to negative emotional material may contribute to vulnerability to MDD [65,68,69].

Abnormal ACC and OFC activity

The analysis of whole-brain and functional connectivity data highlight two more regions showing abnormal activation patterns during emotional face processing in MDD: the cingulate gyrus and the orbitofrontal cortex. Findings in the cingulate gyrus derived by our whole-brain and ROI analysis (see Figure 2) can be broadly subsumed by hyperactivated posterior/middle cingulum, hypoactivated dorsal anterior cingulum and hyperactivated ventral/subgenual anterior cingulum in MDD patients compared to HCs, although findings are less clear for different subregions of the ACC than expected. Several authors postulate a central role particularly for the ACC in the neurobiology of depression, with a special role in therapy response [90-92]. The ACC plays a crucial role for attentional processes that integrate cognitive and emotional processes. While the subgenual ACC seems to be involved in the generation and recognition of emotional states, the supragenual/dorsal ACC seems to be crucial for emotion regulation [25,93,94]. Functional connectivity results between amygdala and subgenual/supragenual ACC on emotional face processing extend the above described neural activation pattern: while (hypoactivated) dorsal regions of the ACC show decreased FC with the amygdala, the rather hyperactivated subgenual parts seem to have increased connectivity with the amygdala ([28,49,50]; see Figure 3). On the one hand, cognitive parts of the ACC are less activated in MDD patients compared to HCs during emotional face processing and show decreased FC to the amygdala, suggesting less capability in MDD patients to modify/suppress emotional salient information crucial for patients' affective states and behavioral responses. On the other hand, connections between subgenual parts of the ACC and the amygdala are increased, maybe mutually enhancing abnormal emotion processing. Future studies should address the direction of influence between different parts of the ACC and the amygdala in more detail, preferably using EC methods and more refined models. A recent example is the EC study by Carballedo et al. [48], pointing to lower connectivity strength from the amygdala to the ACC in patients.

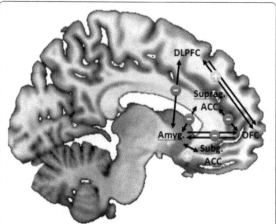

Figure 3 Schematic illustration of main results reported in fMRI connectivity studies on aberrant emotional face processing in major depressive disorder (MDD) patients. Double arrows represent results derived by functional connectivity approaches, whereas the normal arrows present the result derived by effective connectivity analyses. Plus and minus characters indicate increased and decreased connectivity between brain regions in MDD. ACC = anterior cingulate cortex; Amyg = amygdala; DLPFC = dorsolateral prefrontal cortex; OFC = orbitofrontal cortex; suprag = supragenual; subg = subgenual.

Moreover, results on medication effects concerning abnormal ACC activity should also be taken into account and can extend the interpretations. Antidepressant medication reduced ACC activity in HCs during an emotion provoking paradigm [95] and Pizzagalli recently highlighted in his meta-analysis that increased rostral ACC activity at rest is a strong marker of treatment response in depression [96]. Because these data are mainly derived from acutely depressed patients, it is still unknown whether abnormal ACC responses represent state markers of depression or a vulnerability factor [96]. The first evidence supporting the latter notion comes from the previously mentioned study by Cremers et al. [71]. The authors reported a negative correlation between amygdala-ACC connectivity and neuroticism to negative faces compared to neutral faces, possibly indicating that highly neurotic patients are characterized by less inhibitory control of the ACC over the amygdala, which may reflect vulnerability for MDD. A second study in young people at risk for depression would support a possible diminished cortical regulation of negative emotional faces [70].

With respect to the OFC, whole-brain and ROI analyses display remarkably decreased neural activity in MDD patients compared to HCs in medial OFC areas to negative facial stimuli [37,38,42]. In addition, FC between the OFC and other brain areas revealed decreased FC to the amygdala and supragenual ACC as well as increased FC to the DLPFC. The two available EC studies [47,48] in MDD patients further specified the directionality of these brain abnormalities. Both studies indicate reduced left-sided connectivity between the OFC and the amygdala in patients, but show, at first glance, contradictory results with regard to the direction of influence on another (top down vs bottom up). In both paradigms participants were instructed to explicitly label emotions, but different paradigms were used (face-matching task vs morphed facial expression processing paradigm); therefore this may be, next to medication effects, one reason explaining the results. Future studies are needed to further investigate on this issue.

The OFC is a central part of the frontosubcortical circuits, connecting the frontal and limbic systems with each other, and is crucial for mood regulatory processes [97,98]. Relative uncoupling of connections between heightened activity in the limbic system and the OFC during negative facial processing in MDD may account for depressive symptoms such as negative emotional experiences and impaired regulation of emotional and social behavior [41]. Increased FC between OFC and lateral PFC systems could be the neural substrate of a more voluntary compensatory mechanism in MDD [99] for the described altered automatic emotional face processing.

Unresolved questions

To date, it is not clear whether the neurobiological abnormalities described above represent state or trait markers of depression. As highlighted above, a few studies have demonstrated a normalization of abnormal neurobiological response patterns after antidepressant medication (for example, [29,32]). Moreover, these studies are in line with several pharmaco-fMRI studies in healthy subjects, showing that limbic responsiveness to negative facial stimuli can be attenuated even by short-term antidepressant administration [100-102]. However, although it seems that antidepressants modify pathological emotional face processing in depression, it still remains to be clarified whether these functional abnormalities in emotional face processing represent a feature of acute depressed state and would therefore also resolve without medication after remission or whether they represent a risk factor preceding the onset of depression. The first studies in remitted patients and in high-risk subjects [36,65,68,69,71,103], as well as data from imaging genetics and twin studies [73-78] suggest that amygdala responsiveness to emotional faces as well as amygdala-prefrontal and amygdala-ACC connectivity may represent vulnerability factors for MDD.

A second unresolved question concerns possible laterality effects of valence-specific emotion processing in the depressed brain. Although this aspect may be raised by the data, it was not the focus of our analysis and still needs further clarification. As noted above, other unresolved issues concern the heterogeneity of presentation paradigms. For example, studies investigating automatic facial emotion processing are likely to target other brain areas compared to explicit emotion processing paradigms. Obviously, this is particularly important for investigating prefrontal areas and might explain the apparently contradictive results in brain areas involved in emotion regulation, for example the DLPFC. Next to the methodological aspect, variability between patient samples due to different symptom characteristics may be a further critical, influential factor. Age, comorbidity, treatment history, number of prior episodes or age on illness onset may confound the reported results [7]. Unfortunately, information about clinical variables was provided by less than half of the reviewed studies, leaving these variables relatively uncontrolled for in this review and therefore limiting the described results and their interpretation. As described in the Discussion section, differences in medication status and low sample sizes could further contribute to inconsistencies among study results.

The research field would benefit from larger studies with well characterized patient samples (that is, detailed description of clinical variables), particularly multicenter studies. Furthermore, investigators should carry on employing standardized paradigms in order to replicate results and to resolve conflicting findings. For example, the comparison of subliminal and supraliminal stimulus presentation in one patient sample and the influence of attentional mechanisms on a neural level are still rarely investigated. Future studies should explicitly focus on group × valence interactions in factorial designs to explore differential effects of valence and should use connectivity analysis strategies (FC and/or EC) to describe the interplay of core regions such as the amygdala, ACC and OFC more precisely. Longitudinal studies, including relatives or other high-risk subjects are very essential and may ultimately answer the question if the described anomalies represent 'trait' or 'state' marker of depression.

Finally, one should notice that facial processing is only one aspect of altered cognitive/emotional processing among several others in MDD described by behavioral (for review see [104]) and neuroimaging (for review see [7]) studies. Thus, one must caution against overinterpretation of the presented results on altered neural facial processing in MDD.

Conclusions

Based on cognitive models of depression and behavioral studies pointing to an emotion processing bias in acute depression, several neuroimaging studies have investigated the neuronal underpinnings of these emotional processing abnormalities. It has been shown that the use of emotional face processing tasks is a reliable and valid approach to pinpoint most if not all relevant areas. The analysis of neural activation data shows that MDD patients are characterized by abnormalities within the common face processing network, indicating a mood-congruent processing bias particularly in the amygdala, insula and PHG, fusiform face area and putamen responsiveness. Furthermore, abnormalities in the cingulate gyrus and OFC are obvious, which are refined by investigations implementing functional connectivity analysis. A pathologically altered emotion processing and emotion regulation network emerged, including the amygdala, the ACC, OFC and DLPFC as core components. Further neuroimaging studies will be needed to extend these findings, especially by replicating data with same activation paradigms and larger sample sizes in order to enable researchers to make more valid assumptions on neural emotional processing mechanisms, contributing to a better understanding of depressive disorders.

Acknowledgements
The study was supported by grants from Innovative Medizinische Forschung (IMF) of the Medical Faculty of Münster (DA120309 to UD)

Author details
[1]University of Münster, Department of Psychiatry, Albert-Schweitzer-Campus 1, Building, A9, 48149 Münster, Germany. [2]University of Leipzig, Department of Psychosomatic Medicine and Psychotherapy, Semmelweisstraße 10, 04103 Leipzig, Germany.

Authors' contributions
AS performed the literature research and wrote major parts of the article. TS contributed to the Introduction and Discussion sections. UD selected topics, article structure, and inclusion criteria, supervised the literature research, and wrote major parts of the discussion section. All authors read and approved the final manuscript.

Competing interests
The authors declare that they have no competing interests.

References
1. World Health Organization: *Mental Health: New Understanding, New Hope* Geneva, Switzerland: WHO; 2001.
2. Leppänen JM: Emotional information processing in mood disorders: a review of behavioral and neuroimaging findings. *Curr Opin Psychiatry* 2006, 19:34-39.
3. Mathews A, MacLeod C: Cognitive vulnerability to emotional disorders. *Annu Rev Clin Psychol* 2005, 1:167-195.
4. Ridout N, Astell AJ, Reid IC, Glen T, O'Carroll RE: Memory bias for emotional facial expressions in major depression. *Cognition Emotion* 2003, 17:101-122.
5. Williams JMG, Watts FN, MacLeod C, Mathews A: *Cognitive psychology and emotional disorders.* 2 edition. Chichester, UK: John Wiley & Sons; 1997.
6. Bourke C, Douglas K, Porter R: Processing of facial emotion expression in major depression: a review. *Aust N Z J Psychiatry* 2010, 44:681-96.

7. Elliott R, Zahn R, Deakin JFW, Anderson IM: Affective cognition and its disruption in mood disorders. *Neuropsychopharmacol* 2010, 36:153-182.
8. Gotlib IH, Krasnoperova E, Yue DN, Joormann J: Attentional biases for negative interpersonal stimuli in clinical depression. *J Abnorm Psychol* 2004, 113:127-135.
9. Leyman L, De Raedt R, Schacht R, Koster EHW: Attentional biases for angry faces in unipolar depression. *Psychol Med* 2007, 37:393-402.
10. Suslow T, Dannlowski U, Lalee-Mentzel J, Donges U-S, Arolt V: Spatial processing of facial emotion in patients with unipolar depression: a longitudinal study. *J Affect Disord* 2004, 83:59-63.
11. Joormann J, Gotlib IH: Selective attention to emotional faces following recovery from depression. *J Abnorm Psychol* 2007, 116:80-85.
12. Bouhuys AL, Geerts E, Gordijn M: Depressed patients' perceptions of facial emotions in depressed and remitted states are associated with relapse: a longitudinal study. *J Nerv Ment Dis* 1999, 187:595-692.
13. Dannlowski U, Kersting A, Donges U-S, Lalee-Mentzel J, Arolt V, Suslow T: Masked facial affect priming is associated with therapy response in clinical depression. *Eur Arch Psychiatry Clin Neurosci* 2006, 256:215-221.
14. Dannlowski U, Kersting A, Lalee-Mentzel J, Donges U-S, Arolt V, Suslow T: Subliminal affective priming in clinical depression and comorbid anxiety: a longitudinal investigation. *Psychiatry Res* 2006, 143:63-75.
15. Phillips M: Neurobiology of emotion perception I: the neural basis of normal emotion perception. *Biol Psychiatry* 2003, 54:504-514.
16. Blair RJR: Facial expressions, their communicatory functions and neuro-cognitive substrates. *Philos Trans R Soc Lond B Biol Sci* 2003, 358:561-572.
17. Suslow T, Dannlowski U: Detection of facial emotion in depression. In *Mood State and Health*. Edited by: Clark AV. Hauppauge, NY: Nova Biomedical Books; 2005:1-32.
18. Fusar-Poli P, Placentino A, Carletti F, Landi P, Allen P, Surguladze S, Benedetti F, Abbamonte M, Gasparotti R, Barale F, Perez J, McGuire P, Politi P: Functional atlas of emotional faces processing: a voxel-based meta-analysis of 105 functional magnetic resonance imaging studies. *J Psychiatr Neurosci* 2009, 34:418-432.
19. Haxby J, Gobbini MI: The perception of emotion and social cues in faces. *Neuropsychologia* 2007, 45:1.
20. Haxby J, Hoffman E, Gobbini MI: The distributed human neural system for face perception. *Trends Cogn Sci* 2000, 4:223-233.
21. Posamentier MT, Abdi H: Processing faces and facial expressions. *Neuropsychol Rev* 2003, 13:113-143.
22. Haxby J, Hoffman E, Gobbini MI: Human neural systems for face recognition and social communication. *Biol Psychiatry* 2002, 51:59-67.
23. Mayberg HS: Limbic-cortical dysregulation: a proposed model of depression. *J Neuropsychiatry Clin Neurosci* 1997, 9:471-481.
24. Phillips ML, Ladouceur CD, Drevets WC: A neural model of voluntary and automatic emotion regulation: implications for understanding the pathophysiology and neurodevelopment of bipolar disorder. *Mol Psychiatry* 2008, 13:829, 833-857..
25. Phillips ML, Drevets WC, Rauch SL, Lane R: Neurobiology of emotion perception II: Implications for major psychiatric disorders. *Biol Psychiatry* 2003, 54:515-528.
26. Mayberg HS: Defining the neural circuitry of depression: toward a new nosology with therapeutic implications. *Biol Psychiatry* 2007, 61:729-730.
27. Frodl T, Scheuerecker J, Schoepf V, Linn J, Koutsouleris N, Bokde A, Hampel H, Möller H-J, Brückmann H, Wiesmann M, Meisenzahl E: Different effects of mirtazapine and venlafaxine on brain activation: an open randomized controlled fMRI study. *J Clin Psychiatry* 2011, 72:448-457.
28. Matthews SC, Strigo IA, Simmons AN, Yang TT, Paulus MP: Decreased functional coupling of the amygdala and supragenual cingulate is related to increased depression in unmedicated individuals with current major depressive disorder. *J Affect Disord* 2008, 111:13-20.
29. Victor TA, Furey ML, Fromm S, Ohman A, Drevets WC: Relationship between amygdala responses to masked faces and mood state and treatment in major depressive disorder. *Arch Gen Psychiatry* 2010, 67:1128-1138.
30. Suslow T, Konrad C, Kugel H, Rumstaedt D, Zwitserlood P, Schöning S, Ohrmann P, Bauer J, Pyka M, Kersting A, Arolt V, Heindel W, Dannlowski U: Automatic mood-congruent amygdala responses to masked facial expressions in major depression. *Biol Psychiatry* 2010, 67:155-160.
31. Surguladze S, Brammer M, Keedwell P, Giampietro V, Young AW, Travis MJ, Williams SCR, Phillips ML: A differential pattern of neural response toward

sad versus happy facial expressions in major depressive disorder. *Biol Psychiatry* 2005, 57:201-209.

32. Fu CHY, Williams SCR, Cleare AJ, Brammer M, Walsh ND, Kim J, Andrew CM, Pich EM, Williams PM, Reed LJ, Mitterschiffthaler MT, Suckling J, Bullmore ET: Attenuation of the neural response to sad faces in major depression by antidepressant treatment: a prospective, event-related functional magnetic resonance imaging study. *Arch Gen Psychiatry* 2004, 61:877-889.

33. Fu CHY, Williams SCR, Cleare AJ, Scott J, Mitterschiffthaler MT, Walsh ND, Donaldson C, Suckling J, Andrew CM, Steiner H, Murray RM: Neural responses to sad facial expressions in major depression following cognitive behavioral therapy. *Biol Psychiatry* 2008, 64:505-512.

34. Sheline YI, Barch DM, Donnelly JM, Ollinger JM, Snyder AZ, Mintun MA: Increased amygdala response to masked emotional faces in depressed subjects resolves with antidepressant treatment: an fMRI study. *Biol Psychiatry* 2001, 50:651-658.

35. Peluso MAM, Glahn DC, Matsuo K, Monkul ES, Najt P, Zamarripa F, Li J, Lancaster JL, Fox PT, Gao J-H, Soares JC: Amygdala hyperactivation in untreated depressed individuals. *Psychiatry Res* 2009, 173:158-161.

36. Zhong M, Wang X, Xiao J, Yi J, Zhu X, Liao J, Wang W, Yao S: Amygdala hyperactivation and prefrontal hypoactivation in subjects with cognitive vulnerability to depression. *Biol Psychiatry* 2011, 88:233-242.

37. Lawrence NS, Williams AM, Surguladze S, Giampietr V, Brammer M, Andrew CM, Frangou S, Ecker C, Phillips ML: Subcortical and ventral prefrontal cortical neural responses to facial expressions distinguish patients with bipolar disorder and major depression. *Biol Psychiatry* 2004, 55:578-87.

38. Lee B-T, Seok J-H, Lee B-C, Cho SW, Yoon B-J, Lee K-U, Chae J-H, Choi I-G, Ham B-J: Neural correlates of affective processing in response to sad and angry facial stimuli in patients with major depressive disorder. *Prog Neuropsychopharmacol Biol Psychiatry* 2008, 32:778-785.

39. Surguladze S, El-Hage W, Dalgleish T, Radua J, Gohier B, Phillips ML: Depression is associated with increased sensitivity to signals of disgust: a functional magnetic resonance imaging study. *J Psychiatr Res* 2010, 44:894-902.

40. Townsend JD, Eberhart NK, Bookheimer SY, Eisenberger NI, Foland-Ross LC, Cook IA, Sugar CA, Altshuler LL: fMRI activation in the amygdala and the orbitofrontal cortex in unmedicated subjects with major depressive disorder. *Psychiatry Res* 2010, 183:209-217.

41. Scheuerecker J, Meisenzahl EM, Koutsouleris N, Roesner M, Schöpf V, Linn J, Wiesmann M, Brückmann H, Möller H-J, Frodl T: Orbitofrontal volume reductions during emotion recognition in patients with major depression. *J Psychiatr Neurosci* 2010, 35:311-320.

42. Keedwell P, Andrew CM, Williams SCR, Brammer M, Phillips ML: A double dissociation of ventromedial prefrontal cortical responses to sad and happy stimuli in depressed and healthy individuals. *Biol Psychiatry* 2005, 58:495-503.

43. Frodl T, Scheuerecker J, Albrecht J, Kleemann AM, Müller-Schunk S, Koutsouleris N, Möller H-J, Brückmann H, Wiesmann M, Meisenzahl EM: Neuronal correlates of emotional processing in patients with major depression. *World J Biol Psychiatry* 2009, 10:202-208.

44. Mayberg HS, Lozano AM, Voon V, McNeely HE, Seminowicz DA, Hamani C, Schwalb JM, Kennedy S: Deep brain stimulation for treatment-resistant depression. *Neuron* 2005, 45:651-660.

45. Gotlib IH, Sivers H, Gabrieli JDE, Whitfield-Gabrieli S, Goldin P, Minor KL, Canli T: Subgenual anterior cingulate activation to valenced emotional stimuli in major depression. *Neuroreport* 2005, 16:1731-1734.

46. Friston KJ: Functional and effective connectivity in neuroimaging: a synthesis. *Hum Brain Mapp* 1994, 2:56-78.

47. Almeida JRC, Versace A, Mechelli A, Hassel S, Quevedo K, Kupfer DJ, Phillips ML: Abnormal amygdala-prefrontal effective connectivity to happy faces differentiates bipolar from major depression. *Biol Psychiatry* 2009, 66:451-459.

48. Carballedo A, Scheuerecker J, Meisenzahl E, Schoepf V, Bokde A, Möller H-J, Doyle M, Wiesmann M, Frodl T: Functional connectivity of emotional processing in depression. *J Affect Disord* 2011, 134:272-279.

49. Chen C-H, Suckling J, Ooi C, Fu CHY, Williams SCR, Walsh ND, Mitterschiffthaler MT, Pich EM, Bullmore E: Functional coupling of the amygdala in depressed patients treated with antidepressant medication. *Neuropsychopharmacol* 2008, 33:1909-1918.

50. Dannlowski U, Ohrmann P, Konrad C, Domschke K, Bauer J, Kugel H, Hohoff C, Schöning S, Kersting A, Baune BT, Mortensen LS, Arolt V,

Zwitserlood P, Deckert J, Heindel W, Suslow T: Reduced amygdala-prefrontal coupling in major depression: association with MAOA genotype and illness severity. *Int J Neuropsychopharmacol* 2009, 12:11-22.

51. Frodl T, Bokde ALW, Scheuerecker J, Lisiecka D, Schoepf V, Hampel H, Möller H-J, Brückmann H, Wiesmann M, Meisenzahl EM: Functional connectivity bias of the orbitofrontal cortex in drug-free patients with major depression. *Biol Psychiatry* 2010, 67:161-167.

52. Adolphs R, Spezio M: Role of the amygdala in processing visual social stimuli. *Brain* 2006, 156:363-78.

53. Davis M, Whalen PJ: The amygdala: vigilance and emotion. *Mol Psychiatry* 2001, 6:13-34.

54. Phan KL, Wager T, Taylor SF, Liberzon I: Functional neuroanatomy of emotion: a meta-analysis of emotion activation studies in PET and fMRI. *Neuroimage* 2002, 16:331-348.

55. Dannlowski U, Ohrmann P, Bauer J, Kugel H, Arolt V, Heindel W, Kersting A, Baune BT, Suslow T: Amygdala reactivity to masked negative faces is associated with automatic judgmental bias in major depression: a 3 T fMRI study. *J Psychiatr Neurosci* 2007, 32:423-429.

56. Dannlowski U, Ohrmann P, Bauer J, Kugel H, Arolt V, Heindel W, Suslow T: Amygdala reactivity predicts automatic negative evaluations for facial emotions. *Psychiatry Res* 2007, 154:13-20.

57. Siegle GJ, Steinhauer SR, Thase ME, Stenger VA, Carter CS: Can't shake that feeling: event-related fMRI assessment of sustained amygdala activity in response to emotional information in depressed individuals. *Biol Psychiatry* 2002, 51:693-707.

58. Siegle GJ, Thompson WK, Carter CS, Steinhauer SR, Thase ME: Increased amygdala and decreased dorsolateral prefrontal BOLD responses in unipolar depression: related and independent features. *Biol Psychiatry* 2007, 61:198-209.

59. Kessler H, Taubner S, Buchheim A, Münte TF, Stasch M, Kächele H, Roth G, Heinecke A, Erhard P, Cierpka M, Wiswede D: Individualized and clinically derived stimuli activate limbic structures in depression: an fMRI study. *PLoS ONE* 2011, 6:e15712.

60. Abler B, Erk S, Herwig U, Walter H: Anticipation of aversive stimuli activates extended amygdala in unipolar depression. *J Psychiat Res* 2007, 41:511-522.

61. Yang TT, Simmons AN, Matthews SC, Tapert SF, Frank GK, May JE, Bischoff-Grethe A, Lansing AE, Brown G, Strigo IA, Wu J, Paulus MP: Adolescents with major depression demonstrate increased amygdala activation. *J Am Acad Child Psy* 2010, 49:42-51.

62. Almeida JRC, Versace A, Hassel S, Kupfer DJ, Phillips ML: Elevated amygdala activity to sad facial expressions: a state marker of bipolar but not unipolar depression. *Biol Psychiatry* 2010, 67:414-421.

63. Fu CHY, Williams SCR, Brammer M, Suckling J, Cleare AJ, Walsh ND, Mitterschiffthaler MT, Andrew CM, Pich EM, Bullmore ET: Neural responses to happy facial expressions in major depression following antidepressant treatment. *Am J Psychiatry* 2007, 164:599-607.

64. Fitzgerald DA, Angstadt M, Jelsone LM, Nathan PJ, Phan KL: Beyond threat: amygdala reactivity across multiple expressions of facial affect. *Neuroimage* 2006, 30:1441-1448.

65. Neumeister A, Drevets WC, Belfer I, Luckenbaugh DA, Henry S, Bonne O, Herscovitch P, Goldman D, Charney DS: Effects of a alpha 2C-adrenoreceptor gene polymorphism on neural responses to facial expressions in depression. *Neuropsychopharmacol* 2006, 31:1750-1756.

66. Norbury R, Selvaraj S, Taylor MJ, Harmer C, Cowen PJ: Increased neural response to fear in patients recovered from depression: a 3T functional magnetic resonance imaging study. *Psychol Med* 2010, 40:425-432.

67. Thomas EJ, Elliott R, McKie S, Arnone D, Downey D, Juhasz G, Deakin JFW, Anderson IM: Interaction between a history of depression and rumination on neural response to emotional faces. *Psychol Med* 2011, 41:1-11.

68. van der Veen FM, Evers EA, Deutz NE, Schmitt JA: Effects of acute tryptophan depletion on mood and facial emotion perception related brain activation and performance in healthy women with and without a family history of depression. *Neuropsychopharmacol* 2007, 32:216-224.

69. Monk CS, Klein RG, Telzer EH, Schroth EA, Mannuzza S, Moulton JL, Guardino M, Masten CL, McClure EB, Fromm SJ, Blair RJ, Pine DS, Ernst M: Amygdala and nucleus accumbens activation to emotional facial expressions in children and adolescents at risk for major depression. *Am J Psychiatry* 2008, 165:90-98.

70. Mannie ZN, Taylor MJ, Harmer CJ, Cowen PJ, Norbury R: **Frontolimbic responses to emotional faces in young people at familial risk of depression.** *J Affect Disord* 2011, 130:127-132.

71. Cremers HR, Demenescu LR, Aleman A, Renken R, van Tol MJ, van der Wee NJ, Veltman DJ, Roelofs K: **Neuroticism modulates amygdala-prefrontal connectivity in response to negative emotional facial expressions.** *Neurolmage* 2010, 49:963-970.

72. Dannlowski U, Stuhrmann A, Beutelmann V, Zwanzger P, Lenzen T, Grotegerd D, Domschke K, Hohoff C, Ohrmann P, Bauer J, Lindner C, Posterts C, Konrad C, Arolt V, Heindel W, Kugel H: **Limbic scars: Long-term consequences of childhood maltreatment revealed by functional and structural MRI.** *Biol Psychiatry* .

73. Dannlowski U, Ohrmann P, Bauer J, Kugel H, Baune BT, Hohoff C, Kersting A, Arolt V, Heindel W, Deckert J, Suslow T: **Serotonergic genes modulate amygdala activity in major depression.** *Genes Brain Behav* 2007, 6:672-676.

74. Dannlowski U, Konrad C, Kugel H, Zwitserlood P, Domschke K, Schöning S, Ohrmann P, Bauer J, Pyka M, Hohoff C, Zhang W, Baune BT, Heindel W, Arolt V, Suslow T: **Emotion specific modulation of automatic amygdala responses by 5-HTTLPR genotype.** *Neurolmage* 2009, 53:893-898.

75. Dannlowski U, Ohrmann P, Bauer J, Deckert J, Hohoff C, Kugel H, Arolt V, Heindel W, Kersting A, Baune BT, Suslow T: **5-HTTLPR biases amygdala activity in response to masked facial expressions in major depression.** *Neuropsychopharmacol* 2008, 33:418-424.

76. Hariri AR, Weinberger DR: **Imaging genomics.** *Br Med Bull* 2003, 65:259-270.

77. Munafò MR, Brown SM, Hariri AR: **Serotonin transporter (5-HTTLPR) genotype and amygdala activation: a meta-analysis.** *Biol Psychiatry* 2008, 63:852-857.

78. Wolfensberger SPA, Veltman DJ, Hoogendijk WJG, Boomsma DI, Geus EJC de: **Amygdala responses to emotional faces in twins discordant or concordant for the risk for anxiety and depression.** *Neurolmage* 2008, 41:544-552.

79. Delaveau P, Jabourian M, Lemogne C, Jabourian M, Lemogne C, Guionnet S, Bergouignan L, Fossati P: **Brain effects of antidepressants in major depression: a meta-analysis of emotional processing studies.** *J Affect Disord* 2010, 130:66-74.

80. Davidson R, Irwin W: **The functional neuroanatomy of emotion and affective style.** *Trends Cogn Sci* 1999, 3:11-21.

81. Drevets WC: **Neuroimaging studies of mood disorders.** *Biol Psychiatry* 2000, 48:813-829.

82. Drevets WC: **Neuroimaging and neuropathological studies of depression: implications for the cognitive-emotional features of mood disorders.** *Curr Opin Neurobiol* 2001, 11:240-249.

83. Drevets WC, Raichle ME: **Neuroanatomical circuits in depression: implications for treatment mechanisms.** *Psychopharmacol Bull* 1992, 28:261-274.

84. Grady CL, Keightley ML: **Studies of altered social cognition in neuropsychiatric disorders using functional neuroimaging.** *Can J Psychiat* 2002, 47:327-336.

85. Stein JL, Wiedholz LM, Bassett DS, Weinberger DR, Zink CF, Matty VS, Meyer-Lindenberg A: **A validated network of effective amygdala connectivity.** *Neuroimage* 2007, 36:736-745.

86. Calder AJ, Lawrence AD, Young AW: **Neuropsychology of fear and loathing.** *Nat Rev Neurosci* 2001, 2:352-363.

87. Critchley H, Daly E, Phillips ML, Brammer M, Bullmore E, Williams S, Van Amelsvoort T, Robertson D, David A, Murphy D: **Explicit and implicit neural mechanisms for processing of social information from facial expressions: a functional magnetic resonance imaging study.** *Hum Brain Mapp* 2000, 9:93-105.

88. Vuilleumier P, Pourtois G: **Distributed and interactive brain mechanisms during emotion face perception: evidence from functional neuroimaging.** *Neuropsychologia* 2007, 45:174-194.

89. Amaral D: **Topographic organization of projections from the amygdala to the visual cortex in the macaque monkey.** *Neuroscience* 2003, 118:1099-1120.

90. Davidson R, Irwin W, Anderle MJ, Kalin NH: **The neural substrates of affective processing in depressed patients treated with venlafaxine.** *Am J Psychiatry* 2003, 160:64-75.

91. Keedwell P, Drapier D, Surguladze S, Giampietro V, Brammer M, Phillips ML: **Subgenual cingulate and visual cortex responses to sad faces predict clinical outcome during antidepressant treatment for depression.** *J Affect Disord* 2010, 120:120-125.

92. Mayberg HS: **Modulating dysfunctional limbic-cortical circuits in depression: towards development of brain-based algorithms for diagnosis and optimised treatment.** *Br Med Bull* 2003, 65:193-207.

93. Bush G, Luu P, Posner M: **Cognitive and emotional influences in anterior cingulate cortex.** *Trends Cogn Sci* 2000, 4:215-222.

94. Devinsky O, Morrell MJ, Vogt BA: **Contributions of anterior cingulate cortex to behaviour.** *Brain* 1995, 118:279-306.

95. Almeida JRC, Phillips ML, Cerqueira CT, Zilberman M, Lobo D, Henna E, Tavares H, Amaro E, Gorenstein C, Gentil V, Busatto GF: **Neural activity changes to emotional stimuli in healthy individuals under chronic use of clomipramine.** *J Psychopharmacol* 2010, 24:1165-1174.

96. Pizzagalli DA: **Frontocingulate dysfunction in depression: toward biomarkers of treatment response.** *Neuropsychopharmacol* 2010, 36:183-206.

97. Seminowicz DA, Mayberg HS, McIntosh AR, Goldapple K, Kennedy S, Segal Z, Rafi-Tari S: **Limbic-frontal circuitry in major depression: a path modeling metanalysis.** *Neurolmage* 2004, 22:409-418.

98. Tekin S, Cummings JL: **Frontal-subcortical neuronal circuits and clinical neuropsychiatry: an update.** *J Psychosom Res* 2002, 53:647-654.

99. Price JL, Drevets WC: **Neurocircuitry of mood disorders.** *Neuropsychopharmacol* 2010, 35:192-216.

100. Harmer CJ, Mackay CE, Reid CB, Cowen PJ, Goodwin GM: **Antidepressant drug treatment modifies the neural processing of nonconscious threat cues.** *Biol Psychiatry* 2006, 59:816-820.

101. Harmer CJ, Shelley NC, Cowen PJ, Goodwin GM: **Increased positive versus negative affective perception and memory in healthy volunteers following selective serotonin and norepinephrine reuptake inhibition.** *Am J Psychiatry* 2004, 161:1256-1263.

102. Norbury R, Taylor MJ, Selvaraj S, Taylor MJ, Harmer C, Cowen PJ: **Short-term antidepressant treatment modulates amygdala response to happy faces.** *Psychopharmacol* 2009, 206:197-204.

103. Joormann J, Cooney RE, Henry ML, Gotlib IH: **Neural correlates of automatic mood regulation in girls at high risk for depression.** *J Abnorm Psychol* 2011.

104. Gotlib IH, Joormann J: **Cognition and depression: current status and future directions.** *Annu Rev Clin Psychol* 2010, 6:285-312.

The Behavioural Inhibition System, anxiety and hippocampal volume in a non-clinical population

Liat Levita[1*], Catherine Bois[2,3], Andrew Healey[2], Emily Smyllie[2], Evelina Papakonstantinou[2], Tom Hartley[2] and Colin Lever[4]

Abstract

Background: Animal studies have suggested that the hippocampus may play an important role in anxiety as part of the Behavioural Inhibition System (BIS), which mediates reactivity to threat and punishment and can predict an individual's response to anxiety-relevant cues in a given environment. The aim of the present structural magnetic resonance imaging (MRI) study was to examine the relationship between individual differences in BIS and hippocampal structure, since this has not received sufficient attention in non-clinical populations. Thirty healthy right-handed participants with no history of alcohol or drug abuse, neurological or psychiatric disorders, or traumatic brain injury were recruited (16 male, 14 female, age 18 to 32 years). T1-weighted structural MRI scans were used to derive estimates of total intracranial volume, and hippocampal and amygdala gray matter volume using FreeSurfer. To relate brain structure to Gray's BIS, participants completed the Sensitivity to Punishment questionnaire. They also completed questionnaires assessing other measures potentially associated with hippocampal volume (Beck Depression Inventory, Negative Life Experience Survey), and two other measures of anxiety (Spielberger Trait Anxiety Inventory and the Beck Anxiety Inventory).

Results: We found that high scores on the Sensitivity to Punishment scale were positively associated with hippocampal volume, and that this phenomenon was lateralized to the right side. In other words, greater levels of behavioural inhibition (BIS) were positively associated with right hippocampal volume.

Conclusions: Our data suggest that hippocampal volume is related to the cognitive and affective dimensions of anxiety indexed by the Sensitivity to Punishment, and support the idea that morphological differences in the hippocampal formation may be associated with behavioural inhibition contributions to anxiety.

Keywords: Anxiety, Behavioural Inhibition System, Sensitivity to Punishment, Structural MRI, Hippocampus, Amygdala

Background

Lang's tripartite model of anxiety suggests that it consists of three response domains: cognitive, behavioural, and physiological [1], which together result in a state of apprehensive worry, hyperarousal to threat cues, avoidance behaviours and negatively-biased cognitions [2]. Each of these domains is suggested to measure a separate element of response characteristics and potentially independent underlying mechanisms to the construct of anxiety [3]. An influential model of anxiety sees it as reflecting the engagement of the Behavioural Inhibition System (BIS) of which the hippocampus is a key component [4]. Briefly,

in Gray's original account the role of BIS is to govern avoidance behaviours in response to threat and punishment. Excessive activity in BIS when driven by enhanced reactivity to threat/punishment cues manifests as higher proneness to anxiety.

In support of this idea Gray reviewed the evidence in the animal literature that anxiolytic drugs impair hippocampal function, specifically septo-hippocampal theta, to suggest that the hippocampus was the key substrate of BIS [4]. Subsequent revision of the theory has incorporated other regions, most notably the amygdala, as a part of the BIS network, with the amygdala and hippocampus mediating different aspects of anxiety [5,6], and with the BIS interpreted as a conflict mediator system biased toward fight/flight/freeze behaviours and using exploration to resolve conflict. Critically, ensuing empirical work has continued

* Correspondence: l.levita@sheffield.ac.uk
[1]Present address: Department of Psychology, University of Sheffield, Western Bank, Sheffield S10 2TN, UK
Full list of author information is available at the end of the article

to implicate hippocampal theta in anxiety and anxiolytic drug effects (for examples, see [7-14]). For example, Gray and McNaughton [5] observe that anxiolytic drugs, despite their neurochemical dissimilarity, commonly reduce the frequency of reticular-elicited hippocampal theta in the anaesthetised animal. We recently showed that Gray and McNaughton's central observation extends to the awake, freely moving rat, where anxiolytic drugs reduce the frequency of natural theta obtained during locomotion [14].

Two commonly used and well-validated instruments designed to measure individual differences in Gray's BIS are the BIS section of the BIS/Behavioural Activation System scales [15] and the Sensitivity to Punishment (StP) subscale of the Sensitivity to Punishment and Sensitivity to Reward questionnaire [16]. These instruments have been shown to predict clinical anxiety disorders (for examples, see [17,18]), and likely capture cognitive and affective, rather than somatic, aspects of anxiety [16]. Using these instruments and other indicators of BIS activity, neuroimaging studies have begun to implicate the hippocampus and amygdala in behavioural inhibition. Hahn and colleagues [19] found that StP scores predicted hippocampus-amygdala functional connectivity in a monetary loss anticipation task. Further, it is conceivable that hippocampal structure, as well as activity, may be partly heritable. This is supported by a study by Oler and colleagues [20] who investigated 'anxious temperament' in monkeys using a three-part composite measure of anxiety consisting of two behavioural BIS measures and cortisol release. They found that anxiety was clearly heritable, and that both hippocampal and amygdalar activity predicted anxiety, but only the hippocampal anxiety-related activity was heritable.

Together these findings suggest that BIS-related anxiety may be associated with structural variations in the brain. To our knowledge, only three studies have specifically related brain volume measures to BIS self-report [21-23]. Interestingly, two of these found that (para)hippocampal volume positively correlates with behavioural inhibition, one using voxel-based morphometry (VBM) and the StP questionnaire [22], the other using volume measures based on manual tracings and the BIS scale [21]. In the VBM study, the region correlating with StP scores was largely parahippocampal, but reportedly also included the right hippocampus proper [22]. A similar but weaker correlation based on a largely middle-aged sample was found in the manual tracing study [21].

A different approach to the BIS has been to look at neural asymmetry in human scalp electroencephalography (EEG), with right brain dominance, particularly prefrontal, associating with higher behavioural inhibition [24,25] and anxiety [26-29]. Intriguingly, simply being left-handed, and thus more likely to be right-hemisphere dominant, predisposes to higher BIS activity and anxiety [30]. Hippocampal

activity cannot itself be detected by scalp EEG, but animal models suggest that hippocampal influences on prefrontal EEG are important in anxiety [7].

In the present study we used an automated segmentation method to obtain gray matter volumes of both the hippocampus and amygdala in healthy adult students, with no current or past history of any mental health disorder. Restricting our sample to young, well-educated adults may be important in minimising confounding effects of depression, stress and education. Torrubia and colleagues [16] suggest that StP implements Gray's theoretical construct of anxiety more faithfully than Carver and White's BIS scale. Notably, for instance, in Gray's conceptual revision of Eysenck's theory of personality, Gray theorised that anxious people would be both 'introverted' and 'neurotic'. Consistent with this prediction, StP scores are positively correlated with Neuroticism and negatively correlated with Extraversion [16], whereas scores on Carver and White's BIS scale tend only to be positively correlated with Neuroticism [15]. Torrubia and colleagues [16] also suggest that their focus on the response to particular cues was more in line with Gray's theory. Accordingly, in order to relate brain structure to Gray's BIS, we asked participants to complete the StP subscale of the Sensitivity to Punishment and Sensitivity to Reward questionnaire [16]. Participants also completed questionnaires assessing other measures potentially associated with hippocampal volume: depression with the Beck Depression Inventory (BDI)-II [31], negative life events with the Life Experiences Survey (LES) [32]; and two other measures of anxiety: Trait anxiety of the State and Trait Anxiety Inventory (STAI-T) [33] and the Beck Anxiety Inventory (BAI) [34], the latter thought to be particularly sensitive to panic symptomatology [35]. These different measurement instruments approach anxiety differently, which is why we choose to use them in this study. For instance, StP likely captures cognitive and emotional, but not somatic, components of anxiety, while BAI certainly does tap the somatic component [16,35]; trait anxiety as measured by STAI-T is dissociable from anxiety as mediated by BIS [21], and may predict depression and negative affect as much as, or even more than, anxiety *per se* [36,37]. If StP were found to be significantly related to hippocampal volume, we aimed to be able to examine the potential selectivity of this relationship.

Methods
Participants
Thirty healthy right-handed native English speakers (16 male, 14 female, aged 18 to 32 years, (mean ± SD, 24.1 ± 2.66 years)) were recruited from the student population at the University of York. All the participants recruited had previously undergone a structural magnetic resonance imaging (MRI) scan at the York Neuroimaging

Centre. Participants were scanned 0 to 2 years prior to taking part in this study (median, 188 days). None of the participants had a history of alcohol or drug abuse, neurological or psychiatric disorders, or traumatic brain injury. This was determined by a list of questions, verbally administered by the experimenter, about past and present history of drug use and mental health status. The study was approved by the York Neuroimaging Centre Research Ethics and Governance committee. All participants gave written informed consent for participation in the study.

Procedure

Participants were invited to attend a 1-hour test session at the Psychology Department of the University of York. All self-report inventories were administered on-line using LimeSurvey. The on-line questionnaires were administered in a counterbalanced order to control for order of presentation effects. An intelligence quotient (IQ) test was administered between the on-line questionnaires.

Measures

All participants completed the StP scale, which is a revision of the Susceptibility to Punishment scale that was first published by Torrubia and Tobena [38] designed to measure individual differences in the Behavioural Inhibition system (BIS). The StP scale is a 24-item scale, with high internal consistency ($\alpha = 0.83$) and test-retest reliability coefficients ranging up to 0.85, indicating that scores on this scale are indicative of a long-lasting aspect of anxiety [16]. The items included in this version were devised to measure individual differences in functions dependent on the BIS in situations involving the possibility of aversive consequences or novelty as well as items that assess cognitive processes produced by threat of punishment of failure.

In order to obtain comparative measures of potentially different aspects of anxiety, participants also completed the BAI and the STAI-T. The BAI is a 21-item self-report inventory used to assess primarily the intensity of somatic (hands trembling, face flushed) anxiety symptoms experienced over the last week, with each item having a scale value of 0 to 3. A score of 0 to 7 is considered minimal, 8 to 15 indicates mild anxiety, 16 to 25 reflects moderate anxiety, and 26 to 63 is considered severe anxiety. The BAI scale has high internal consistency ($\alpha = 0.92$) and high discriminant validity against depression [34]. The State and Trait Anxiety Inventory consists of both a measure of State anxiety (STAI-S) and a measure of Trait anxiety (STAI-T) [33,39]. Each scale has 20 items. The STAI-T scale has been found to have high internal consistency ($\alpha = 0.9$) [40].

Further, all participants were matched on IQ, as measured by the Wechsler Abbreviated Scale of Intelligence-III two-test subscales, vocabulary and matrix-reasoning,

respectively [41]. In addition, BDI-II was administered [31] as depression has also been shown to affect hippocampal volume (for examples, see [42,43]). Since trauma and negative life events have been shown to be positively associated with anxiety [32], participants also filled in the LES [32], where participants are required to indicate which positive and negative events listed in the survey they had experienced in the last year. Our sample experienced very low levels of negative life events (range 1 to 27), and scores of negative life events were not correlated with StP scores ($r = -0.162$, $P = 0.144$), or any other of our measures of emotionality. None of these psychometric measures correlated with age, except BAI (see Additional file 1: Table S1).

Automated segmentation analysis

T1-weighted structural MRI images were obtained from our participants at the York Neuroimaging Centre on a GE 3 T HD Excite MRI Scanner (General Electric Medical Systems, Milwaukee, WI). Whole-brain T1-weighted data sets were acquired in the sagittal plane using fast spoiled gradient reaction echo (3DFSPGR) sequence to collect data from 176 continuous slices (repetition time = 7.8 ms, echo time = 3 ms, inversion time = 450 ms, field of view = $290 \times 290 \times 176$, matrix size = $256 \times 256 \times 176$, slice thickness = 1.0 mm, resolution = $1.13 \times 1.1.3 \times 1.0$ mm, flip angle = $20°$)[a]. Automated subcortical and cortical segmentation was performed using Freesurfer version 5.1 [44]. Parcellation of the subcortical and cortical anatomy, and calculations of the total subcortical gray matter volume, total gray matter volume and intracranial volume were performed by delineating anatomical divisions via FreeSurfer's automatic parcellation methods, in which the statistical knowledge base derives from a training set incorporating the anatomical landmarks and conventions described by Duvernoy [45]. This procedure assigns a neuroanatomical label to each voxel in an MRI volume based on probabilistic information estimated from a manually labelled training set. This classification technique employs a non-linear registration procedure that is robust to anatomical variability [46]. The segmentation uses three pieces of information to disambiguate labels: (1) the prior probability of a given tissue class occurring at a specific atlas location; (2) the likelihood of the image given what tissue class; and (3) the probability of the local spatial configuration of labels given the tissue class. The technique has shown comparable accuracy to manual labelling [46]. The hippocampus and amygdala were identified as regions of interest based on previous literature on the neural bases of anxiety [5]. This, as well as volumes (mm^3) for total subcortical gray matter volume, total gray matter volume and intracranial volume, were obtained from the statistics output file (aseg. stats). An example of the parcellation results is shown for a representative participant in Figure 1.

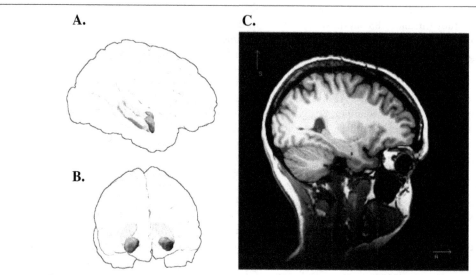

Figure 1 Parcellation of hippocampus and amygdala in a representative participant (female, right hippocampal volume ranked 15/30). Left: "glass brain" renderings showing three-dimensional volumes of right and left hippocampi (yellow) and right and left amygdalae (cyan) viewed from participant's right **(A)** and front **(B)**; the outline of the pial surface is shown in black. **C**. Right labelled voxels overlaid on a T1 image, sagittal section passing through right hippocampus (yellow) and amygdala (cyan).

Data analysis

On initial analysis of the data we found two major consistent predictors of hippocampal volume (age and sex), which can potentially confound estimation of the relationship of hippocampal volume with anxiety traits. Previous developmental studies of hippocampal volume show that hippocampal volume peaks in middle age (approximately 45 years, [47]). Consistent with these findings, age had a positive significant correlation with hippocampal volume in our young sample (Pearson's r, total hippocampal volume versus age, $r(30) = 0.41$, $P = 0.025$) and men were found to have larger hippocampi than women (bilateral raw hippocampal volume, independent t-test, two-tailed, $t(28) = -2.72$, $P = 0.011$). This was also the case for the amygdala; age had a positive correlation with amygdala volume (Pearson's $r = 0.36$ $P = 0.051$), and men were found to have larger amygdala volume than women (bilateral raw amygdala volume, independent t-test, two-tailed, $t(28) = -4.02$, $P = 0.001$). In addition, we found a general effect of sex on brain volume such that, in comparison to females, males had greater total gray matter volume ($t(28) = 4.374$, $P = 0.001$), total subcortical gray matter volume ($t(28) = 4.315$, $P = 0.001$), and intracranial volume ($t(28) = 3.394$, $P = 0.002$).

In order to establish the extent to which StP predicted brain volumes, and to control for sex- and age-related potential confounds mentioned above, we incorporated intracranial volume, age, and sex as co-regressors alongside StP into multiple regression models. All the beta values that we report are standardised beta values. A recent methodological study [48] addressing volume correction in structural MRI studies has specifically recommended the use of intracranial volume, age, and sex as covariates in multiple regression models relating variables of interest to specific brain region volumes. To investigate effects of hippocampal lateralisation, we calculated a laterality index specific to that structure using the formula: Right - Left hippocampal volume)/total hippocampal volume; that is, a unit-less measure. One advantage of this measure is that it obviates the need for co-regressors controlling for whole volume. Essentially, this measure sacrifices information about the absolute volume of each hippocampus in order to obtain a well-controlled measure of laterality. Analysis using this measure makes fewer assumptions about linearity and stability of association between variables. For instance, the average relationship between hippocampal volume and intracranial volume may not be expected to be constant across a sample of different ages. Each analytic approach yielded convergent results regarding the association between right hippocampal volume and Gray's BIS as indexed by the StP scale. All statistical analyses were conducted using SPSS version 20.0 (SPSS Inc., Chicago, IL, USA).

Results

Participant characteristics

Participant demographics and self-report measure scores are summarized in Table 1. StP scores did not differ between males and females in the sample (independent t-test, two-tailed $t(28) = 1.12$, $P = 0.27$). There were also

Table 1 Participants demographics and self-report measure scores

	Female		Male		Total	
	Range	Mean (SD)	Range	Mean (SD)	Range	Mean (SD)
Age	20-27	23.29 (1.73)	22-32	24.81 (3.15)	20-32	24.10 (2.66)
Intelligence quotient	100-129	117.86 (9.04)	90-131	118.5 (10.15)	90-131	118.20 (9.48)
Life experiences survey positive	3-29	12.93 (7.91)	3-24	16.19 (6.71)	3-29	14.67 (7.35)
Life experiences survey negative	2-27	9.86 (6.87)	1-11	4.38 (2.73)	1-27	6.93 (5.72)
Beck depression inventory	0-18	4.86 (4.91)	0-8	2.69 (2.18)	0-18	3.70 (3.81)
Beck anxiety inventory	5-20	9.43 (4.72)	0-17	5.00 (4.63)	0-20	7.07 (5.11)
Trait anxiety	44-79	54.64 (9.95)	37-65	50.13 (8.22)	37-79	52.23 (9.20)
Sensitivity to Punishment	1-16	9.29 (4.97)	2-19	7.38 (4.41)	1-19	8.27 (4.70)

no gender differences in STAI-T scores in this sample (independent t-test, two-tailed, $t(28) = 1.36$, $P = 0.18$). Since the Shapiro-Wilks test indicated that BAI, BDI and negative LES scores were not normally distributed, they were analysed using the Mann–Whitney test. This analysis revealed a gender differences in BAI and negative LES scores, where females had higher BAI scores, and reported a greater number of negative life events (BAI, $U = 47.50$, $z = -2.70$, $P = 0.007$; negative life events, $U = 43.50$, $z = -2.86$, $P = 0.004$). There were no gender differences in scores for depression as measured by BDI ($U = 84.00$, $z = -1.17$, $P = 0.24$).

Volumetric brain measures

Bilateral, right and left hippocampal and amygdala volumes (Figure 1), and intracranial volume, total gray matter volume, and subcortical gray matter volumes are shown in Table 2. In this study our specific aim was to investigate the relationship between hippocampal volume and behavioural inhibition. One potentially important predictor of hippocampal volume is depression; however, in our healthy sample we found no evidence that depression

scores co-varied with hippocampal volume (Spearman's rho = 0.034, $P = 0.858$).

Right hippocampal volume is correlated with Sensitivity to Punishment

Using multiple regression to examine the relationship between right hippocampal volume and StP, we controlled for age, sex, and intracranial volume (ICV) by including these variables as co-regressors alongside StP scores. A significant model emerged ($F(4,29) = 4.789$, $P = 0.005$, adjusted $R^2 = 0.343$), whereby StP ($\beta = 0.334$, $P = 0.040$) and age ($\beta = 0.379$, $P = 0.024$) but not the other variables (sex, $\beta = -0.148$, $P = 0.440$; ICV, $\beta = 0.305$, $P = 0.10$) predicted right hippocampal volume.

Furthermore, we ran an additional analysis using a two-step approach in a hierarchical regression model, where step 1 included sex, age and ICV, and step 2 added StP. This analysis showed that StP explains a further 11% of the variance in right hippocampal volume over and above the initial model including sex, age and ICV, and the significance of the change in F from the first to second model was $P = 0.04$ (step 1, R^2 change = 0.327; step 2, R^2 change = 0.107).

Table 2 Volumetric brain measures

	Female		Male		Total	
Volume (mm³)	Range	Mean (SD)	Range	Mean (SD)	Range	Mean (SD)
Intracranial volume	1,066,529.5-1,581,389.1	1,365,722.9 (187,852.801)	1,079,697.4-1,945,463.8	1,628,006.319 (229,462.0061)	1,066,529.5-1,945,463.8	1,505,607.39 (246,506.369)
Total gray matter	576,015-735,158	652850 (49,290)	657,592.1-875,048	739,810 (59,634)	576,015-875,048	699,230 (69,827)
Subcortical gray matter	156,112-210,381	182988 (14,859)	185,983-252,345	209,839 (18,269)	156,112-252,345	197,309 (21,383)
Bilateral hippocampus	8,083-10,763	8,860 (775)	7,786-11,605	9,826 (1,114)	7,786-11,605	9,375 (1,073)
Right hippocampus	3,568-5,345	4,395 (430)	3,814-5,688	4,760 (551)	3,568-5,688	4,590 (524)
Left hippocampus	3,993-5,418	4,464 (417)	3,972-6,150	5,065 (613)	3,972-6,150	4,785 (604)
Bilateral amygdala	2,443-3,282	2,777 (236)	2,427-4,240	3,266 (397)	2,427-4,240	3,038 (410)
Right amygdala	1,294-1,660	1,442 (105)	1,404-2,248	1,663 (194)	1,294-2,248	1,560 (192)
Left amygdala	1,065-1,622	1,334 (152)	1,023-2,113	1,603 (236)	1,023-2,113	1,478 (240)

Right/left hippocampal laterality is correlated with Sensitivity to Punishment

To investigate the right hippocampus laterality effect further, we next calculated a ratio measure of hippocampal laterality, by dividing the right minus the left hippocampal volume by the total hippocampal volume, where a zero score would reflect a perfectly symmetric hippocampus (laterality ratio scores: range = −0.14 to 0.04; mean = −0.02 SD = 0.038). One advantage of this measure is that it obviates the need for co-regressors controlling for whole volume (see Methods). We performed a multiple regression analysis controlling for age and sex by including these variables as co-regressors alongside hippocampal laterality scores. Using this approach, a significant model emerged $(F(3,29) = 3.238, P = 0.038,$ adjusted $R^2 = 0.188)$, where only StP significantly predicted right/left hippocampal laterality (StP, $\beta = 0.383, P = 0.034$; age, $\beta = 0.211, P = 0.239$; sex, $\beta = 0.285, P = 0.122$). Furthermore, we ran an additional analysis using a two-step approach in a hierarchical regression model, where step 1 included sex, age and ICV, and step 2 added StP. This analysis showed that StP explains a further 15% of the variance in right/left hippocampal laterality, over and above the initial model (step 1), with the significance of the change in F from the first to second model being $P = 0.019$ (step 1, R^2 change = 0.248; step 2, R^2 change = 0.151, StP $\beta = 0.397$). For illustrative purposes, Figure 2 shows the relationship between right/left hippocampal laterality and StP scores.

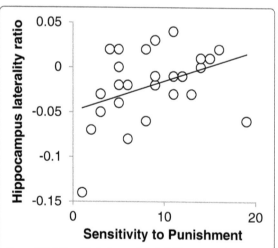

Figure 2 Relationship between right/left hippocampal laterality and StP scores. Individuals where the right hemisphere may be approaching symmetry with the left or overtaking it in terms of size have higher scores on the Sensitivity to Punishment scale suggestive of a more hyperactive Behavioural Inhibition System. Hippocampus laterality ratio = (right − left hippocampal volume)/total hippocampal volume; a zero score would reflect a perfectly symmetric hippocampus.

Sensitivity to Punishment was not significantly correlated with either left hippocampal or amygdala volumes

When we replaced the volume of the right hippocampus in the multiple regression analysis with the volume of the left hippocampus or either the left or right amygdala, again controlling for known associations of age, sex, and ICV, we found no relationship between these regions and StP (Additional file 2: Table S2).

No significant relationship between hippocampal volume and other anxiety constructs

Although our focus was on the animal literature-based behavioural inhibition approach to anxiety conceptualised by Gray, and implemented through the StP instrument of Torrubia and colleagues [16], we also examined whether the relationship observed between right hippocampal volume and StP was specific to the BIS construct of anxiety, or whether a similar relationship existed for other constructs of anxiety. Using the same regressions performed for the StP scores, we asked to what extent hippocampal volume could be predicted by two additional and well-established anxiety constructs, STAI-T and BAI. One multiple regression analysis was run with STAI-T and a second multiple regression analysis with BAI (both controlling for age, sex, and ICV). These revealed that neither STAI-T nor BAI predicted either right or left hippocampal volumes (right hippocampus: STAI-T, $\beta = 0.215, P = 0.205$; BAI, $\beta = 0.114, P = 0.580$; left hippocampus: STAI-T, $\beta = 0.199, P = 0.172$; BAI, $\beta = −0.0110 P = 0.953$; for the other relationships see Additional file 3: Table S3). To gain some idea of the overlap and specificity of these measures, we tested for correlations among the three different anxiety measures (StP, STAI-T, BAI) and the BDI (Table 3). We note that, firstly, STAI-T scores were, but StP and BAI scores were not, significantly correlated with depression scores and, secondly, that StP scores were significantly correlated with STAI-T scores, but not with BAI scores.

Discussion

In this study we examined whether a relationship exists between hippocampal volume and behavioural inhibition, as measured by the StP scale. We found that high scores on the StP scale were positively associated with hippocampal

Table 3 Correlations between self-report inventories of depression and anxiety

Measure	BDI	BAI	STAI-T
Beck Depression Inventory (BDI)	-		
Beck Anxiety Inventory (BAI)	0.266	-	
Trait anxiety of the State and Trait Anxiety Inventory (STAI-T)	0.490**	0.446*	-
Sensitivity to Punishment	0.306	0.341	0.536**

Spearman's rho (n = 30) two-tailed; **P < 0.01, *P < 0.05.

volume, when controlling for both sex, age and ICV, and that this phenomenon was lateralized to the right side.

The Behavioural Inhibition System, anxiety, and the hippocampus

Our findings contribute to a growing body of work showing that the hippocampus plays a critical role in anxiety-related behaviour as part of the BIS [6]. Including our own, there are now three studies that show a positive relationship between hippocampal volume and BIS activity in non-clinical populations [21,22]. These results lend support to Gray's theory of the neurobiological basis of anxiety [4]. However, although motivated by pre-existing theory, such correlational findings cannot directly suggest whether such anatomical variations precede or follow from the behavioural, cognitive and affective effects of BIS related activity. Indeed, it seems possible that both genetic and experiential factors as well as their interactions may contribute to the observed association. Genetic factors are very likely to be important. For instance, while both hippocampal and amygdalar activity (as measured by positron emission tomography imaging) predicted behavioural inhibition in a study on monkeys, only hippocampal activity was found to be heritable [20]. Although gray matter volume in the hippocampus is not as strongly genetically determined as it is in regions such as the lateral prefrontal cortex, its heritability still appears to be moderate to high, at 40 to 69% [49].

That experiential factors are important is suggested by human longitudinal structural neuroimaging studies, which show that repeated activation of a brain region, either whilst learning new skills [50-52] or through transcranial magnetic stimulation [53], can lead to an increase in the corresponding region's gray matter volume. Thus, it is plausible that the increased gray matter volume we observed in the right hippocampus may reflect an increase in activity of this region, associated with higher levels of BIS-based anxiety. Further, the positive relationship between BIS activity and hippocampal volume observed in this study and by others complements neuroimaging studies that have found that BIS-related measures are associated with greater activation of the hippocampus to aversive stimuli [54,55]. Moreover, consistent with the right-side relationship between BIS and hippocampal volume we found in this study, Mathews and colleagues [54] found that enhanced activation by fear-related versus neutral pictures was more pronounced in those individuals with high BIS scores specifically in the right hippocampus.

Interestingly, the correlation we and others report regarding BIS and hippocampal volume is a positive correlation. A classic problem of investigating anxiety in clinical populations is that it is often associated with depression. Estimates reported in Van Tol and colleagues [56] indicate that the comorbidity of anxiety disorders and depression ranges from 10% to over 50%, and have shown that major depressive episodes are associated with a significantly smaller gray matter volume of both the hippocampus and amygdala. Notably, other pathologies, such as seen in psychopathy [57] and schizophrenia [58], are often associated with smaller hippocampi. Since anxiety may often precede depression [59], it remains possible that smaller hippocampal and amygdalar volumes primarily occur after depression sets in. Some studies have shown reduced hippocampal volume in post-traumatic stress disorder (PTSD) [60,61]. PTSD is associated with high levels of trauma and stress, both of which are known to increase levels of corticosteroids [62,63] which in turn reduce both amygdalar [64] and hippocampal volumes [65,66]. Some researchers [67] have argued that trauma, rather than anxiety or PTSD *per se*, is associated with smaller gray matter volume, supported by their study of severe burn victims without PTSD who had significantly smaller hippocampal volumes than patients with no experience of trauma [67]. Notably, StP, unlike STAI-T, was not significantly correlated with depression scores on the BDI in our sample.

In all, this suggests that different aspects of anxiety may have dissociable and potentially opposing relationships with hippocampal volume. Our observation of increased hippocampal volume in BIS anxiety may have been facilitated by our relatively restricted sample - young, well-educated people who had not experienced many negative and stressful life events. Although it was not the main focus of our study, we note that STAI-T measure and anxiety measured by BAI were not significantly positively correlated with hippocampal volume while the BIS anxiety measure was. We caution against prematurely interpreting this as a dissociation, but this would be consistent with the view that different anxiety scales measure somewhat different forms of anxiety or negative emotionality, with potentially distinct neurobiological bases, and that a multidimensional rather than unitary approach to anxiety is appropriate. For instance, it has been suggested that the STAI-T measure may predict depression and negative affect as much as, or even more than, anxiety *per se* [36,37]. Consistent with this we also found that the STAI-T measure was highly positively correlated with BDI.

Brain laterality effects and the Behavioural Inhibition System

Our findings suggest that aspects of anxiety associated with the BIS may be lateralized to the right hemisphere, and/or depend on the relative asymmetry of the left and right hippocampus. Interestingly, a number of studies of individuals with severe psychiatric disorders have found that asymmetry of the hippocampus is normative, whilst symmetry is not [68-70]. In our sample, we found overall that the left hippocampus was larger than the right; hence, our hippocampal laterality ratio indicates that participants where the right hemisphere may be approaching symmetry with the left or overtaking it in terms of size may have a more hyperactive BIS. Consistent with this, some researchers have suggested that some aspects of anxiety may be lateralized to the right hemisphere [71-73], and heightened right hemisphere activity [74], and structural changes [75] in general has been reported for clinical anxiety populations.

The Behavioural Inhibition System and the amygdala

Three studies, including ours, that could have observed a relationship between amygdala volume and BIS activity did not find any such relationship [21,23]. To our knowledge, one study to date, Barros-Loscertales and colleagues [22], has found a positive relationship between amygdala volume and StP scores (using VBM analysis). We have no obvious explanation for these differences, but note that we, like Barros-Loscertales and colleagues [22], did observe a positive correlation between StP scores and hippocampal volume. Whether this implies that the association between the BIS and hippocampal volume is more reliable (and perhaps more heritable) than that between the BIS and amygdala remains speculative at this point, and deserving of study. Further studies would be required to investigate if there is a difference between hippocampal and amygdalar volume relationships to StP, as would be consistent with the view of Gray and McNaughton [5] that they contribute differently to anxiety. Briefly, for instance, these authors posit that the hippocampus plays a greater role in behavioural inhibition and risk assessment aspects of anxiety, while the amygdala plays a greater role in increased arousal and active avoidance. It must be noted that our sample was relatively small (n = 30). Importantly, then, we cannot rule out the possibility that a larger number of participants might have revealed an association between StP scores and amygdala volumes. Because of this, we would caution against interpreting our findings as positive evidence of the lack of an association between amygdala volume and StP.

Limitations of study

It is worth noting that a limitation of our study was our relatively small sample size, which was also restricted to young, well-educated people, which might limit the generalisability of the results. Therefore, replication of our results using larger samples is necessary. Our focus was on Gray's conception of anxiety, based originally on the role of the hippocampus in behavioural inhibition as seen in the animal literature, including the highly replicable observation that anxiolytic drugs reliably disrupt not only behavioural inhibition but also hippocampal theta. Notably, we have recently extended this observation to freely-moving animals [14]. Thus, our focus was on StP,

an instrument designed specifically to assess Gray's construct of behavioural inhibition. We compared results using StP to two other standard measures of anxiety (STAI-T and BAI) for illustrative purposes, but did not perform a correction for multiple comparisons. In our sample, StP scores were significantly correlated with STAI-T scores, but not BAI scores or BDI scores. We caution that these are only suggestive hints of the potential selectivity of the StP measure and its positive correlation with hippocampal volume. Larger studies and meta-analyses will be required to definitively disentangle shared and separate contributions to anxiety, and to incorporate any direct and secondary effects relating to stress and depression.

Larger studies should also examine the possibility that there may be interactions between sex and other variables, which our study is underpowered to detect. For instance, it remains a possibility that associations between hippocampal volume measures and StP vary between sexes, and/or that these associations are related to age. Our results clearly point to an association between right hippocampal volume and StP in our sample. However, our limited methodology did not allow us to test whether a larger absolute volume of the right hippocampus is most predictive of StP scores, or rather, a relatively large right hippocampus with respect to the left hippocampus, conceivably reflecting a tendency away from left hemispheric dominance towards right hemispheric dominance which has previously been associated with measures of Gray's BIS [24,25,30].

Conclusions

We investigated the relationship between participants' self-report of behavioural inhibition and the volume of two brain regions, the hippocampus and amygdala, previously linked to anxiety in research in rodents, non-human primates and humans. Behavioural inhibition was measured by the StP scale designed to implement Gray's construct of anxiety. Brain volume was measured by structural MRI using FreeSurfer's automatic segmentation method to obtain gray matter volume estimates of the hippocampus and amygdala. Results revealed a positive association between behavioural inhibition and right hippocampal volume. These findings suggest that structural variation or change affecting hippocampal volume, and the relative size of left and right hippocampi in particular, may reflect a predisposition to, or play a part in mediating BIS-related anxiety, and support the idea that morphological differences in the hippocampal formation may reflect a risk factor for developing anxiety.

Endnote

[a]One participant was scanned using a different protocol with 1.0 × 1.0 mm in-plane resolution, repetition time = 8.06 ms; echo time = 3 ms; inversion time = 600 ms; flip angle = 12°.

Additional files

Additional file 1: Table S1. Correlations of psychometric measures with age.

Additional file 2: Table S2. Multiple regression to examine the relationship between left hippocampal volume and StP, and the left and right amygdala volumes and StP.

Additional file 3: Table S3. Multiple regression to examine the relationship between right and left hippocampal volumes and anxiety as measured by STAI-T and BAI.

Abbreviations

BAI: Beck Anxiety Inventory; BDI: Beck Depression Inventory; BIS: Behavioural Inhibition System; EEG: electroencephalography; ICV: intracranial volume; IQ: intelligence quotient; LES: Life Experiences Survey; MRI: magnetic resonance imaging; PTSD: post-traumatic stress disorder; STAI-T: Trait anxiety of the State and Trait Anxiety Inventory; StP: Sensitivity to Punishment; VBM: voxel-based morphometry.

Competing interests

The authors declare that they have no competing interests.

Authors' contributions

LL, TH and CL designed the study and performed the statistical analysis, and were involved in the writing of the manuscript. CB made a significant contribution to the laterality analysis and first draft. CB, AH, ES and EP collected the data, contributed to the initial data analysis and to the first draft of the paper. LL wrote the first draft of the manuscript. All authors read and approved the final manuscript.

Acknowledgments

The research was funded by a BBSRC (BB/G01342X/2) grant to CL. We would also like to thank the York Neuroimaging Centre for help and assistance while conducting the study.

Author details

[1]Present address: Department of Psychology, University of Sheffield, Western Bank, Sheffield S10 2TN, UK. [2]Department of Psychology, University of York, York YO10 5DD, UK. [3]Department of Psychiatry, University of Edinburgh, Edinburgh EH10 5HF, UK. [4]Department of Psychology, University of Durham, Durham DH1 3LE, UK.

References

1. Lang PJ: **Fear reduction and fear behavior: problems in treating a construct.** In *Research in psychotherapy.* Edited by Lang PJ, Shlien JM. Washington, DC, US: American Psychological Association; 1968:90–102. vii, 615 pp.
2. Risbrough V: **Behavioral correlates of anxiety.** *Curr Top Behav Neurosci* 2010, **2:**205–228.
3. Turner SM, Michelson L: **Conceptual, methodological, and clinical issues in the assessment of anxiety disorders.** *J Behav Assess* 1984, **6:**265–279.
4. Gray JA: **The neuropsychology of anxiety - an inquiry into the functions of the septo-hippocampal system.** *Behav Brain Sci* 1982, **5:**469–484.
5. Gray JA, McNaughton N: *The Neuropsychology of Anxiety: an Enquiry into the Function of the Septo-Hippocampal System.* 2nd edition. Oxford: Oxford University Press; 2000.
6. McNaughton N, Corr PJ: **A two-dimensional neuropsychology of defense: fear/anxiety and defensive distance.** *Neurosci Biobehav Rev* 2004, **28:**285–305.
7. Adhikari A, Topiwala MA, Gordon JA: **Single units in the medial prefrontal cortex with anxiety-related firing patterns are preferentially influenced by ventral hippocampal activity.** *Neuron* 2011, **71:**898–910.
8. Adhikari A, Topiwala MA, Gordon JA: **Synchronized activity between the ventral hippocampus and the medial prefrontal cortex during anxiety.** *Neuron* 2010, **65:**257–269.
9. Engin E, Stellbrink J, Treit D, Dickson CT: **Anxiolytic and antidepressant effects of intracerebroventricularly administered somatostatin: behavioral and neurophysiological evidence.** *Neuroscience* 2008, **157:**666–676.
10. Cornwell BR, Arkin N, Overstreet C, Carver FW, Grillon C: **Distinct contributions of human hippocampal theta to spatial cognition and anxiety.** *Hippocampus* 2012, **22:**1848–1859.
11. McNaughton N, Kocsis B, Hajos M: **Elicited hippocampal theta rhythm: a screen for anxiolytic and procognitive drugs through changes in hippocampal function?** *Behav Pharmacol* 2007, **18:**329–346.
12. Seidenbecher T, Laxmi TR, Stork O, Pape HC: **Amygdalar and hippocampal theta rhythm synchronization during fear memory retrieval.** *Science* 2003, **301:**846–850.
13. Yeung M, Treit D, Dickson CT: **A critical test of the hippocampal theta model of anxiolytic drug action.** *Neuropharmacology* 2012, **62:**155–160.
14. Wells CE, Amos DP, Jeewajee A, Douchamps V, Rodgers RJ, O'Keefe J, Burgess N, Lever C: **Novelty and anxiolytic drugs dissociate two components of hippocampal theta in behaving rats.** *J Neurosci* 2013, **33:**8650–8667.
15. Carver CS, White TL: **Behavioral-inhibition, behavioral activation, and affective responses to impending reward and punishment - the BIS BAS Scales.** *J Pers Soc Psychol* 1994, **67:**319–333.
16. Torrubia R, Avila C, Molto J, Caseras X: **The Sensitivity to Punishment and Sensitivity to Reward Questionnaire (SPSRQ) as a measure of Gray's anxiety and impulsivity dimensions.** *Pers Indiv Differ* 2001, **31:**837–862.
17. Vervoort L, Wolters LH, Hogendoorn SM, de Haan E, Boer F, Prins PJM: **Sensitivity of Gray's Behavioral Inhibition System in clinically anxious and non-anxious children and adolescents.** *Pers Indiv Differ* 2010, **48:**629–633.
18. Maack DJ, Tull MT, Gratz KL: **Examining the incremental contribution of behavioral inhibition to generalized anxiety disorder relative to other Axis I disorders and cognitive-emotional vulnerabilities.** *J Anxiety Disord* 2012, **26:**689–695.
19. Hahn T, Dresler T, Plichta MM, Ehlis AC, Ernst LH, Markulin F, Polak T, Blaimer M, Deckert J, Lesch KP, Jakob PM, Fallgatter AJ: **Functional amygdala-hippocampus connectivity during anticipation of aversive events is associated with Gray's trait "Sensitivity to Punishment".** *Biol Psychiatry* 2010, **68:**459–464.
20. Oler JA, Fox AS, Shelton SE, Rogers J, Dyer TD, Davidson RJ, Shelledy W, Oakes TR, Blangero J, Kalin NH: **Amygdalar and hippocampal substrates of anxious temperament differ in their heritability.** *Nature* 2010, **466:**864–868.
21. Cherbuin N, Windsor TD, Anstey KJ, Maller JJ, Meslin C, Sachdev PS: **Hippocampal volume is positively associated with behavioural inhibition (BIS) in a large community-based sample of mid-life adults: the PATH through life study.** *Soc Cogn Affect Neurosci* 2008, **3:**262–269.
22. Barros-Loscertales A, Meseguer V, Sanjuan A, Belloch V, Parcet MA, Torrubia R, Avila C: **Behavioral Inhibition System activity is associated with increased amygdala and hippocampal gray matter volume: a voxel-based morphometry study.** *Neuroimage* 2006, **33:**1011–1015.
23. Fuentes P, Barros-Loscertales A, Bustamante JC, Rosell P, Costumero V, Avila C: **Individual differences in the Behavioral Inhibition System are associated with orbitofrontal cortex and precuneus gray matter volume.** *Cogn Affect Behav Neurosci* 2012, **12:**491–498.
24. Sutton SK, Davidson RJ: **Prefrontal brain asymmetry: a biological substrate of the behavioral approach and inhibition systems.** *Psychol Sci* 1997, **8:**204–210.
25. Shackman AJ, McMenamin BW, Maxwell JS, Greischar LL, Davidson RJ: **Right dorsolateral prefrontal cortical activity and behavioral inhibition.** *Psychol Sci* 2009, **20:**1500–1506.
26. Davidson RJ, Saron CD, Senulis JA, Ekman P, Friesen WV: **Approach withdrawal and cerebral asymmetry - emotional expression and brain physiology. 1.** *J Pers Soc Psychol* 1990, **58:**330–341.
27. Davidson RJ: **Cerebral asymmetry, emotion and affective style.** *J Clin Exp Neuropsychol* 1990, **12:**62–62.
28. Nitschke JB, Heller W, Palmieri PA, Miller GA: **Contrasting patterns of brain activity in anxious apprehension and anxious arousal.** *Psychophysiology* 1999, **36:**628–637.
29. Blackhart GC, Minnix JA, Kline JP: **Can EEG asymmetry patterns predict future development of anxiety and depression? A preliminary study.** *Biol Psychol* 2006, **72:**46–50.
30. Wright L, Hardie SM, Wilson K: **Handedness and behavioural inhibition: left-handed females show most inhibition as measured by BIS/BAS self-report.** *Pers Indiv Differ* 2009, **46:**20–24.

31. Beck AT, Steer RA, Ball R, Ranieri W: Comparison of Beck Depression Inventories-IA and -II in psychiatric outpatients. *J Pers Assess* 1996, **67**:588–597.

32. Sarason IG, Johnson JH, Siegel JM: Assessing the impact of life changes: development of the Life Experiences Survey. *J Consult Clin Psychol* 1978, **46**:932–946.

33. Spielberger CD: *State–Trait Anxiety Inventory: a Comprehensive Bibliography.* Palo Alto, CA: Consulting Psychologists Press; 1989.

34. Beck AT, Brown G, Epstein N, Steer RA: An inventory for measuring clinical anxiety - psychometric properties. *J Consult Clin Psychol* 1988, **56**:893–897.

35. Leyfer OT, Ruberg JL, Woodruff-Borden J: Examination of the utility of the Beck Anxiety Inventory and its factors as a screener for anxiety disorders. *J Anxiety Disord* 2006, **20**:444–458.

36. Gros DF, Antony MM, Simms LJ, McCabe RE: Psychometric properties of the State-Trait Inventory for Cognitive and Somatic Anxiety (STICSA): comparison to the State-Trait Anxiety Inventory (STAI). *Psychol Assess* 2007, **19**:369–381.

37. Bados A, Gomez-Benito J, Balaguer G: The state-trait anxiety inventory, trait version: does it really measure anxiety? *J Pers Assess* 2010, **92**:560–567.

38. Torrubia R, Tobena A: A scale for the assessment of susceptibility to punishment as a measure of anxiety - preliminary-results. *Pers Indiv Differ* 1984, **5**:371–375.

39. Spielberger CD: *State-Trait Anxiety Inventory for Adults.* Palo Alto, CA: Mind Garden; 1983.

40. Spielberger CD, Gorsuch RL, Lushene R, Vagg PR, Jacobs GA: *Manual for the State-Trait Anxiety Inventory.* Palo Alto, CA: Consulting Psychologists Press; 1983.

41. Wechsler D: *Manual for the Wechsler Adult Intelligence Scale-Third Edition.* San Antonio, TX: The Psychological Cooperation; 1997.

42. Rao U, Chen LA, Bidesi AS, Shad MU, Thomas MA, Hammen CL: Hippocampal changes associated with early-life adversity and vulnerability to depression. *Biol Psychiatry* 2010, **67**:357–364.

43. Campbell S, Macqueen G: The role of the hippocampus in the pathophysiology of major depression. *J Psychiatry Neurosci* 2004, **29**:417–426.

44. Reuter M, Schmansky NJ, Rosas HD, Fischl B: Within-subject template estimation for unbiased longitudinal image analysis. *Neuroimage* 2012, **61**(4):1402–1418.

45. Duvernoy HM: *The Human Brain: Surface, Three-dimensional Sectional Anatomy and MRI.* New York: Springer-Verlag; 1991.

46. Fischl B, Salat DH, Busa E, Albert M, Dieterich M, Haselgrove C, van der Kouwe A, Killiany R, Kennedy D, Klaveness S, Montillo A, Makris N, Rosen B, Dale AM: Whole brain segmentation: automated labeling of neuroanatomical structures in the human brain. *Neuron* 2002, **33**:341–355.

47. Li W, van Tol MJ, Li M, Miao W, Jiao Y, Heinze HJ, Bogerts B, He H, Walter M: Regional specificity of sex effects on subcortical volumes across the lifespan in healthy aging. *Hum Brain Mapp* 2012. Published online ahead of print.

48. Barnes J, Ridgway GR, Bartlett J, Henley SM, Lehmann M, Hobbs N, Clarkson MJ, MacManus DG, Ourselin S, Fox NC: Head size, age and gender adjustment in MRI studies: a necessary nuisance? *Neuroimage* 2010, **53**:1244–1255.

49. Peper JS, Brouwer RM, Boomsma DI, Kahn RS, Hulshoff Pol HE: Genetic influences on human brain structure: a review of brain imaging studies in twins. *Hum Brain Mapp* 2007, **28**:464–473.

50. Woollett K, Maguire EA: Acquiring "the Knowledge" of London's layout drives structural brain changes. *Curr Biol* 2011, **21**:2109–2114.

51. Bangert M, Peschel T, Schlaug G, Rotte M, Drescher D, Hinrichs H, Heinze HJ, Altenmuller E: Shared networks for auditory and motor processing in professional pianists: evidence from fMRI conjunction. *Neuroimage* 2006, **30**:917–926.

52. Taubert M, Villringer A, Ragert P: Learning-related gray and white matter changes in humans: an update. *Neuroscientist* 2012, **18**:320–325.

53. May A, Hajak G, Ganssbauer S, Steffens T, Langguth B, Kleinjung T, Eichhammer P: Structural brain alterations following 5 days of intervention: dynamic aspects of neuroplasticity. *Cereb Cortex* 2007, **17**:205–210.

54. Mathews A, Yiend J, Lawrence AD: Individual differences in the modulation of fear-related brain activation by attentional control. *J Cogn Neurosci* 2004, **16**:1683–1694.

55. Cools R, Calder AJ, Lawrence AD, Clark L, Bullmore E, Robbins TW: Individual differences in threat sensitivity predict serotonergic modulation of amygdala response to fearful faces. *Psychopharmacology (Berl)* 2005, **180**:670–679.

56. van Tol MJ, van der Wee NJ, van den Heuvel OA, Nielen MM, Demenescu LR, Aleman A, Renken R, van Buchem MA, Zitman FG, Veltman DJ: Regional brain volume in depression and anxiety disorders. *Arch Gen Psychiatry* 2010, **67**:1002–1011.

57. Ermer E, Cope LM, Nyalakanti PK, Calhoun VD, Kiehl KA: Aberrant paralimbic gray matter in criminal psychopathy. *J Abnorm Psychol* 2012, **121**:649–658.

58. Nelson MD, Saykin AJ, Flashman LA, Riordan HJ: Hippocampal volume reduction in schizophrenia as assessed by magnetic resonance imaging: a meta-analytic study. *Arch Gen Psychiatry* 1998, **55**:433–440.

59. Bishop SJ: Neurocognitive mechanisms of anxiety: an integrative account. *Trends Cogn Sci* 2007, **11**:307–316.

60. Pavic L, Gregurek R, Rados M, Brkljacic B, Brajkovic L, Simetin-Pavic I, Ivanac G, Pavlisa G, Kalousek V: Smaller right hippocampus in war veterans with posttraumatic stress disorder. *Psychiatry Res* 2007, **154**:191–198.

61. Smith ME: Bilateral hippocampal volume reduction in adults with post-traumatic stress disorder: a meta-analysis of structural MRI studies. *Hippocampus* 2005, **15**:798–807.

62. Eriksson PS, Perfilieva E, Bjork-Eriksson T, Alborn AM, Nordborg C, Peterson DA, Gage FH: Neurogenesis in the adult human hippocampus. *Nat Med* 1998, **4**:1313–1317.

63. Lupien SJ, McEwen BS, Gunnar MR, Heim C: Effects of stress throughout the lifespan on the brain, behaviour and cognition. *Nat Rev Neurosci* 2009, **10**:434–445.

64. Brown ES, Woolston DJ, Frol AB: Amygdala volume in patients receiving chronic corticosteroid therapy. *Biol Psychiatry* 2008, **63**:705–709.

65. McEwen BS: Effects of adverse experiences for brain structure and function. *Biol Psychiatry* 2000, **48**:721–731.

66. Brown ES, J Woolston D, Frol A, Bobadilla L, Khan DA, Hanczyc M, Rush AJ, Fleckenstein J, Babcock E, Cullum CM: Hippocampal volume, spectroscopy, cognition, and mood in patients receiving corticosteroid therapy. *Biol Psychiatry* 2004, **55**:538–545.

67. Winter H, Irle E: Hippocampal volume in adult burn patients with and without posttraumatic stress disorder. *Am J Psychiatry* 2004, **161**:2194–2200.

68. Zaidel DW: Regional differentiation of neuron morphology in human left and right hippocampus: comparing normal to schizophrenia. *Int J Psychophysiol* 1999, **34**:187–196.

69. Sapolsky RM: Glucocorticoids and hippocampal atrophy in neuropsychiatric disorders. *Arch Gen Psychiatry* 2000, **57**:925–935.

70. Qiu AQ, Wang L, Younes L, Harms MP, Ratnanather JT, Miller MI, Csernansky JG: Neuroanatomical asymmetry patterns in individuals with schizophrenia and their non-psychotic siblings. *Neuroimage* 2009, **47**:1221–1229.

71. Wager TD, Phan KL, Liberzon I, Taylor SF: Valence, gender, and lateralization of functional brain anatomy in emotion: a meta-analysis of findings from neuroimaging. *Neuroimage* 2003, **19**:513–531.

72. Heller W, Nitschke JB: The puzzle of regional brain activity in depression and anxiety: the importance of subtypes and comorbidity. *Cogn Emotion* 1998, **12**:421–447.

73. Mogg K, Bradley BP: Selective orienting of attention to masked threat faces in social anxiety. *Behav Res Ther* 2002, **40**:1403–1414.

74. Reiman EM, Raichle ME, Butler FK, Herscovitch P, Robins E: A focal brain abnormality in panic disorder, a severe form of anxiety. *Nature* 1984, **310**:683–685.

75. Brambilla P, Como G, Isola M, Taboga F, Zuliani R, Goljevscek S, Ragogna M, Brondani G, Baiano M, Perini L, Ferro A, Bazzocchi M, Zuiani C, Balestrieri M: White-matter abnormalities in the right posterior hemisphere in generalized anxiety disorder: a diffusion imaging study. *Psychol Med* 2011, **42**:427–434.

Individual differences in cognitive reappraisal usage modulate the time course of brain activation during symptom provocation in specific phobia

Andrea Hermann[1,2*], Verena Leutgeb[3], Wilfried Scharmüller[3], Dieter Vaitl[2], Anne Schienle[3] and Rudolf Stark[1,2]

Abstract

Background: Extinction learning is proposed to be one key mechanism of action underlying exposure-based cognitive-behavioral therapy (CBT) in specific phobia. Beyond that, cognitive reappraisal, one important strategy to regulate negative emotions, is a crucial component of CBT interventions, but has been disregarded in previous studies investigating neural change processes in specific phobia. The aim of this study was to investigate the association of individual differences in habitual/dispositional cognitive reappraisal usage and the time course of brain activation during phobic stimulation in specific phobia.

Methods: Dental phobic patients and healthy control subjects participated in a functional magnetic resonance imaging (fMRI) study whilst being confronted with phobic, disgust, fear and neutral pictures. Individual differences in cognitive reappraisal usage were assessed via a self-report questionnaire and correlated with activation decreases over the course of time.

Results: Phobic individuals with higher dispositional cognitive reappraisal scores showed a more pronounced activation decline in the right dorsomedial prefrontal cortex (dmPFC) which might be associated with a diminution of explicit cognitive emotion regulation over the course of time. Less decrease of activation in the right ventromedial prefrontal cortex (vmPFC) and the lateral orbitofrontal cortex (lOFC) over time in subjects with higher cognitive reappraisal scores might be related to a stronger automatic regulation of emotions or even emotional relearning. Additionally, phobic subjects compared with healthy controls showed a stronger habituation of the left dmPFC over the course of symptom provocation.

Conclusions: The results of this study show for the first time that individual differences in cognitive reappraisal usage are associated with the time course of brain activation during symptom provocation in specific phobia. Additionally, the present study gives first indications for the importance of considering individual differences in cognitive reappraisal usage in the treatment of specific phobia.

Keywords: Specific phobia, Emotion regulation, Cognitive reappraisal, vmPFC, Insula, Habituation, Extinction, fMRI, CBT

* Correspondence: andrea.hermann@psychol.uni-giessen.de
[1]Department of Psychotherapy and Systems Neuroscience, Bender Institute of Neuroimaging, Justus Liebig University, Otto-Behaghel-Strasse 10H, Giessen 35394, Germany
[2]Bender Institute of Neuroimaging, Justus Liebig University, Giessen, Germany
Full list of author information is available at the end of the article

Background

Dental phobia - one form of specific phobia - is characterized by an excessive fear in response to and a strong avoidance of phobic situations [1] as for instance dental treatment. Regarding the development of dental phobia, individuals with high levels of dental anxiety report distressing dental experiences up to 18 times more often than low-anxious individuals [2,3]. Classical conditioning is considered as one important mechanism underlying the development of phobic fear in response to distressing events [4,5]. Thereby, a former neutral stimulus (e.g. dentist) acquires a negative affective value by being paired with an unconditioned stimulus (e.g. pain during dental treatment) that elicits an unconditioned response (e.g. fear response). Subsequently, the former neutral stimulus (conditioned stimulus) elicits a conditioned response (e.g. fear) that is similar to the unconditioned response, without being paired with the unconditioned stimulus again. Numerous studies have been conducted in recent years trying to elucidate the neural mechanisms underlying the acquisition of fear in healthy individuals as well as the neural basis underlying phobic fear responses (for an overview see [6]). Supporting a learning theory-based perspective on specific phobia, fear conditioning in healthy subjects and symptom provocation in specific phobia seem to be characterized by similar neural correlates including enhanced amygdala, insula, and dorsal anterior cingulate cortex (dACC) activation (for an overview see [6]). In dental phobia, activation has also been found in basal ganglia and prefrontal cortex regions [7,8].

Based on learning theory, the extinction of conditioned responses is supposed to be the central process underlying exposure based treatments in anxiety disorders as for instance specific phobia [9]. Extinction is defined as the repeated confrontation with a conditioned stimulus without subsequent presentation of the unconditioned stimulus, leading to a reduction of conditioned responding over time. Especially the ventromedial prefrontal cortex (vmPFC) has been emphasized as a key structure underlying extinction learning and retrieval (for an overview see [10]). Correspondingly, reduced vmPFC activation has been shown in patients with specific phobias during symptom provocation [11-13]. Studies investigating the effects of cognitive-behavioral therapy (CBT) on neural correlates of symptom provocation in spider phobia indicate reduced activation of the insula and the dACC [14] as well as increased activation of the vmPFC [13] as a result of successful CBT. All in all, these findings demonstrate that fear acquisition and symptom provocation as well as fear extinction and symptom modification via CBT are characterized by similar neural circuits.

Despite the vast literature on the neural correlates of symptom provocation in specific phobia and the few studies on the effects of CBT on these neural correlates, little is known about the mechanisms of action (e.g. habituation, extinction) underlying such processes of change in phobic patients. There is one H2 15O-positron emission tomography study showing habituation of several brain regions including the amygdala and the insula during prolonged exposure to phobic compared with non-phobic stimuli in spider phobic subjects [15]. These results give first evidence for the neural basis underlying habituation or extinction processes in specific phobia. Generally, it has been claimed that fear extinction in humans comprises more than mere passive learning, namely cognitive processes [16], which might additionally influence conditioned responding during extinction. In line with this, cognitive interventions are important components of CBT [17]. Moreover, it has been shown that adding guided threat reappraisal to exposure treatment in specific phobia led to enhanced between-trial habituation [18] as well as decreased return of fear [19].

Cognitive reappraisal is one prominent form of cognitive emotion regulation defined as reinterpreting a stimulus or situation in a way that reduces its emotional impact [20]. Several functional magnetic resonance imaging (fMRI) studies investigating the neural basis of emotion regulation via cognitive reappraisal found enhanced activation of lateral and medial prefrontal cortical control regions accompanied by reduced activation of emotional arousal-related brain structures like the amygdala and the insula during (successful) emotion regulation (for an overview see [21]). One of our own studies investigated cognitive reappraisal of phobic compared with general aversive stimuli in specific phobia [12]. Results of this study show that cognitive down-regulation of emotional responses to phobic pictures led to reduced activation of insula and dACC compared with just looking at the pictures. In addition, down-regulation of phobic compared with general aversive emotional responses was associated with an increased regulation effort and diminished activation of the right rostral ACC (rACC) and the dorsomedial PFC (dmPFC), regions crucially involved in the cognitive regulation of emotions [21]. Altogether, these results indicate that patients with specific phobia exhibit a phobia-specific regulation deficit reflected in a dysfunctional recruitment of rACC and dmPFC.

Beyond that, previous research has shown that individuals vary in their habitual use of cognitive reappraisal (dispositional cognitive reappraisal) as a strategy to regulate emotions. This individual tendency has been shown to be stable in time [20]. A more frequent use of cognitive reappraisal has been related to better interpersonal functioning, enhanced psychological well-being, and reduced depressive symptoms [20]. On the neurobiological level, dispositional cognitive reappraisal has been found to be correlated with reduced insula activation during the anticipation of negative affective stimuli [22], with reduced amygdala and stronger dACC responses while viewing negative emotional faces [23], and with stronger dACC and dorsolateral prefrontal cortex (dlPFC) responses during response inhibition towards negative emotional material (sad vs. happy faces; [24]). Moreover, studies investigating brain structural correlates found an association of dispositional cognitive reappraisal with dACC [25] and vmPFC [26] gray matter volumes. In sum, these numerous findings regarding individual differences in cognitive reappraisal usage indicate a pivotal role of this factor in the modulation of emotional responses.

Despite generally large effect sizes of exposure-based treatments in specific phobia [27], one challenging future task is to figure out possible factors contributing to individual differences in treatment response and return of fear at follow-up. Considering the abovementioned correlates of dispositional cognitive reappraisal, this factor might be a promising candidate for modulating treatment responses in specific phobia. Individuals might differ in the extent they use cognitive reappraisal to regulate their emotions during an exposure session. This might moreover result in different outcomes of exposure therapy at the end of treatment or at follow-up. Previous results on mechanisms of change in CBT have shown that the 'performance' during exposure (e.g. rate of habituation, initial fear responding) is not a good predictor for final therapy success [28]. Furthermore, Craske and colleagues assume that the toleration of fear during exposure is far more important to exposure therapy than the reduction of fear. This general ability to manage ones own emotions is also represented in the strategy of cognitive reappraisal. However, until now there are no studies investigating the influence of individual differences in cognitive reappraisal usage on the neural correlates of extinction-related processes in anxiety disorders, as for instance specific phobia. Because it is difficult to conduct typical exposure therapy during scanning, one first approximation is to investigate the time course of brain activation during symptom provocation. The repeated presentation of phobic stimuli without negative consequences (e.g. pain) might be a plausible equivalent to emotional relearning/extinction learning, habituation as well as to a first exposure session in the treatment of specific phobias.

Hence, we investigated a sample of 27 dental phobic patients and 21 healthy control subjects who underwent fMRI during symptom provocation with phobia-specific, generally disgust and fear inducing as well as affectively neutral pictures. The aim of the study was to identify brain structures showing differential activation over time for phobic compared with neutral stimuli depending on the extent of habitual cognitive reappraisal usage in phobic patients. The emotion regulation questionnaire (ERQ,

[20]. German version [29]) was used to measure individual differences in habitual cognitive reappraisal usage. A stronger dispositional use of cognitive reappraisal is supposed to lead to enhanced habituation or emotional relearning (e.g. extinction) because these individuals might be better at spontaneously using reappraisal during symptom provocation. This is expected to result in a stronger reduction of activation in brain regions associated with phobia specific processing (amygdala, insula, dACC, basal ganglia). In addition, extinction-related structures as for instance the vmPFC should exhibit less activation decrease over time because individuals with more pronounced habitual reappraisal use are supposed to show stronger emotional relearning respectively extinction learning. Furthermore, cortical control-related areas (rACC, dmPFC, vlPFC, dlPFC) involved in cognitive reappraisal processes are assumed to exhibit a different time course as a function of habitual cognitive reappraisal usage. It is conceivable that subjects high in cognitive reappraisal are characterized by enhanced activation in these areas over time due to sustained cognitive reappraisal of phobic stimuli during the course of symptom provocation. On the other hand, these individuals might be more effective in reducing emotional responses and therefore might show a stronger reduction of activation in these PFC structures over time because regulation might take place faster automatically rather than by explicit and effortful cognitive reappraisal processes. Additionally, we were interested in the specificity of the effects and therefore compared phobic with general affective responses (fear and disgust) as well as phobic individuals with healthy control subjects.

Methods

Subjects and procedure

Twenty-seven individuals (15 females/12 males) with dental phobia according to DSM-IV-TR [1] and 21 healthy control subjects (12 females/9 males) participated in a functional magnetic resonance imaging study (mostly overlapping with the sample from [8]). Three further subjects in the phobia group were excluded due to problems in stimulus timing. This study is part of a larger project investigating the functional and structural basis of dental phobia. The main results of this fMRI study have recently been published by [8]. The phobic participants had a mean age of 31 years (SD = 11.56 years) and the healthy controls of 29.81 years (SD = 9.13). They completed the Dental Anxiety Scale (DAS; [30] range: 4-20; cut-off: 15 for highly anxious or phobic individuals), a questionnaire assessing the experienced anxiety during dental treatment. All subjects were right-handed. The participants were recruited via announcements in local newspapers and at the university campus. All subjects gave written informed consent. The local ethics committee of the department 06 of the Justus Liebig University Giessen (Germany) approved the study procedure and the study was conducted according to the Declaration of Helsinki. Subjects received 10euro/h for participation.

In a first session, a standardized clinical interview [31] was conducted in order to make a clinical diagnosis of dental phobia and to screen for comorbid disorders in the phobia group. Exclusion criteria consisted of substance dependence (except nicotine), psychotic disorder, bipolar disorder, obsessive-compulsive disorder, posttraumatic stress disorder, major depressive disorder, blood phobia with fainting symptoms, intake of psychotropic medication, and any MRI contraindications. Six patients had a further diagnosis of another specific phobia (e.g. height phobia). For control participants exclusion criteria consisted of any diagnosis according to DSM-IV-TR.

During the second session, the subjects participated in an fMRI study, in which they were confronted with phobic, disgust, fear, and neutral pictures. The main results concerning the neural correlates of symptom provocation have been reported by [8].

The present study focused on the effects of individual differences in cognitive reappraisal usage on the neural correlates of habituation processes in dental phobics and healthy controls. For this purpose, participants completed the emotion regulation questionnaire (ERQ [20] German version [29]). This questionnaire is a 10-item measure to assess the habitual use of "cognitive reappraisal" and "expressive suppression" on a 7-point Likert scale ('1' = "strongly disagree" to '7' = "strongly agree"). One example item for the cognitive reappraisal scale is for instance "When I want to feel less negative emotion, I change the way I'm thinking about the situation". The mean score of the six reappraisal items was calculated for the purpose of the present study.

Experimental design

During the fMRI session, participants were presented with 120 pictures representing the four emotional categories 'Phobia', 'Fear', 'Disgust', and 'Neutral' (30 pictures in each category). The pictures were taken from the International Affective Picture System (IAPS [32]) and from two other sets [33,34]. The phobic category consisted of pictures showing dental treatment (e.g. physician holding a dental drill in his hand). Fear stimuli depicted predators and attacks by humans, whereas disgust pictures showed e.g. repulsive animals and scenes from the domain 'poor hygiene'. Neutral pictures consisted of household articles. During the experiment the pictures were randomly presented for 3 s each. The inter-stimulus intervals varied between 3 and 6 s and participants were presented with a white fixation cross on a black background. In addition, 30 null events (fixation cross) with a mean duration of 6s were presented throughout the experiment. After the experiment, subjects gave valence, arousal, fear and disgust ratings (9-point Likert scales) for each picture category block-wise.

Data acquisition and analysis

Magnetic resonance imaging was carried out with a 1.5 Tesla whole-body tomograph (Siemens Symphony with a quantum gradient system) with a standard head coil. A total of 530 volumes was registered using a T2*-weighted gradient echo-planar imaging sequence (EPI) with 30 slices covering the whole brain (slice thickness = 4 mm; 1 mm gap; descending slice order; TA = 100 ms; TE = 55 ms; TR = 3 s; flip angle = 90°; field of view = 192 mm × 192 mm; matrix size = 64 pixel × 64 pixel; 3×3×4 mm voxel size). Due to an incomplete steady state of magnetization, the first three volumes were discarded. The orientation of the axial slices was parallel to the OFC tissue - bone transition. An anatomical T1-weighted scan (3D-MPRAGE, 1.4×1×1 mm voxel, FoV: 250 mm; TI: 1,100 ms, TE: 4.18 ms, TR: 1,990 ms, flip angle: 15°) was carried out to get highly resolved structural information for the normalization procedure and a gradient echo field map sequence to get information for unwarping B_0 distortions (gre_fieldmap; 30 slices, 4 mm + 1 mm gap, in-plane: 3×3 mm, TE1: 10 ms, TE2: 14.76 ms, FoV: 192 mm, flip angle: 90°; comparable parameters to the echo-planar images).

Data analysis was done with the Statistical Parametric Mapping software (SPM8, Wellcome Department of Cognitive Neurology, London) implemented in MatLab R2007b (Mathworks Inc., Sherborn, MA). Unwarping and realignment, slice time correction, and normalization to the standard space of the Montreal Neurological Institute brain (MNI brain) were carried out. Smoothing was executed with an isotropic three dimensional Gaussian filter with a full width at half maximum (FWHM) of 9 mm. The four conditions were each modeled by one regressor and its time modulation (1st order; models increasing activation across trials) in order to investigate the time course of brain activation. All regressors were modeled by a stick function convolved with the canonical hemodynamic response function (hrf) in the general linear model. The duration was set to 3 s for each event. Furthermore, the six movement parameters of the rigid body transformation applied by the realignment procedure were introduced as covariates in the model. A high-pass filter of 128 s was applied.

The contrasts 'activation decrease (Phobia) vs. activation decrease (Neutral)', 'activation decrease (Phobia) vs. activation decrease (Fear)' and 'activation decrease (Phobia) vs. activation decrease (Disgust)' were calculated on an individual level. One-sample t-tests were calculated for the analysis of habituation effects within the phobia group for these contrasts and two-sample t-tests for comparison of the phobic and the control group for the 'activation decrease (Phobia) vs. activation decrease (Neutral)' contrast. The correlation of cognitive reappraisal and symptom severity (Dental Anxiety Scale) with neural responses (activation decrease for phobic vs. neutral pictures) and of cognitive reappraisal with activation for phobic vs. neutral pictures was tested via t-contrasts in multiple regression analyses (second-level analyses), with the reappraisal or DAS score entered as the covariate of interest. Regions of interest (ROI) were the amygdala, insula, basal ganglia (pallidum, putamen, caudate nucleus), SMA, lateral orbitofrontal cortex (lOFC), dACC, rACC, dmPFC, vmPFC, dlPFC, and vlPFC. The significance threshold was set to $\alpha = 0.05$ on voxel-level, corrected for multiple testing (family wise error (FWE) correction) in the respective search volume (ROI, whole brain) with an intensity threshold of $p = .001$ for ROI analyses. For exploratory whole brain analyses, an inclusive gray matter mask was used. ROI analyses were performed using the small volume correction option of SPM8. Amygdala and insula masks were maximum probability masks (probability threshold set to .50) taken from the current "Harvard-Oxford cortical and subcortical structural atlases" provided by the Harvard Center for Morphometric Analysis (http://www.cma.mgh.harvard.edu/), included in the FSL software package (http://www.fmrib.ox.ac.uk/fsl/). The dACC mask consisted of a 10 mm sphere surrounding a peak voxel for phobia specific neural responses in the anterior cingulate/mid-cingulate gyrus (MNI: x = 0, y = 0, z = 40) as indicated in a meta-analysis of symptom provocation studies in specific phobia [6]. The remaining masks were created by the MARINA software package [35].

Results

Questionnaire and rating data

For the cognitive reappraisal scale, the phobic patients reported a mean score of 4.75 ($SD = 0.95$; range: 2.17.-6.17) and for the Dental Anxiety Scale (DAS) a mean score of 17.37 ($SD = 2.24$; range: 11-20). There was no significant correlation of cognitive reappraisal with symptom severity as measured by the Dental Anxiety Scale in this group ($r = .10$, $p = .62$). The control group had a mean score of 4.65 on the reappraisal scale ($SD = .70$; range: 3.17-6.00) and for the DAS a mean score of 6.29 ($SD = 1.65$; range: 4-10), with no significant correlation between the reappraisal and the DAS score ($r = -.19$, $p = .41$). Additionally, there was no significant difference between the phobic group and the control group in dispositional cognitive reappraisal ($T(46) = .39$, $p = .70$).

The phobic group reported a mean score of $M = 2.40$ for valence ($SD = 1.08$), $M = 6.00$ for arousal ($SD = 2.27$),

$M = 6.15$ for fear ($SD = 1.94$) and $M = 3.89$ for disgust ratings ($SD = 2.31$) of the phobic picture category. There was no significant association of cognitive reappraisal or DAS with valence, arousal, fear and disgust ratings of the phobic stimuli in the phobic group (all $p > .2$).

The control group reported a mean score of $M = 5.63$ for valence ($SD = 1.57$), $M = 2.32$ for arousal ($SD = 1.49$), $M = 1.76$ for fear ($SD = 1.26$) and $M = 1.76$ for disgust ratings ($SD = 0.89$) of the phobic picture category. Furthermore, there was no significant association of the cognitive reappraisal score with valence, arousal, fear and disgust ratings of the phobic stimuli in the control group (all $p > .45$). The same applies for the association of the DAS score with arousal, fear and disgust ratings (all p > .14), whereas the DAS was significantly (negatively) correlated with the valence ratings of the phobic pictures in the control group ($r = -.503$, $p = .028$).

fMRI data

Activation decreases and increases

For phobic compared with neutral stimuli, several brain regions showed a decrease in activation over time in the phobic group. Especially the right middle temporal gyrus (exploratory analysis), right caudate nucleus, bilateral vmPFC, dmPFC, rACC, and left vlPFC showed a significant activation decline (see Table 1). Marginally significant responses were found for the left insula ($Z_{max} = 3.30$, $p = .069$), the left dlPFC ($Z_{max} = 3.74$, $p = .071$), and a further cluster in the right dmPFC ($Z_{max} = 3.33$, $p = .098$) and the left vlPFC ($Z_{max} = 3.57$, $p = .071$) (see Table 1). There were no activation increases for phobic compared with neutral pictures over time. Compared with the fear category, phobic patients showed a stronger activation decline during phobic stimulation in the insula (marginally significant; $Z_{max} = 3.18$, $p = .097$) and the left and (tendentially) right vlPFC ($Z_{max} = 3.57$, $p = .076$) (see Table 1). There were no stronger activation decreases for fear vs. phobic pictures. However, phobic compared with disgust pictures led to a stronger activation decrease in the right rACC, whereas less decrease for this contrast was observed in the right vmPFC (see Table 1). In order to investigate the specificity of the results we further conducted a comparison of the phobic and the healthy control group for phobic vs. neutral pictures. As the only result a (marginally significant) stronger activation decrease appeared in the left dmPFC (MNI coordinates: x = -6, y = 29, z = 40; $Z_{max} = 3.54$; $p_{fwe} = .058$) in phobic compared with control participants (see Figure 1).

Correlations with dispositional cognitive reappraisal and symptom severity

In the phobic group, dispositional cognitive reappraisal was correlated with a stronger activation decrease in the right dmPFC (marginally significant; $Z_{max} = 3.56$, $p = .052$)

Table 1 Neural activation decrease over time in the phobic group

Structure	H	x	y	z	Z_{max}	p_{fwe}
Phobia gt neutral						
Middle temporal gyrus	L	−45	14	−29	4.92	.029E
insula	L	−30	20	−8	3.30	.069[+]
caudate nucleus	R	21	−16	22	3.45	.037
dlPFC	L	−24	32	46	3.74	.071[+]
dmPFC	L	−6	29	40	4.79	.001
						.050E[+]
dmPFC	L	−3	53	7	3.99	.017
dmPFC	R	6	47	4	4.33	.004
dmPFC	R	6	32	43	3.33	.098[+]
rACC	L	−3	50	7	4.00	.006
rACC	R	6	44	4	3.87	.009
vlPFC	L	−39	29	13	4.14	.011
vlPFC	L	−45	17	13	3.57	.071[+]
vmPFC	L	−3	56	−11	4.05	.008
vmPFC	R	9	59	−14	3.76	.021
Neutral gt phobia						
no significant results						
Phobia gt fear						
insula	L	−39	−1	4	3.18	.097[+]
vlPFC	L	−45	8	10	3.94	.023
vlPFC	R	48	17	1	3.57	.076[+]
Fear gt phobia						
no significant results						
Phobia gt disgust						
rACC	R	6	38	13	3.94	.031
Disgust gt phobia						
vmPFC	R	9	29	−23	3.57	.034
vmPFC	R	3	23	−23	3.52	.039

Neural activation decrease over the course of symptom provocation for phobic compared with neutral pictures for exploratory whole brain analyses (marked with [E]) and regions of interest analyses ($p_{fwe} < .05$); tendentially significant results $p_{fwe} < .1$ are marked with [+]; all coordinates (x, y, z) are given in MNI space. H, hemisphere; L, left R, right; Z_{max}, maximum Z-value p_{fwe}, fwe-corrected p-value (small-volume correction).

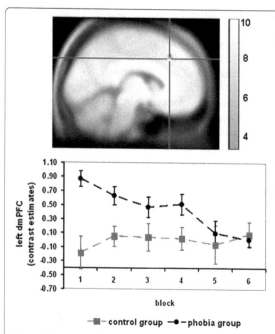

Figure 1 Stronger activation decrease in the left dmPFC (MNI coordinate: -6, 29, 40; marginally significant: $p_{fwe} = .058$) for phobic vs. neutral pictures in the phobia group compared with the control group. For illustration purposes, contrast estimates were averaged across 5 consecutive trials, respectively, resulting in 6 blocks for 30 trials. Color bar indicates T-values; for illustration reasons, data were thresholded at $p < .001$ and superimposed on the MNI305-T1 template.

for phobic compared with neutral pictures (see Table 2a and Figure 2). A negative correlation of cognitive reappraisal with activation decreases for phobic vs. neutral pictures was observed for the right lOFC and two clusters in the right vmPFC (marginally significant; $Z_{max} = 3.45$, $p = .053$ and $Z_{max} = 3.33$, $p = .076$) (see Table 2a and Figure 2). Furthermore, the correlation of symptom severity with activation decreases in response to phobic vs. neutral stimuli in the phobic group yielded no significant results.

In order to assess the generalizability of the results, a correlation of dispositional cognitive reappraisal and activation decreases was calculated within the control group. Hereby, we observed a positive correlation of dispositional cognitive reappraisal with activation decreases in the left dlPFC and marginally significant with the SMA (left: $Z_{max} = 3.38$, $p = .074$; right: $Z_{max} = 3.43$, $p = .069$) and left vlPFC ($Z_{max} = 4.46$, $p = .055$) (see Table 2b).

For comparability with previous studies, we further conducted a correlation of dispositional cognitive reappraisal with neural activation in response to phobic compared with neutral stimuli. In the phobic group, we observed a negative correlation with cognitive reappraisal in the left SMA, the right vlPFC, bilateral dmPFC and marginally significant in the left dlPFC ($Z_{max} = 3.55$, $p = .091$), lOFC ($Z_{max} = 3.56$, $p = .056$), rACC ($Z_{max} = 3.10$, $p = .074$) and two clusters in the vlPFC ($Z_{max} = 3.57$, $p = .051$ and $Z_{max} = 3.43$, $p = .075$) (see Table 3a). No positive correlation with dispositional cognitive reappraisal was found for this group. The control group showed a positive correlation of reappraisal with the left amygdala and the left insula as well as marginally significant with right insula ($Z_{max} = 3.37$, $p = .060$) and left lOFC ($Z_{max} = 3.70$, $p = .055$) activation (see Table 3b).

Table 2 Correlation of dispositional cognitive reappraisal with neural activation decrease for phobic vs. neutral pictures

Structure	H	x	y	z	Z_{max}	p_{fwe}
a) Phobic group						
positive correlation with dispositional cognitive reappraisal						
dmPFC	R	9	53	34	3.56	.052[+]
negative correlation with dispositional cognitive reappraisal						
lOFC	R	27	59	−5	4.27	.008
vmPFC	R	12	23	−14	3.45	.053[+]
vmPFC	R	6	62	−17	3.33	.076[+]
b) Control group						
positive correlation with dispositional cognitive reappraisal						
dlPFC	L	−39	26	43	3.99	.031
SMA	L	−3	8	43	3.38	.074[+]
SMA	R	6	−16	73	3.43	.069[+]
vlPFC	L	−45	17	7	4.46	.055[+]
negative correlation with dispositional cognitive reappraisal						

no significant results

Correlation of dispositional cognitive reappraisal with neural activation decrease over the course of symptom provocation for phobic compared with neutral pictures in the a) phobic and b) control group for exploratory whole brain analyses (marked with [E]) and regions of interest analyses ($p_{fwe} < .05$); tendentially significant results $p_{fwe} < .1$ are marked with [+]; all coordinates (x, y, z) are given in *MNI* space. *H* hemisphere, *L* left, *R* right, Z_{max} maximum Z-value, p_{fwe} fwe-corrected p-value (small-volume correction).

Discussion

The aim of this fMRI study was to investigate the association of dispositional cognitive reappraisal with neural temporal dynamics during phobic stimulation in dental phobia. For this purpose, the time course of brain activation during symptom provocation with visual phobic stimuli was investigated in a sample of 27 dental phobic patients and 21 healthy controls. The habitual use of cognitive reappraisal was assessed with the Emotion Regulation Questionnaire (ERQ [20] German version [29]) in order to investigate the association of dispositional reappraisal with activation decreases over the course of symptom provocation.

A general decrease of activation for phobic compared with neutral stimuli was observed in several brain regions including the insula (marginally significant), the middle temporal gyrus, and the caudate nucleus. Some of these regions have previously been shown to be overactive during symptom provocation in specific phobia [6,8] and might therefore be associated with reduced emotional responding respectively stronger habituation over time in the present study. Concerning the specificity of the results, our data mainly demonstrate that the activation decrease in most of the reported brain regions does not differ from the time course of activation in response to fear and disgust pictures as well as when comparing phobic patients

with healthy control subjects. However, a stronger activation decrease in the insula (marginally significant) was also observed in response to phobic compared with fear pictures. As mentioned above, several studies reported a hyperactivation of the insula during symptom provocation in specific phobia (for an overview see [6]). Moreover, the insula is a central structure in interoceptive perception and awareness [36]. One study has even demonstrated an anatomical overlap of insula activation during interoception and symptom provocation in patients with specific phobia [37]. Stronger activation decrease in the insula might therefore be associated with enhanced habituation of bodily arousal in response to phobic compared with fear stimuli, probably due to heightened responding in the insula during early confrontation with phobic stimuli. Habituation of insula and middle temporal gyrus activation, as found in our study, has already been demonstrated in spider phobic subjects [15]. However, it needs to be emphasized that activation decrease in the insula was only marginally significant and needs to be interpreted with caution. Further studies are needed to replicate the current results.

In addition, several regulation-related prefrontal and anterior cingulate cortex areas showed a reduction of activation over the time course of the experiment. Stronger habituation was found in the vlPFC even for phobic compared with fear pictures and in the rACC for phobic compared with disgust pictures. This might be interpreted as a reduction of cognitive control processes over the course of symptom provocation. On the one hand, this might be due to a reduced need for cognitive control based on a decline of emotional responding, and thus might be adaptive. On the other hand, the activation decrease might be associated with reduced (although necessary) cognitive control or extinction processes, and thus might be non-adaptive. This might be more pronounced in response to phobic stimuli in the vlPFC and the rACC due to a higher salience of phobic stimuli that require stronger cognitive processing and regulation especially in the beginning of confrontation.

The main goal of the present study was to investigate the association of dispositional cognitive reappraisal with neural temporal dynamics during processing of phobic stimuli in dental phobia.

As a main result a stronger activation decrease in the right dmPFC (marginally significant) was found in frequent reappraisers in the phobia group. This could possibly be explained by diminished cognitive regulation of negative emotions over time. Additionally, an enhanced activation decrease in the left dmPFC over the course of symptom provocation was also observed in phobic compared with healthy control subjects in the present study and points further to the important role of this region.

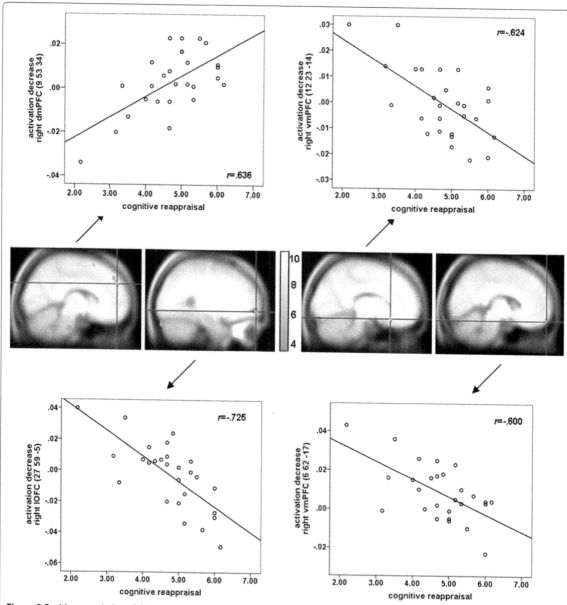

Figure 2 Positive association of dispositional cognitive reappraisal with activation decrease in the right dmPFC (MNI coordinate: 9, 53, 34; marginally significant: $p_{fwe} = .052$) in the phobic group; negative associations of dispositional cognitive reappraisal with activation decrease in the right lOFC (MNI coordinate: 27, 59, -5; $p_{fwe} = .008$), the right vmPFC (MNI coordinate: 12, 23, -14; marginally significant: $p_{fwe} = .053$), and a further cluster in the right vmPFC (MNI coordinate: 6, 62, -17; marginally significant: $p_{fwe} = .076$) in the phobic group. Color bar indicates T-values; for illustration reasons, data were thresholded at $p < .001$ and superimposed on the MNI305-T1 template.

The dmPFC is crucially involved in emotion regulation processes via cognitive reappraisal (for an overview see [21]). Additionally, previously observed reduced dmPFC activation during phobia-specific cognitive reappraisal points to an important role of this region in phobia-specific cognitive emotion regulation [12]. A stronger activation decrease over time might be related to a stronger

decline of explicit cognitive emotion regulation over the course of the experiment. This might be due to a reduced need to effortfully down-regulate negative emotions because of a more effective automatic regulation or reduced emotional responding.

In line with this interpretation, dispositional reappraisal has been shown to be associated with a diminished

Table 3 Correlation of dispositional cognitive reappraisal with neural activation for phobic vs. neutral pictures

Structure	H	x	y	z	Z_{max}	p_{fwe}
a) Phobic group						
positive correlation with dispositional cognitive reappraisal						
no significant results						
negative correlation with dispositional cognitive reappraisal						
dlPFC	L	−42	8	46	3.55	.091[+]
SMA	L	−12	14	64	3.93	.011
dmPFC	L	−9	53	25	3.75	.027
dmPFC	R	12	29	52	3.59	.035
lOFC	L	−54	23	−8	3.56	.056[+]
rACC	L	−9	38	10	3.10	.074[+]
vlPFC	L	−33	5	28	3.57	.050[+]
vlPFC	L	−45	29	13	3.57	.051[+]
vlPFC	L	−48	20	25	3.43	.075[+]
vlPFC	R	51	17	31	4.05	.011
b) Control group						
positive correlation with dispositional cognitive reappraisal						
insula	L	−39	2	−14	3.69	.024
insula	R	39	16	10	3.37	.060[+]
amygdala	L	−30	−1	−23	3.14	.035
lOFC	L	−27	29	−8	3.70	.055[+]
negative correlation with dispositional cognitive reappraisal						
no significant results						

Correlation of dispositional cognitive reappraisal with neural activation for phobic compared with neutral pictures in the a) phobic and b) control group for exploratory whole brain analyses (marked with [E]) and regions of interest analyses ($p_{fwe} < .05$); tendentially significant results $p_{fwe} < .1$ are marked with [+]; all coordinates (x, y, z) are given in MNI space. H hemisphere, L left, R right, Z_{max} maximum, Z-value p_{fwe}, fwe-corrected p-value (small-volume correction).

activation decrease in the vmPFC over time in the present study. The vmPFC has previously been found to exhibit reduced activation during symptom provocation in patients with specific phobia [11-13]. Moreover, reduced activation of the vmPFC along with amygdala hyperactivation has been observed during the acquisition of conditioned fear responses [38] most likely indicating reduced cognitive control of emotional reactions. In addition, vmPFC activation has previously been found during extinction learning and recall [38] as well as a result of successful CBT in specific phobia [13]. Regarding these results, the observed reduced decrease of vmPFC activation in the present study in individuals more frequently using cognitive reappraisal might be related to a decreased fear recall or stronger extinction learning over the course of symptom provocation. This interpretation fits well with the observed reduced activation decrease in the vmPFC in response to phobic compared with disgust stimuli in phobic subjects.

In addition, lateral OFC activation showed a diminished decline in individuals with a higher habitual use of cognitive reappraisal. This region has frequently been found to be activated during symptom provocation in specific phobia [39,40] and seems to be especially involved in the processing of negative affective states [41]. Hence, the association of dispositional reappraisal with sustained lOFC activation during symptom provocation might be related to prolonged negative affective processing. This interpretation seems to contradict the hypothesis of stronger extinction learning in individuals high in dispositional cognitive reappraisal. However, the OFC has also been found to play a crucial role in the regulation of emotions via cognitive reappraisal (for an overview see [21]). Therefore, OFC activation might more likely reflect the activation and reinterpretation of negative appraisals in response to phobic stimuli, which is more sustained in subjects high in dispositional reappraisal over the course of symptom provocation.

The results for the correlation of cognitive reappraisal with activation decreases for phobic vs. neutral pictures in control subjects differ from the results of the phobia group. In the control group, a stronger activation decrease for frequent reappraisers was observed in the dlPFC, vlPFC and SMA and might be interpreted as a reduced employment of cognitive control strategies over the course of the experiment. The differences to the phobia group, however, indicate that there might be differences in the underlying processes. On the one hand, phobic and control subjects differ in the extent of emotional responding towards phobic stimuli which might result in different correlations with dispositional cognitive reappraisal. On the other hand phobics and controls might use different tactics of cognitive reappraisal (i.e. distancing vs. reinterpretation) leading to distinct activation patterns. Further studies are needed in order to disentangle the underlying mechanism by investigating for instance instructed rather than dispositional cognitive reappraisal.

Additional analyses focused on the association of dispositional cognitive reappraisal and activation rather than on the activation decrease during symptom provocation. A number of regulation-related prefrontal, anterior cingulate and orbitofrontal cortex areas were found to be negatively correlated with cognitive reappraisal in the phobic group. This supports the hypothesis that individuals with higher reappraisal abilities do not need to recruit these regulation-related brain areas as much as individuals with lower reappraisal abilities to control their emotions during symptom provocation. Enhanced insula, amygdala and lOFC responses in frequent reappraisers in the control group indicate, however, a more pronounced emotional processing in these individuals. This might probably derive from a stronger engagement with emotional aspects of the stimuli during reappraisal and needs to be further investigated in future studies.

Because there was no association of cognitive reappraisal and symptom severity as well as symptom severity and time course of brain activation one might speculate that cognitive reappraisal is a better predictor of habituation or even emotional relearning during exposure than symptom severity. Therefore, it might be of special importance to assess the general cognitive reappraisal abilities of phobic patients prior to exposure sessions and to improve these abilities if necessary in order to strengthen the (long-term) outcome of CBT.

Conclusions

In conclusion, the results of this study indicate that individual differences in cognitive reappraisal usage differentially modulate the time course of brain activation during symptom provocation in distinct brain areas. A stronger decline of dmPFC activation might be related to a diminished (need for) explicit emotion regulation over the course of symptom provocation. This result is in line with a diminished habituation of the vmPFC and the lOFC, regions important in more automatic emotion regulation processes like extinction learning. The vmPFC has even been shown to be associated with successful CBT in spider phobic patients [13]. Individuals high in dispositional cognitive reappraisal might be faster or even better at regulating their emotional responses with less effort, leading to a more successful emotional relearning. Due to the assumed stronger habituation and probably enhanced extinction learning, one could speculate that individuals high in dispositional cognitive reappraisal might be more able to benefit from CBT interventions. Or the other way round, strengthening cognitive reappraisal abilities in individuals low in dispositional cognitive reappraisal might be a promising way to enhance therapy success for a larger number of individuals in the short- and the long-term.

Limitations

Some limitations of our study need to be mentioned. As we used a correlational approach, it is not clear if dispositional cognitive reappraisal leads to stronger habituation/extinction or if individual differences in these habituation/extinction processes preceded and influenced the habitual use of cognitive reappraisal. In addition, the present study investigated processes taking place during one single exposure session. In order to evaluate the association of individual differences in cognitive reappraisal with long-lasting neural changes, the recall of the extinction memory needs to be studied. Future studies investigating cognitive reappraisal and the neural correlates of extinction processes in specific phobia over the course of 'real' exposure therapy are important further steps in order to validate the current findings and optimize existing psychological interventions in specific phobia.

Competing interests
All authors declare no financial or non-financial competing interests.

Authors' contributions
AS and AH designed this study. VL and WS conducted diagnostics and data acquisition. AH conducted the statistical analyses and AH, DV and RS interpreted the data. AH drafted the manuscript. DV and RS edited and revised the manuscript. All authors read and approved the final manuscript.

Acknowledgements
This research was funded by a grant to RS and AS from the German Research Foundation (STA 475/10-1).

Author details
[1]Department of Psychotherapy and Systems Neuroscience, Bender Institute of Neuroimaging, Justus Liebig University, Otto-Behaghel-Strasse 10H, Giessen 35394, Germany. [2]Bender Institute of Neuroimaging, Justus Liebig University, Giessen, Germany. [3]Department of Clinical Psychology, University of Graz, Graz, Austria.

References
1. American Psychiatric Association: *Diagnostic and Statistical Manual of Mental Disorders DSM-IV-TR.* 4th edition. Washington DC: American Psychiatric Press; 2000.
2. de Jongh A, Fransen J, Oosterink-Wubbe F, Aartman I: **Psychological trauma exposure and trauma symptoms among individuals with high and low levels of dental anxiety.** *Eur J Oral Sci* 2006, **114**:286–292.
3. Oosterink FMD, de Jongh A, Hoogstraten J, Aartman IHA: **The Level of Exposure-Dental Experiences Questionnaire (LOE-DEQ): a measure of severity of exposure to distressing dental events.** *Eur J Oral Sci* 2008, **116**:353–361.
4. Mineka S, Zinbarg R: **A contemporary learning theory perspective on the etiology of anxiety disorders: It's not what you thought it was.** *Am Psychol* 2006, **61**:10–26.
5. Mineka S, Oehlberg K: **The relevance of recent developments in classical conditioning to understanding the etiology and maintenance of anxiety disorders.** *Acta Psychol* 2008, **127**:567–580.
6. Etkin A, Wager TD: **Functional neuroimaging of anxiety: a meta-analysis of emotional processing in PTSD, social anxiety disorder, and specific phobia.** *Am J Psychiatry* 2007, **164**:1476–1488.
7. Lueken U, Kruschwitz JD, Muehlhan M, Siegert J, Hoyer J, Wittchen H: **How specific is specific phobia? Different neural response patterns in two subtypes of specific phobia.** *Neuroimage* 2011, **56**:363–372.
8. Schienle A, Scharmüller W, Leutgeb V, Schäfer A, Stark R: **Sex differences in the functional and structural neuroanatomy of dental phobia.** *Brain Struct Funct* 2013, **218**:779–787.
9. Graham BM, Milad MR: **The study of fear extinction: implications for anxiety disorders.** *Am J Psychiatry* 2011, **168**:1255–1265.
10. Diekhof EK, Geier K, Falkai P, Gruber O: **Fear is only as deep as the mind allows.** *Neuroimage* 2011, **58**:275–285.
11. Hermann A, Schäfer A, Walter B, Stark R, Vaitl D, Schienle A: **Diminished medial prefrontal cortex activity in blood-injection-injury phobia.** *Biol Psychol* 2007, **75**:124–130.
12. Hermann A, Schafer A, Walter B, Stark R, Vaitl D, Schienle A: **Emotion regulation in spider phobia: role of the medial prefrontal cortex.** *Soc Cogn Affect Neurosci* 2009, **4**:257–267.
13. Schienle A, Schäfer A, Hermann A, Rohrmann S, Vaitl D: **Symptom provocation and reduction in patients suffering from spider phobia.** *Eur Arch Psychiatry Clin Neurosc* 2007, **257**:486–493.
14. Straube T, Glauer M, Dilger S, Mentzel H, Miltner WH: **Effects of cognitive-behavioral therapy on brain activation in specific phobia.** *Neuroimage* 2006, **29**:125–135.
15. Veltman DJ, Tuinebreijer WE, Winkelman D, Dolan RJ, Emmelkamp PMG: **Neurophysiological correlates of habituation during exposure in spider phobia.** *Psychiatry Res* 2004, **132**:149–158.

16. Hofmann S: Cognitive processes during fear acquisition and extinction in animals and humans: Implications for exposure therapy of anxiety disorders. *Clin Psychol Rev* 2008, **28**:199–210.

17. Beck AT: *Cognitive therapy and the emotional disorders*. NY: International Universities Press; 1976.

18. Sloan T, Telch MJ: The effects of safety-seeking behavior and guided threat reappraisal on fear reduction during exposure: an experimental investigation. *Behav Res Ther* 2002, **40**:235–251.

19. Kamphuis JH, Telch MJ: Effects of distraction and guided threat reappraisal on fear reduction during exposure-based treatments for specific fears. *Behav Res Ther* 2000, **38**:1163–1181.

20. Gross JJ, John OP: Individual differences in two emotion regulation processes: Implications for affect, relationships, and well-being. *J Pers Soc Psychol* 2003, **85**:348–362.

21. Ochsner K, Gross J: The cognitive control of emotion. *Trends Cogn Sci* 2005, **9**:242–249.

22. Carlson JM, Mujica-Parodi L: A disposition to reappraise decreases anterior insula reactivity during anxious anticipation. *Biol Psychol* 2010, **85**:383–385.

23. Drabant EM, McRae K, Manuck SB, Hariri AR, Gross JJ: Individual differences in typical reappraisal Use predict amygdala and prefrontal responses. *Biol Psychiatry* 2009, **65**:367–373.

24. Vanderhasselt M, Baeken C, van Schuerbeek P, Luypaert R, de Raedt R: Inter-individual differences in the habitual use of cognitive reappraisal and expressive suppression are associated with variations in prefrontal cognitive control for emotional information: An event related fMRI study. *Biol Psychol* 2013, **92**:433–439.

25. Giuliani NR, Drabant EM, Gross JJ: Anterior cingulate cortex volume and emotion regulation: Is bigger better? *Biol Psychol* 2011, **86**:379–382.

26. Welborn BL, Papademetris X, Reis DL, Rajeevan N, Bloise SM, Gray JR: Variation in orbitofrontal cortex volume: relation to sex, emotion regulation and affect. *Soc Cogn Affect Neurosci* 2009, **4**:328–339.

27. Wolitzky-Taylor KB, Horowitz JD, Powers MB, Telch MJ: Psychological approaches in the treatment of specific phobias: A meta-analysis. *Clin Psychol Rev* 2008, **28**:1021–1037.

28. Craske MG, Kircanski K, Zelikowsky M, Mystkowski J, Chowdhury N, Baker A: Optimizing inhibitory learning during exposure therapy. *Behav Res and Ther* 2008, **46**:5–27.

29. Abler B, Kessler H: Emotion Regulation Questionnaire – Eine deutschsprachige Fassung des ERQ von Gross und John. *Diagnostica* 2009, **55**:144–152.

30. Corah NL: Development of a dental anxiety scale. *J Dent Res* 1969, **48**:596.

31. Wittchen H-U, Zaudig M, Fydrich T: *Strukturiertes Klinisches Interview für DSM-IV*. Göttingen: Hogrefe; 1997.

32. Lang PJ, Bradley MM, Cuthbert BN: *International affective picture system (IAPS): instruction manual and affective ratings*, Technical report A-4. The center for research in psychophysiology. Gainsville: University of Florida; 1999.

33. Schienle A, Stark R, Walter B, Blecker C, Ott U, Kirsch P, Sammer G, Vaitl D: The insula is not specifically involved in disgust processing: an fMRI study. *Neuroreport* 2002, **13**:2023–2026.

34. Schienle A, Köchel A, Leutgeb V: Frontal late positivity in dental phobia: A study on gender differences. *Biol Psychol* 2011, **88**:263–269.

35. Walter B, Blecker C, Kirsch P, Sammer G, Schienle A, Stark R, Vaitl D: MARINA: An easy to use tool for the creation of MAsks for Region of INterest Analyses. *Neuroimage* 2003, **19**: . CD-Rom.

36. Critchley HD, Wiens S, Rotshtein P, Öhman A, Dolan RJ: Neural systems supporting interoceptive awareness. *Nat Neurosci* 2004, **7**:189–195.

37. Caseras X, Murphy K, Mataix-Cols D, López-Solà M, Soriano-Mas C, Ortriz H, Pujol J, Torrubia R: Anatomical and functional overlap within the insula and anterior cingulate cortex during interoception and phobic symptom provocation. *Hum Brain Mapp* 2013, **34**:1220–1229.

38. Milad MR, Wright CI, Orr SP, Pitman RK, Quirk GJ, Rauch SL: Recall of fear extinction in humans activates the ventromedial prefrontal cortex and hippocampus in concert. *Biol Psychiatry* 2007, **62**:446–454.

39. Dilger S, Straube T, Mentzel H, Fitzek C, Reichenbach JR, Hecht H, Krieschel S, Gutberlet I, Miltner WHR: Brain activation to phobia-related pictures in spider phobic humans: an event-related functional magnetic resonance imaging study. *Neurosci Lett* 2003, **348**:29–32.

40. Paquette V, Lévesque J, Mensour B, Leroux J, Beaudoin G, Bourgouin P, Beauregard M: "Change the mind and you change the brain": effects of cognitive-behavioral therapy on the neural correlates of spider phobia. *Neuroimage* 2003, **18**:401–409.

41. Kringelbach M, Rolls ET: The functional neuroanatomy of the human orbitofrontal cortex: evidence from neuroimaging and neuropsychology. *Prog Neurobiol* 2004, **72**:341–372.

Area-dependent time courses of brain activation during video-induced symptom provocation in social anxiety disorder

Stephanie Boehme[1*], Alexander Mohr[1], Michael PI Becker[2], Wolfgang HR Miltner[1] and Thomas Straube[2*]

Abstract

Background: Previous functional imaging studies using symptom provocation in patients with social anxiety disorder (SAD) reported inconsistent findings, which might be at least partially related to different time-dependent activation profiles in different brain areas. In the present functional magnetic resonance imaging study, we used a novel video-based symptom provocation design in order to investigate the magnitude and time course of activation in different brain areas in 20 SAD patients and 20 healthy controls.

Results: The disorder-related videos induced increased anxiety in patients with SAD as compared to healthy controls. Analyses of brain activation to disorder-related *versus* neutral video clips revealed amygdala activation during the first but not during the second half of the clips in patients as compared to controls. In contrast, the activation in the insula showed a reversed pattern with increased activation during the second but not during the first half of the video clips. Furthermore, a cluster in the anterior dorsal anterior cingulate cortex showed a sustained response for the entire duration of the videos.

Conclusions: The present findings suggest that different regions of the fear network show differential temporal response patterns during video-induced symptom provocation in SAD. While the amygdala is involved during initial threat processing, the insula seems to be more involved during subsequent anxiety responses. In accordance with cognitive models of SAD, a medial prefrontal region engaged in emotional-cognitive interactions is generally hyperactivated.

Keywords: Social anxiety disorder, Symptom provocation, Functional magnetic resonance imaging (fMRI), Amygdala, Insula, Medial prefrontal cortex

Background

Individuals suffering from social anxiety disorder (SAD), classified as 'social phobia' in DSM-IV-TR [1], show exaggerated fear responses in social or performance situations. In particular, patients are excessively concerned about being evaluated negatively by others. In search of the neural basis of SAD, different brain areas have been identified that seem to be involved in SAD. By means of functional brain imaging, heightened activation of the amygdala has been found during the processing of disorder-related

stimuli (for example, [2-9]) as well as during symptom provocation in SAD patients (for example, [10-14]), supporting the assumed role of the amygdala in threat processing [15,16]. Furthermore, several other regions have been associated with increased activation in SAD, including medial prefrontal areas, for example, dorsal anterior cingulate cortex (ACC) and dorsomedial prefrontal cortex (dmPFC), and the insular cortex (for example, [3,5,8,10,17-20]). Medial prefrontal cortex areas have been proposed to be linked to explicit emotional evaluation, emotional-cognitive interactions, self-referential processing, and emotion-regulation [21-26]. The insula seems to be involved in interoception and representation of bodily states [27-29] and might support aversive feelings by evaluating arousal responses [28,30,31].

* Correspondence: stephanie.boehme@uni-jena.de; thomas.straube@uni-muenster.de
[1]Department of Biological and Clinical Psychology, Friedrich Schiller University Jena, Am Steiger 3 // 1, Jena D-07743, Germany
[2]Institute of Medical Psychology and Systems Neuroscience, University of Muenster, Von-Esmarch-Str. 52, Muenster D-48149, Germany

However, although these areas have been repeatedly shown to be associated with the processing of disorder-relevant stimuli in SAD and other anxiety disorders [32], reported brain activation patterns are rather inconsistent across studies with most studies describing different areas to be involved. Furthermore, there are only few symptom provocation studies as compared to the large number of studies that investigated the neural correlates during the processing of social stimuli such as facial expressions in SAD patients. Remarkably, even though disorder-related stimuli such as emotional faces do not induce reliable anxiety symptoms in patients, they seem to activate parts of an emotional network. However, findings are variable and strongly depend on task conditions [8,9] and time course parameters [18,33].

Reliable anxiety responses are induced by symptom provocation designs such as actual or anticipated public performance. Furthermore, findings from anxiety symptom provocation studies should provide stronger evidence which regions are involved in anxiety symptoms in SAD. While some symptom provocation studies reported increased amygdala activation during public speaking in patients with SAD [11-14,34], studies using other symptom provocation tasks did not [35-37]. Similarly, there are also inconsistencies regarding the involvement of the insula (see [10,12,13,35-38]) and prefrontal regions in SAD [12-14,34,36,37].

Obviously, threat-related brain activation in SAD depends on various factors, which are not well understood yet. For example, some symptom provocation tasks such as overt speaking tasks are associated with active performance but are also inherently susceptible to brain imaging-relevant artefacts such as head movements and performance differences between patients and controls. Moreover, in different tasks, different functions of the threat-processing network might be involved. Furthermore and most importantly, brain activation was shown to vary over time in response to anticipatory anxiety in social anxiety (see [10]) and some variability in previous findings may be due to different time courses of brain activation. Accordingly, there is general evidence that indicates different time courses of several brain areas within the defense cascade (for example, [39,40]). Thus, while the amygdala has been suggested to be primarily relevant during the initial period of threat processing in healthy participants and patients with phobias (for example, [39-42]), the insula and prefrontal areas were shown to be associated with explicit and more sustained fear responses [39,40,42-44]. In SAD, the time course of activation in different brain areas during symptom provocation is largely unknown. A recent study found increased amygdala activation only during the first half of an anticipatory threat interval in SAD [10].

In the present study, we used a novel symptom provocation design in SAD by presenting disorder-related and neutral video clips. We developed a new set of video stimuli for symptom provocation in SAD, based on evidence that the use of short film clips represents one of the most effective and reliable methods to induce emotions in laboratory settings [45-47]. The study aimed to investigate increased brain activation in several areas that have been identified to be important in SAD during symptom provocation (amygdala, insula, ACC, and dmPFC). Activation was modelled to account (a) for the full time course of the video clips, and (b) specifically, for the first and (c) second half of the clips. If the amygdala bears specific relevance for initial threat processing, effects should be most pronounced during the first half of the video clips. In contrast, responses in other areas should also be manifest during the second half of the video clips or may occur specifically during the second half of the clips.

Methods

Participants

Twenty-one patients with a primary diagnosis of SAD of the generalized subtype and 20 healthy control participants (HC) took part in the study. Due to strong head movement (>3 mm) one patient had to be excluded from analyses. Therefore, the final sample comprised 20 SAD and 20 HC participants. All were right-handed with normal or corrected-to-normal vision. They were recruited via public announcement and provided written informed consent for participation. The study was approved by the ethics committee of the University of Jena. Diagnoses were confirmed by clinical psychologists administering the Structured Clinical Interview for DSM-IV Axis I and II disorders (SCID I and II [48,49]). Exclusion criteria were any of the following: (1) A diagnosis of panic disorder and/or agoraphobia, current alcohol/substance abuse, psychotic disorder, dementia, primary or secondary major depression; (2) a history of seizures or head injury with loss of consciousness; (3) a severe uncontrollable medical condition; and (4) the use of any psychotropic medication within the preceding 6 months. HC were free of any psychopathology and medication. In the SAD sample, co-morbidities were specific phobia (n = 3), obsessive-compulsive disorder (n = 1), bulimia nervosa (recurrent in full remission; n = 1), and depressive episodes in the past (n = 5). Six patients also met the criteria of an Axis II personality disorder (anxious (avoidant) personality disorder, dependent personality disorder). Patients with SAD and HC participants were matched for age (SAD: 23.85 years, HC: 24.20 years, $t[38] = 0.45$, $P >0.05$), gender (SAD: 10 women, HC: 10 women, $\chi^2[1] = 0.00$, $P >0.05$) and education (all participants had high school graduation with a minimum school period of 12 years). Before scanning, all participants completed the LSAS (Liebowitz Social Anxiety Scale, German version, [50]) and the BDI (Beck

Depression Inventory, German version, [51]) question-naire. SAD patients scored significantly higher on both LSAS (SAD: LSAS = 71.95, HC: LSAS = 10.65, $t[38]$ = 18.23, P <0.05) and BDI (SAD: BDI = 11.90, HC: BDI = 3.05, $t[38]$ = 8.33, P <0.05) questionnaires than HC participants.

Paradigm

Stimuli consisted of disorder-related (social) and disorder-unrelated (neutral) video clips that lasted 24 s each. The clips were developed by our group and filmed with the help of experienced actors who belonged to student or layman theater groups. The clips showed a man or woman (counter-balanced) acting either in a social (social activity) or in a corresponding neutral situation (same environment but actor is alone and engaged in a non-social activity). Prototypically feared situations for the generalized subtype of SAD were subsumed in four broad categories: (1) formal interaction situations (for example, oral examinations); (2) informal interaction situations (for example, asking someone for directions); (3) situations that require self-assurance (for example, complaints about goods); and (4) situations where the actor's behavior is observed by others (for example, during social eating; see Additional file 1: Table S1: Description of the used video clips). Eighteen disorder-related and 18 neutral video clips were chosen from an initial pool of 36 social and 36 neutral clips by five leading German experts on SAD with extensive experience in diagnosis and therapy of SAD (see Acknowledgments) who judged the anxiety-inducing potential and social phobia-relevance of the clips on nine-point Likert scales. Based on these ratings, a final set of maximally anxiety-inducing and SAD-related videos was chosen which comprised five videos for the categories (1) and (4) and four videos for the categories (2) and (3), respectively. All disorder-related videos had to exceed a rating cutoff score of κ_s = 5 and neutral videos had to fall below κ_s. On average, phobia-relevance of disorder-related videos used in the present study was rated M = 7.10 (SD = ±.52), and anxiety-inducing potential was rated M = 7.03 (SD = ±.81), while neutral videos were rated only minimally anxiety-inducing (M = 2.10 (SD = ±0.54)) and phobia-relevant (M = 2.04 (SD = ±0.52)). The order of clips was pseudo-randomized with no more than two clips of the same category (social or neutral) succeeding each other. Inter-stimulus interval (white fixation cross in front of a black screen) was set to 16 s. Participants were asked to focus on the main actor of the scene, to take his/her perspective and to empathize as much as possible with her/his behavior.

After magnetic resonance imaging (MRI), participants were re-exposed to the clips and were asked to rate valence, arousal, and anxiety which were induced by each clip on a nine-point Likert scale (valence: 1 = very pleasant to 9 = very unpleasant, whereas 5 = neutral; arousal: 1 = not arousing to 9 = very arousing; anxiety: 1 = not anxious to 9 = very anxious). Behavioral data were analyzed by repeated measures analyses of variance (ANOVA) and subsequent t-tests using SPSS software (Version 19.0.0.1, SPSS, Inc.). For ANOVAs and t-tests a probability level of P <0.05 was considered statistically significant.

Functional magnetic resonance imaging

Scanning was performed in a 1.5 Tesla magnetic resonance scanner ('Magnetom VISION Plus', Siemens, Medical Solutions, Erlangen, Germany). After a T1-weighted anatomical scan, two runs with 184 volumes (each video clip appeared once in a run) were conducted using a T2*-weighted echo-planar sequence (TE, 50 ms; flip angle, 90°; matrix, 64 × 64; field of view, 192 mm; TR, 3.9 s). Each volume consisted of 40 axial slices (thickness, 3 mm; gap, 0 mm; in plane resolution, 3 × 3 mm). The first four volumes were discarded from analysis to ensure steady-state tissue magnetization.

Functional magnetic resonance imaging (fMRI) data preprocessing and analyses were realized by BrainVoyager QX software (Version 1.10.4; Brain Innovation BV). As a first step of preprocessing, all volumes were realigned to the first volume in order to minimize artifacts due to head movements. Afterwards, spatial (8 mm full-width half-maximum isotropic Gaussian kernel) and temporal filter were applied (high pass filter: 3 cycles per run; low pass filter: 2.8 s; linear trend removal). Then, the anatomical and functional images were co-registered and normalized to the Talairach space [52].

Statistical analyses of blood oxygen-level-dependent (BOLD) data were performed by multiple linear regression of its signal time course at each voxel. The expected signal change of BOLD response for each event type (predictor) was modeled by a canonical hemodynamic response function. First, the whole duration intervals of the video clips were defined as predictors. Second, for investigating the time course of activation, the period of brain activation to social and neutral video clips was divided into two succeeding parts of 12 s each and a new general linear model (GLM) was computed. Both GLMs comprised motion correction parameters as events of no interest. Statistical comparisons were realized using a mixed effect analysis, which considers inter-subject variance and permits population-level inferences. Then, voxel-wise statistical maps were generated and the relevant, planned contrasts of predictor estimates (beta-weights) were computed for each individual. After that, a random effects group analysis of these individual contrasts was performed.

First, analyses were conducted for specific regions of interest (ROIs). Following the approach recommended by Eickhoff et al. [53], we extracted the amygdala ROI consisting of three bilateral amygdala maximum probability maps (laterobasal, centromedial, and superficial; 9,077 mm³ in total) of the anatomy toolbox [54]. ROIs for the bilateral insula (32,822 mm³), ACC (23,963 mm³), and dmPFC (medial division of the superior frontal cortex; 44,945 mm³) were extracted from the AAL atlas included in WFU PickAtlas software [55-57]. Using MATLAB (Version 7.8; The MathWorks, Inc) all maps were transformed into BrainVoyager-compatible Talairach coordinates via ICBM2tal [58]. Second, whole brain analyses were conducted.

Statistical parametric maps resulting from voxel-wise analyses were considered statistically significant for clusters that survived a correction for multiple comparisons. For this purpose, we used the approach as implemented in BrainVoyager (based on a 3D extension of the randomization procedure described by Forman et al. [59]). First, voxel-level threshold was set to $P < 0.005$ (uncorrected) for the ROI-based and to $P < 0.001$ (uncorrected) for the whole brain analyses. Then, threshold maps were submitted to a correction for multiple comparisons that was firstly calculated for each ROI and secondly for the whole brain. The correction is based on the estimation of the cluster threshold that is the minimal number of voxels necessary to control for multiple comparisons. The cluster threshold criterion was based on an estimate of each map's spatial smoothness [59] and on an iterative procedure (Monte Carlo simulation). The Monte-Carlo simulation used 1,000 iterations in order to estimate the minimum cluster size threshold that yielded a cluster-level false-positive rate of 5%. The cluster size thresholds (full length: amygdala, 88 mm³; insula, 180 mm³; ACC, 142 mm³; dmPFC, 167; first and second half: amygdala, 79 mm³; insula, 162 mm³; ACC, 108 mm³; dmPFC, 156 mm³) were applied to the statistical maps. Finally, activation of peak voxels in the ROIs was correlated with symptom severity as measured by LSAS. For this purpose SPSS was used.

Results

Rating data
Analyses of post scanning stimulus ratings showed that both SAD patients and HC participants rated social video clips as more negative ($F[1,38] = 170.61$, $P < 0.05$), more arousing ($F[1,38] = 222.71$, $P < 0.05$), and more anxiety-inducing ($F[1,38] = 185.69$, $P < 0.05$) than neutral video clips. Additionally, SAD patients as compared to controls rated all video clips as more unpleasant ($F[1,38] = 24.23$, $P < 0.05$), more arousing ($F[1,38] = 24.68$, $P < 0.05$), and anxiety inducing ($F[1,38] = 32.97$, $P < 0.05$). Furthermore, there was a significant group by condition interaction (valence: $F[1,38] = 37.65$, $P < 0.05$; arousal: $F[1,38] = 11.16$, $P < 0.05$; anxiety: $F[1,38] = 76.46$, $P < 0.05$) with

increased ratings for social *versus* neutral video clips in SAD patients as compared to HC participants. Figure 1 shows rating data for SAD and HC participants.

fMRI data
Interaction group by video valence
We investigated BOLD activation during the full length of video clips and during the first and second period of clip presentation. When analyzing the full length of the social *versus* neutral video clips in SAD as compared to HC participants, we only detected significant activation differences in the prefrontal cortex. There was a cluster of activated voxels in the right anterior dorsal ACC (peak voxel Talairach coordinates: x = 14; y = 20; z = 28; size = 1,026 mm³; $t[38] = 4.45$; see Figure 2).

However, when analyzing BOLD activation during the first and second half of the video clips separately, we observed a hyperactivation of the left amygdala in response to social *versus* neutral video clips during the first half of the video clips in SAD patients as compared to HC participants (peak voxel Talairach coordinates: x = -23; y = 0; z = -19; size = 81 mm³; $t[38] = 2.93$; probability = 50%; see Figure 3). In contrast, activation in the left insula differed significantly during the second half of the social *versus* neutral video clips in SAD as compared to HC participants. There were two clusters of hyperactivated voxels in the left (anterior cluster: peak voxel Talairach coordinates: x = -24; y = 23; z = 13; size = 756 mm³; $t[38] = 3.61$; mid-insula cluster: peak voxel Talairach coordinates: x = -36; y = 5; z = 16; size = 648 mm³; $t[38] = 4.31$; see Figure 4) and in the right insula (anterior cluster: peak voxel Talairach coordinates: x = 36; y = 20; z = 13; size = 999 mm³; $t[38] = 4.11$; mid-insula cluster: peak

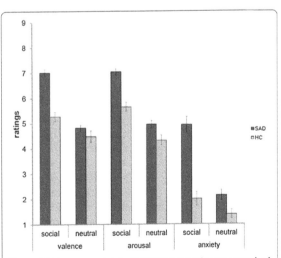

Figure 1 Valence, arousal, and anxiety ratings (mean ± standard error) for social and neutral video clips in patients with social anxiety disorder (SAD) and healthy control participants (HC).

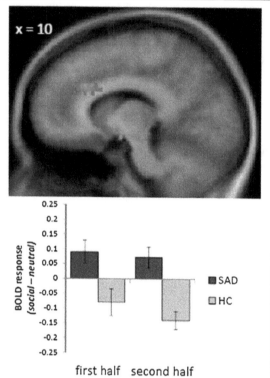

Figure 2 Differential brain activation in the anterior dorsal ACC during the social vs. neutral video clip presentation. Patients with social anxiety disorder (SAD) displayed an enhanced activation as compared to healthy control participants (HC) during the first as well as during the second part of the video clips (social > neutral). Statistical parametric maps are overlaid on a T1 scan (radiological convention: left = right). The plot at the bottom displays contrasts of parameter estimates (social vs. neutral video clips for first and second half separately; mean ± standard error for maximally activated voxel).

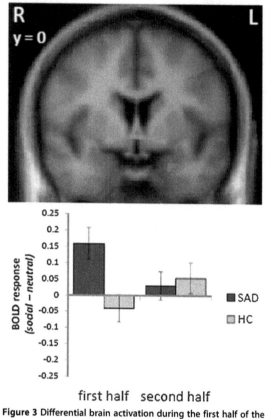

Figure 3 Differential brain activation during the first half of the social vs. neutral video clips. Patients with social anxiety disorder (SAD) displayed an enhanced activation in the left amygdala as compared to healthy control participants (HC; social > neutral video clips). Statistical parametric maps are overlaid on a T1 scan (radiological convention: left = right). The plot shows contrasts of parameter estimates (social vs. neutral video clips for first and second half separately; mean ± standard error for maximally activated voxel).

voxel Talairach coordinates: x = 42; y = -1; z = 13; size = 324 mm³; $t[38] = 3.83$; see Figure 4) for social *versus* neutral video clips during the second half in SAD *versus* HC subjects.

Furthermore, a cluster in the anterior dorsal ACC was found to be stronger activated in SAD *versus* HC participants during both halves of the social *versus* neutral video clips. The clusters were almost at the same location with similar peak voxels (first half: peak voxel Talairach coordinates: x = 14; y = 21; z = 29; size = 108 mm³; $t[38] = 3.22$; second half: peak voxel Talairach coordinates: x = 9; y = 27; z = 29; size = 1,431 mm³; $t[38] = 4.44$). Within the ROIs, there were no clusters of greater activation during neutral > social video clips in SAD *versus* HC subjects. For the sake of completeness, results of the whole brain analysis are shown in Table 1, indicating primarily additional increased activations in

SAD patients in (pre)frontal cortex during both halves of the videos.

Correlational analysis

Finally, correlations between activation of significant peak voxels within the ROIs and symptom severity in SAD as measured by LSAS was investigated. This revealed no significant correlation in SAD patients (for all analyses $P > 0.05$).

Discussion

The present study investigated brain activation in response to disorder-related and anxiety-provoking video clips *versus* neutral video clips in patients with SAD and healthy controls. Results showed that brain activation varies over time during symptom provocation in SAD as compared to HC subjects. The left amygdala was

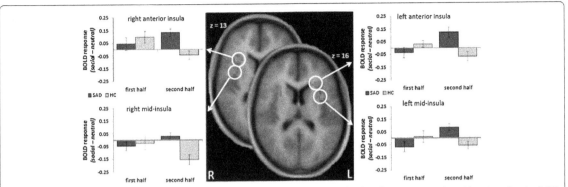

Figure 4 Differential brain activation during the second half of the social *vs.* neutral video clips. Patients with social anxiety disorder (SAD) displayed enhanced activation within the left and right anterior and mid-insula as compared to healthy control participants (HC; social > neutral video clips). Statistical parametric maps are overlaid on a T1 scan (radiological convention: left = right). The bar graphs show contrasts of parameter estimates (social *vs.* neutral video clips for first and second half separately; mean ± standard error for maximally activated voxel).

hyperactivated in SAD patients compared to controls specifically during the first part of the disorder-related video clips. Specifically during the second part of the video clips, SAD patients showed stronger insula activation than controls in response to social *versus* neutral video clips. Finally, increased activation of the anterior dorsal ACC to social *versus* neutral video clips was found during the whole time course of video presentation in patients with SAD compared to HC participants.

The hyperactivation of the amygdala during disorder-related video clips in SAD is in accordance with previous studies that reported increased amygdala responses during threat processing in SAD patients (for example, [3-8,60-65]; but see [20,35-37,66,67]). The amygdala, due to its interconnections to various cortical regions and to the brain stem and the hypothalamus additionally, is

suggested to be of essential relevance for mediation of automatic, bottom-up processing of emotional, and particularly threatening stimuli [15,68-70]. Furthermore, the present amygdala hyperactivation in SAD patients was found during the first half of the video presentation only. This implies a temporally restricted role of the amygdala at least during some forms of symptom provocation in SAD. The current finding is in accordance with a recent study on anticipatory anxiety in social anxiety [10] and allocates the amygdala a central role within a transient threat detection system [71,72], which affects both regulation of the autonomic nervous system as well as modulation of perceptual and emotional processing of relevant stimuli [9,68-70,73].

Repeatedly, the insula was shown to be involved in the processing of aversive emotional cues in SAD and other

Table 1 Whole brain analysis of group differences in activation between social and neutral videos (SAD > HC)

	Hemisphere	Social > neutral			t-value	Size (mm³)	Neutral > social			t-value	Size (mm³)
		Talairach					Talairach				
		x	y	z			x	y	z		
Whole video											
Superior frontal gyrus (BA 10)	R	23	62	27	4.54	621					
First half											
Globus pallidus	R						15	-1	6	4.49	216
Second half											
Middle frontal gyrus (BA 46)	L	-50	24	19	3.66	297					
Inferior frontal gyrus (BA 44)	R	57	11	10	4.52	1350					
Superior frontal gyrus (BA 8)	L	-15	50	39	4.18	513					
Superior frontal gyrus (BA 9)	R	19	60	24	4.54	1215					
Inferior parietal gyrus (BA 40)	R						55	-48	42	3.64	162
Inferior temporal gyrus (BA 20)	R						46	-7	-34	3.77	567

Peak coordinates obtained at a threshold of P <0.001 and cluster size ≥143 mm³ voxels.
BA: Brodmann Area.

anxiety disorders [32]. Especially the anterior insula has been shown to play an important role in the processing of visceral and autonomic responses to emotional stimuli (for example, [30,74]) and the integration of affective arousal responses with the perception of current physiological states [75]. Although several studies found a differential activation between SAD patients and controls in the insula (for example, [5,8,10,63,66]) others did not (for example, [3,6,13,60,61]). The delayed emergence of insula hyperactivation in SAD patients in the present study might indicate an increased monitoring of bodily states that follows after an initial phase of arousal and hypervigilance during the confrontation with disorder-related video clips. Bodily responses might in turn be monitored in more detail and assessed as well as integrated into cached models of physiological response patterns and stimulus related autobiographic and declarative information about the particular threat. These processes were proposed to contribute to the maintenance of social anxiety [76].

The response pattern of anterior dorsal ACC supports previous findings of increased activation in medial prefrontal cortex areas in response to threatening stimuli or situations in patients with anxiety disorders [32], including SAD patients (for example, [6,8,66], but see [19,37,62]). Our results suggest a time-independent, constant affective-cognitive processing of threat in SAD due to the assumed role of midline regions of prefrontal cortex. This may reflect the special characteristics of the video stimuli used in the present study, but it might in part also indicate greater self-referential and self-regulative processes [23-25] in SAD patients. Generally, individuals suffering from SAD are excessively self-focused [76], which may strongly rely on prefrontal functions [21,77-79]. Heightened self-focused attention seems to cause exaggerated negative self-evaluation, anxiety and arousal, and even social withdrawal [80] and is therefore a potentially relevant mediator for the development and maintenance of SAD.

We would like to note several limitations of our study. We decided to analyze the video-related time courses based on a split-half method and refrained from using finer-grained time scale resolutions for the sake of parsimony. Further studies should investigate the time course of different brain areas with higher temporal resolutions. Furthermore, additional analyses did not reveal significant correlations between enhanced brain activation in the ROIs and symptom severity in SAD patients, suggesting limited clinical relevance of the present findings. The lack of significant correlations might be due to BOLD ceiling effects in SAD during processing of social video clips or varying effectiveness of different categories of video clips for different patients. These points should be investigated with increased sample sizes. Finally, we investigated only one method of symptom provocation.

Our findings might be restricted to the stimuli used here. Future studies should compare different methods of symptom provocation in order to investigate whether similar effects are also present with other designs. Nevertheless, our results suggest that responses in the amygdala, the insula, and other areas might be associated with a specific time course during symptom provocation.

Conclusions

In summary, using a newly developed symptom provocation design, we found different phases of brain activation in SAD patients as compared to controls when exposed to disorder-related and anxiety-provoking *versus* neutral video clips. We found increased amygdala activation during the first half of the video clips and increased insula activation during the second half in SAD patients compared to controls. Activation in medial prefrontal areas was significantly enhanced during the whole exposure period. Our findings support the prominent role of the amygdala in a transient threat detection system and the importance of the insula for prolonged and sustained processing of threat, while the time invariant hyperactivation pattern of anterior dorsal ACC is in accordance with current cognitive models of SAD.

Additional file

Additional file 1: Table S1. Description of the used video clips.

Abbreviations

ANOVA: Analysis of variance; BDI: Beck depression inventory; BOLD: Blood oxygen-level-dependent; ACC: Anterior cingulate cortex; dmPFC: Dorsomedial prefrontal cortex; DSM-IV-TR: Diagnostic and statistical manual of mental disorders, 4. Ed., text revision; fMRI: Functional magnetic resonance imaging; GLM: General linear model; HC: Healthy control; LSAS: Liebowitz social anxiety scale; ROI: Region of interest; SAD: Social anxiety disorder; SCID: Structured clinical interview for DSM-IV; TE: Echo time; TR: Repetition time.

Competing interests

The authors declare that they have no competing interests.

Authors' contributions

SB participated in data collection, data preprocessing, performed the statistical analysis, and drafted the manuscript. AM participated in the design of the study, conducted the study, and was involved in data preprocessing and analysis. MPlB helped in the analysis of the data and to draft the manuscript. WHRM participated in the design of the study and helped to draft the manuscript. TS participated in the design and analysis of the study and drafted the manuscript. All authors read and approved the final manuscript.

Acknowledgments

We are grateful to the actors and the German experts in Clinical Psychology that helped to create the used set of video stimuli (Prof. Ulrich Stangier, Prof. Alexander Gerlach, Prof. Nina Heinrichs, and Prof. Thomas Heidenreich, and Prof. Ulrike Willutzki), and to all participants of the study. This work was partly supported by grants from the Deutsche Forschungsgemeinschaft (Project No. STR 987/3-2; SFB/ TRR 58: C06, C07).

Area-dependent time courses of brain activation during video-induced symptom provocation...

99

References

1. American Psychiatric Association: *Diagnostic and statistical manual of mental disorders (DSM-IV-TR)*. Washington, DC: APA; 2000.
2. Gentili C, Ricciardi E, Gobbini MI, Santarelli MF, Haxby JV, Pietrini P, Guazzelli M: Beyond amygdala: default mode network activity differs between patients with social phobia and healthy controls. *Brain Res Bull* 2009, 79:409–413.
3. Yoon KL, Fitzgerald DA, Angstadt M, McCarron RA, Phan KL: Amygdala reactivity to emotional faces at high and low intensity in generalized social phobia: a 4-Tesla functional MRI study. *Psychiatry Res* 2007, 154:93–98.
4. Blair K, Geraci M, Devido J, McCaffrey D, Chen G, Vythilingam M, Ng P, Hollon N, Jones M, Blair RJ, Pine DS: Neural response to self- and other referential praise and criticism in generalized social phobia. *Arch Gen Psychiatry* 2008, 65:1176–1184.
5. Straube T, Mentzel H, Miltner W: Common and distinct brain activation to threat and safety signals in social phobia. *Neuropsychobiology* 2005, 52:163–168.
6. Phan KL, Fitzgerald DA, Nathan PJ, Tancer ME: Association between amygdala hyperactivity to harsh faces and severity of social anxiety in generalized social phobia. *Biol Psychiatry* 2006, 59:424–429.
7. Schmidt S, Mohr A, Miltner WHR, Straube T: Task-dependent neural correlates of the processing of verbal threat-related stimuli in social phobia. *Biol Psychol* 2010, 84:304–312.
8. Straube T, Kolassa IT, Glauer M, Mentzel H, Miltner W: Effect of task conditions on brain responses to threatening faces in social phobics: an event-related functional magnetic resonance imaging study. *Biol Psychiatry* 2004, 56:921–930.
9. Schulz C, Mothes-Lasch M, Straube T: Automatic neural processing of disorder-related stimuli in social anxiety disorder (SAD): faces and more. *Front Psychol* 2013, 4:282.
10. Boehme S, Ritter V, Tefikow S, Stangier U, Strauss B, Miltner WHR, Straube T: Brain activation during anticipatory anxiety in social anxiety disorder. *Soc Cogn Affect Neurosci* 2013, [Epub ahead of print].
11. Furmark T, Appel L, Henningsson S, Åhs F, Faria V, Linnman C, Pissiota A, Frans Ö, Bani M, Bettica P, Pich EM, Jacobbson E, Wahlstedt K, Oreland L, Langstrom B, Eriksson E, Fredrikson M: A link between serotonin-related gene polymorphisms, amygdala activity, and placebo-induced relief from social anxiety. *J Neurosci* 2008, 28:13066–13074.
12. Furmark T, Appel L, Michelgard A, Wahlstedt K, Ahs F, Zancan S, Jacobsson E, Flyckt K, Grohp M, Bergstrom M, Pich EM, Nilsson LG, Bani M, Langstrom B, Fredrikson M: Cerebral blood flow changes after treatment of social phobia with the neurokinin-1 antagonist GR205171, citalopram, or placebo. *Biol Psychiatry* 2005, 58:132–142.
13. Tillfors M, Furmark T, Marteinsdottir I, Fischer H, Pissiota A, Langstrom B, Fredrikson M: Cerebral blood flow in subjects with social phobia during stressful speaking tasks: a PET study. *Am J Psychiatry* 2001, 158:1220–1226.
14. Furmark T, Tillfors M, Marteinsdottir I, Fischer H, Pissiota A, Langstrom B, Fredrikson M: Common changes in cerebral blood flow in patients with social phobia treated with citalopram or cognitive-behavioral therapy. *Arch Gen Psychiatry* 2002, 59:425–433.
15. Öhman A: The role of the amygdala in human fear: automatic detection of threat. *Psychoneuroendocrinology* 2005, 30:953–958.
16. LeDoux J: The emotional brain, fear, and the amygdala. *Cell Mol Neurobiol* 2003, 23:727–738.
17. Phan KL, Fitzgerald DA, Cortese BM, Seraji-Bozorgzad N, Tancer ME, Moore GJ: Anterior cingulate neurochemistry in social anxiety disorder: 1H-MRS at 4 Tesla. *Neuroreport* 2005, 16:183–186.
18. Campbell DW, Sareen J, Paulus MP, Goldin PR, Stein MB, Reiss JP: Time-varying amygdala response to emotional faces in generalized social phobia. *Biol Psychiatry* 2007, 62:455–463.
19. Blair KS, Geraci M, Smith BW, Hollon N, DeVido J, Otero M, Blair JR, Pine DS: Reduced dorsal anterior cingulate cortical activity during emotional regulation and top-down attentional control in generalized social phobia, generalized anxiety disorder, and comorbid generalized social phobia/generalized anxiety disorder. *Biol Psychiatry* 2012, 72:476–482.
20. Goldin PR, Manber T, Hakimi S, Canli T, Gross JJ: Neural bases of social anxiety disorder: emotional reactivity and cognitive regulation during social and physical threat. *Arch Gen Psychiatry* 2009, 66:170–180.
21. Pessoa L: On the relationship between emotion and cognition. *Nat Rev Neurosci* 2008, 9:148–158.

22. Etkin A, Egner T, Peraza DM, Kandel ER, Hirsch J: Resolving emotional conflict: a role for the rostral anterior cingulate cortex in modulating activity in the amygdala. *Neuron* 2006, 51:871–882.
23. Kalisch R, Wiech K, Critchley HD, Dolan RJ: Levels of appraisal: a medial prefrontal role in high-level appraisal of emotional material. *Neuroimage* 2006, 30:1458–1466.
24. Phan KL, Wager T, Taylor SF, Liberzon I: Functional neuroanatomy of emotion: a meta-analysis of emotion activation studies in PET and fMRI. *Neuroimage* 2002, 16:331–348.
25. Ochsner KN, Beer JS, Robertson ER, Cooper JC, Gabrieli JDE, Kihsltrom JF, D'Esposito M: The neural correlates of direct and reflected self-knowledge. *NeuroImage* 2005, 28:797–814.
26. Northoff G, Heinzel A, de Greck M, Bermpohl F, Dobrowolny H, Panksepp J: Self-referential processing in our brain–a meta-analysis of imaging studies on the self. *NeuroImage* 2006, 31:440–457.
27. Craig AD: How do you feel? Interoception: the sense of the physiological condition of the body. *Nat Rev Neurosci* 2002, 3:655–666.
28. Critchley HD, Mathias CJ, Josephs O, O'Doherty J, Zanini S, Dewar BK, Cipolotti L, Shallice T, Dolan RJ: Human cingulate cortex and autonomic control: converging neuroimaging and clinical evidence. *Brain* 2003, 126:2139–2152.
29. Critchley HD, Wiens S, Rotshtein P, Ohman A, Dolan RJ: Neural systems supporting interoceptive awareness. *Nat Neurosci* 2004, 7:189–195.
30. Critchley HD: The human cortex responds to an interoceptive challenge. *Proc Natl Acad Sci U S A* 2004, 101:6333–6334.
31. Straube T, Miltner WHR: Attention to aversive emotion and specific activation of the right insula and right somatosensory cortex. *NeuroImage* 2011, 54:2534–2538.
32. Etkin A, Wager TD: Functional neuroimaging of anxiety: a meta-analysis of emotional processing in PTSD, social anxiety disorder, and specific phobia. *Am J Psychiatry* 2007, 164:1476–1488.
33. Sladky R, Höflich A, Atanelov J, Kraus C, Baldinger P, Moser E, Lanzenberger R, Windischberger C: Increased neural habituation in the amygdala and orbitofrontal cortex in social anxiety disorder revealed by fMRI. *PLoS One* 2012, 7:e50050.
34. Åhs F, Furmark T, Michelgård Å, Långström B, Appel L, Wolf OT, Kirschbaum C, Fredrikson M: Hypothalamic blood flow correlates positively with stress-induced cortisol levels in subjects with social anxiety disorder. *Psychosom Med* 2006, 68:859–862.
35. Ziv M, Goldin P, Jazaieri H, Hahn K, Gross J: Is there less to social anxiety than meets the eye? behavioral and neural responses to three socio-emotional tasks. *Biol Mood Anxiety Disord* 2013, 3:5.
36. Kilts CD, Kelsey JE, Knight B, Ely TD, Bowman FD, Gross RE, Selvig A, Gordon A, Newport DJ, Nemeroff CB: The neural correlates of social anxiety disorder and response to pharmacotherapy. *Neuropsychopharmacology* 2006, 31:2243–2253.
37. Van Ameringen M, Mancini C, Szechtman H, Nahmias C, Oakman JM, Hall GBC, Pipe B, Farvolden P: A PET provocation study of generalized social phobia. *Psychiatry Res Neuroimaging* 2004, 132:13–18.
38. Furmark T: Social phobia: overview of community surveys. *Acta Psychiatr Scand* 2002, 105:84–93.
39. Wendt J, Lotze M, Weike A, Hosten N, Hamm A: Brain activation and defensive response mobilization during sustained exposure to phobia-related and other affective pictures in spider phobia. *Psychophysiology* 2008, 45:205–215.
40. Wendt J, Schmidt LE, Lotze M, Hamm AO: Mechanisms of change: effects of repetitive exposure to feared stimuli on the brain's fear network. *Psychophysiology* 2012, 49:1319–1329.
41. Wright CI, Fischer H, Whalen PJ, McInerney SC, Shin LM, Rauch SL: Differential prefrontal cortex and amygdala habituation to repeatedly presented emotional stimuli. *NeuroReport* 2001, 12:379–383.
42. Straube T, Mentzel H, Miltner W: Neural mechanisms of automatic and direct processing of phobogenic stimuli in specific phobia. *Biol Psychiatry* 2006, 59:162–170.
43. Stein MB, Simmons AN, Feinstein JS, Paulus MP: Increased amygdala and insula activation during emotion processing in anxiety-prone subjects. *Am J Psychiatry* 2007, 164:318–327.
44. Rauch SL, Savage CR, Alpert NM, Fischman AJ, Jenike MA: The functional neuroanatomy of anxiety: a study of three disorders using positron emission tomography and symptom provocation. *Biol Psychiatry* 1997, 42:446–452.

45. Feinstein JS, Adolphs R, Damasio A, Tranel D: **The human amygdala and the induction and experience of fear.** Curr Biol 2011, **21**:34–38.

46. Rottenberg J, Ray RD, Gross JJ: **Emotion elicitation using films.** In Handbook of emotion elicitation and assessment. Edited by Coan JA, Allen JJB. New York: Oxford University Press; 2007:9–28.

47. Gerrards-Hesse A, Spies K, Hesse FW: **Experimental inductions of emotional states and their effectiveness: a review.** Br J Psychol 1994, **85**:55–78.

48. Fydrich T, Renneberg B, Schmitz B, Wittchen HU: Strukturiertes klinisches interview für DSM-IV, Achse II (Persönlichkeitsstörungen). Göttingen: Hogrefe; 1997.

49. Wittchen H-U, Wunderlich U, Gruschwitz S, Zaudig M: Strukturiertes klinisches interview für DSM-IV, Achse-I (SKID-I). Göttingen: Hogrefe; 1997.

50. Stangier U, Heidenreich T: **Liebowitz social anxiety scale.** In Internationale Skalen für psychiatrie (Internatioal scales for psychiatry). Edited by Scalarum CIP. Weinheim: Beltz; 2005:299–306.

51. Hautzinger M, Bailer M, Worall H, Keller F: Beck-depressions-inventar (BDI). Testhandbuch der deutschen Ausgabe. Bern: Huber; 1995.

52. Talairach J, Tournoux P: Co-planar stereotaxic atlas of the human brain: 3-dimensional proportional system: an approach to cerebral imaging. Stutgart: Thieme; 1988.

53. Eickhoff SB, Heim S, Zilles K, Amunts K: **Testing anatomically specified hypotheses in functional imaging using cytoarchitectonic maps.** Neuroimage 2006, **32**:570–582.

54. Eickhoff SB, Stephan KE, Mohlberg H, Grefkes C, Fink GR, Amunts K, Zilles K: **A new SPM toolbox for combining probabilistic cytoarchitectonic maps and functional imaging data.** Neuroimage 2005, **25**:1325–1335.

55. Maldjian JA, Laurienti PJ, Burdette JH: **Precentral gyrus discrepancy in electronic versions of the Talairach atlas.** Neuroimage 2004, **21**:450–455.

56. Maldjian JA, Laurienti PJ, Kraft RA, Burdette JH: **An automated method for neuroanatomic and cytoarchitectonic atlas-based interrogation of fMRI data sets.** Neuroimage 2003, **19**:1233–1239.

57. Tzourio-Mazoyer N, Landeau B, Papathanassiou D, Crivello F, Etard O, Delcroix N, Mazoyer B, Joliot M: **Automated anatomical labeling of activations in SPM using a macroscopic anatomical parcellation of the MNI MRI single-subject brain.** Neuroimage 2002, **15**:273–289.

58. Lancaster JL, Tordesillas-Gutiérrez D, Martinez M, Salinas F, Evans A, Zilles K, Mazziotta JC, Fox PT: **Bias between MNI and Talairach coordinates analyzed using the ICBM-152 brain template.** Hum Brain Mapp 2007, **28**:1194–1205.

59. Forman SD, Cohen JD, Fitzgerald M, Eddy WF, Mintun MA, Noll DC: **Improved assessment of significant activation in functional magnetic resonance imaging (fMRI): use of a cluster-size threshold.** Magn Reson Med 1995, **33**:636–647.

60. Cooney RE, Atlas LY, Joormann J, Eugene F, Gotlib IH: **Amygdala activation in the processing of neutral faces in social anxiety disorder: is neutral really neutral?** Psychiatry Res 2006, **148**:55–59.

61. Stein M, Goldin P, Sareen J, Zorrilla L, Brown G: **Increased amygdala activation to angry and contemptuous faces in generalized social phobia.** Arch Gen Psychiatry 2002, **59**:1027–1034.

62. Gentili C, Gobbini MI, Ricciardi E, Vanello N, Pietrini P, Haxby JV, Guazzelli M: **Differential modulation of neural activity throughout the distributed neural system for face perception in patients with social phobia and healthy subjects.** Brain Res Bull 2008, **77**:286–292.

63. Shah SG, Klumpp H, Angstadt M, Nathan PJ, Luan Phan K: Amygdala and insula response to emotional images in patients with generalized social anxiety disorder. Ottawa, ON: Canadian Medical Association; 2009.

64. Blair KS, Geraci M, Otero M, Majestic C, Odenheimer S, Jacobs M, Blair RJR, Pine DS: **Atypical modulation of medial prefrontal cortex to self-referential comments in generalized social phobia.** Psychiatry Res Neuroimaging 2011, **193**:38–45.

65. Klumpp H, Angstadt M, Phan KL: **Insula reactivity and connectivity to anterior cingulate cortex when processing threat in generalized social anxiety disorder.** Biol Psychol 2012, **89**:273–276.

66. Amir N, Klumpp H, Elias J, Bedwell JS, Yanasak N, Miller LS: **Increased activation of the anterior cingulate cortex during processing of disgust faces in individuals with social phobia.** Biol Psychiatry 2005, **57**:975–981.

67. Quadflieg S, Mohr A, Mentzel H, Miltner W, Straube T: **Modulation of the neural network involved in the processing of anger prosody: the role of task-relevance and social phobia.** Biol Psychol 2008, **78**:129–137.

68. Tamietto M, de Gelder B: **Neural bases of the non-conscious perception of emotional signals.** Nat Rev Neurosci 2010, **11**:697–709.

69. LeDoux J: **Emotion circuits in the brain.** Annu Rev Neurosci 2000, **23**:155–184.

70. Pessoa L, Adolphs R: **Emotion processing and the amygdala: from a 'low road' to 'many roads' of evaluating biological significance.** Nat Rev Neurosci 2010, **11**:773–783.

71. LeDoux J: **Fear and the brain: where have we been, and where are we going?** Biol Psychiatry 1998, **44**:1229–1238.

72. Öhman A, Mineka S: **Fears, phobias, and preparedness: toward an evolved module of fear and fear learning.** Psychol Rev 2001, **108**:483–522.

73. Lipka J, Miltner W, Straube T: **Vigilance for threat interacts with amygdala responses to subliminal threat cues in specific phobia.** Biological Psychiatry 2011 2011, **70**:472–478.

74. Damasio AR, Grabowski TJ, Bechara A, Damasio H, Ponto LL, Parvizi J, Hichwa RD: **Subcortical and cortical brain activity during the feeling of self-generated emotions.** Nat Neurosci 2000, **3**:1049–1056.

75. Craig AD: **How do you feel – now? The anterior insula and human awareness.** Nat Rev Neurosci 2009, **10**:59–70.

76. Clark DM, Wells A: **A cognitive model of social phobia.** In Social phobia: diagnosis, assessment, and treatment. Edited by Heimberg RG, Liebowitz MR, Hope DA, Schneier FR. New York: Guilford Press; 1995:69–93.

77. Northoff G, Bermpohl F: **Cortical midline structures and the self.** Trends Cogn Sci 2004, **8**:102–107.

78. van der Meer L, Costafreda S, Aleman A, David AS: **Self-reflection and the brain: a theoretical review and meta-analysis of neuroimaging studies with implications for schizophrenia.** Neurosci Biobehav Rev 2010, **34**:935–946.

79. Mitchell JP, Banaji MR, Macrae CN: **The link between social cognition and self-referential thought in the medial prefrontal cortex.** J Cogn Neurosci 2005, **17**:1306–1315.

80. Clark DM, McManus F: **Information processing in social phobia.** Biol Psychiatry 2002, **51**:92–100.

Sex differences in the neurobiology of fear conditioning and extinction: a preliminary fMRI study of shared sex differences with stress-arousal circuitry

Kelimer Lebron-Milad[1*], Brandon Abbs[2], Mohammed R Milad[1], Clas Linnman[1,3], Ansgar Rougemount-Bücking[1,4], Mohammed A Zeidan[1], Daphne J Holt[1] and Jill M Goldstein[1,2]

Abstract

Background: The amygdala, hippocampus, medial prefrontal cortex (mPFC) and brain-stem subregions are implicated in fear conditioning and extinction, and are brain regions known to be sexually dimorphic. We used functional magnetic resonance imaging (fMRI) to investigate sex differences in brain activity in these regions during fear conditioning and extinction.

Methods: Subjects were 12 healthy men comparable to 12 healthy women who underwent a 2-day experiment in a 3 T MR scanner. Fear conditioning and extinction learning occurred on day 1 and extinction recall occurred on day 2. The conditioned stimuli were visual cues and the unconditioned stimulus was a mild electric shock. Skin conductance responses (SCR) were recorded throughout the experiment as an index of the conditioned response. fMRI data (blood-oxygen-level-dependent [BOLD] signal changes) were analyzed using SPM8.

Results: Findings showed no significant sex differences in SCR during any experimental phases. However, during fear conditioning, there were significantly greater BOLD-signal changes in the right amygdala, right rostral anterior cingulate (rACC) and dorsal anterior cingulate cortex (dACC) in women compared with men. In contrast, men showed significantly greater signal changes in bilateral rACC during extinction recall.

Conclusions: These results indicate sex differences in brain activation within the fear circuitry of healthy subjects despite similar peripheral autonomic responses. Furthermore, we found that regions where sex differences were previously reported in response to stress, also exhibited sex differences during fear conditioning and extinction.

Keywords: Sex differences, Fear extinction, Fear conditioning, fMRI, Stress response circuitry

Background

A substantial literature implicates the amygdala, hippocampus, hypothalamus, medial prefrontal cortex (mPFC) and brain-stem nuclei in the generation of fear responses and in the inhibition and extinction of fear. Recent work has suggested that these regions are dysregulated in anxiety disorders [1-4]. Interestingly, these regions have also been shown to be sexually dimorphic [5-7] and to activate differentially in healthy men and women under stress [4] and during learning paradigms [8-10]. Therefore, understanding sex differences could provide some insight into the differences between men and women in the incidence of anxiety disorders.

Sex differences in the fear circuitry have been reported in both animal studies [11-15] and human studies [16-18] using fear conditioning paradigms. However, these results are inconsistent. Although some studies have reported no sex differences [19,20], others have reported that in humans and rodents, males tend to exhibit higher conditioning responses relative to females [21,22]. As for fear extinction, we recently reported data showing that

* Correspondence: kmilad@nmr.mgh.harvard.edu
[1]Department of Psychiatry, Harvard Medical School & Massachusetts General Hospital, 149 13th St, Charlestown, MA, 02129, USA
Full list of author information is available at the end of the article

estradiol significantly enhances extinction recall in fe-male rats and in women [23]. We have also previously reported sex differences during fear conditioning and fear extinction in humans [17] and in rodents [24]. The modulation of arousal by estradiol is consistent with Goldstein and colleagues' finding of sex differences in the stress response circuitry of the healthy brain [4], which shares brain regions with fear circuitry. However, the neurobiological mechanisms underlying sex differences shared in fear and stress response circuitries have not been previously reported.

Sex differences in the function of the healthy adult brain during a visual stress challenge in a functional magnetic resonance imaging (fMRI) environment has been studied by Goldstein and colleagues. These authors reported that men, compared with women in the late follicular menstrual phase, showed greater blood-oxygenation-level-dependent [25] signal changes in the amygdala, anterior cingulate cortex (ACC), orbi-tofrontal cortex (OFC), medial prefrontal cortex (mPFC), hippocampus, anterior hypothalamus and periaqueductal gray [4]. These findings were distinct from comparisons of the same women imaged during the early follicular phase [26], suggesting that circulating sex-steroid hormones par-tially accounted for sex differences in brain activity in these regions [4], which is consistent with other fMRI studies using arousing stimuli [27]. Goldstein's reported BOLD-signal differences [4] were in the same ventral mPFC (vmPFC) region as our previous study of the fear circuitry [28], suggesting anatomical overlap between sex differences in arousal due to stress and fear.

In the present study, we used fMRI and a fear condition-ing and extinction paradigm to investigate sex differences in the fear circuitry of healthy subjects, extending regions of interest [29] to include those that previous work has identified as part of the stress-response circuitry [4]. Our rationale is based on the idea that arousal is a component of fear and stress, suggesting that they share brain circuitry that is highly sexually dimorphic. Thus, we predict similar sex differences in this circuitry whether arousal is caused by fear or stress-related stimuli. The approach of investi-gating shared brain circuitry across behavioral domains and psychiatric illnesses is in line with the recent NIMH strategic plan associated with the development of the Re-search Domain Criteria [30,31].

Subjects participated in a previously established 2-day fear conditioning and extinction paradigm [32]. Condi-tioning and extinction took place on day 1, and extinc-tion recall took place on day 2. Skin conductance response (SCR) was measured as an autonomic index of fear responses, and all testing took place in a 3T fMRI scanner. Based on previous studies, we hypothesized sig-nificant sex differences in brain activity in fear responses in the amygdala, vmPFC, and hippocampus during fear

conditioning, extinction learning, and extinction recall. We predicted that healthy men would exhibit greater ac-tivity in these arousal-mediating regions than women. More specifically, we predicted that men would exhibit greater activation in the vmPFC and hippocampus and less activation in the amygdala and dACC during extinc-tion recall. Regarding fear conditioning, we predicted greater amygdala and dACC activations in women com-pared with men and greater vmPFC activation in men compared with women.

Methods
Subjects
The sample consisted of 12 healthy women and 12 healthy men who were recruited from the local commu-nity via advertisements for two previously published neu-roimaging studies [28,33] and reanalyzed to test our hypotheses. One of the original studies was not initially designed to investigate sex differences in fear extinction, therefore women were in different phases of the men-strual cycle (4 follicular phase, 4 late luteal phase, 4 un-known). Table 1 shows that subjects are right-handed and primarily Caucasian with a relatively high education level (at least some college, on average). Men were older and had more years of education. We controlled for these differences when comparing males and females (see below).

Subjects were excluded if they had neurologic, endocri-nologic, or other medical conditions affecting central nervous system function. Subjects were also screened for Axis-I psychiatric disorders, including substance-use dis-orders, using the Structured Clinical Interview for DSM-IV [34]. There were no significant sex differences in anx-iety measures (see Table 1). No participant was using psychoactive or other potentially confounding drugs or

Table 1 Demographics information about the study subjects

	Female (n = 12)	Males (n = 12)	P=
Age	22.1(SD: 2.6)	26(SD: 5.0)	0.02
Years of Education	15.4(SD: 1.4)	16.8(SD: 1.8)	0.04
Ethnicity			
Caucasian	10	11	
Asian	2	0	
Hisp/Black	0	1	
Behavioral measure of anxiety			
STAI T	30.6(SD: 6.1)	33.1(SD: 1.8)	0.5
STAI S	31.5(SD: 9.4)	29.8(SD: 6.2)	0.6
Phases of menstrual cycle			
Luteal	4	N/A	
Follicular	4	N/A	
unknown	4		

medications, and women had abstained from oral contraceptives or hormone replacement for at least three months. After a complete description of the procedures, written informed consent was obtained from all subjects in accordance with the requirements of the Partners Healthcare Human Research Committee.

Conditioning and extinction procedure

The two-day fear conditioning and extinction procedures have been described elsewhere [35] (see Figure 1). Briefly, two digital photographs of rooms (an office and a library) were the visual contexts in which a lamp was switched from the off position (no color) to one of three colored lights (red, yellow, blue), constituting the conditioned stimuli (CSs). All images were displayed on a computer monitor located approximately two feet behind the subject and viewed on a mirror while the subject was in a 3 T MRI scanner. The unconditioned stimulus (US) was a 500 ms electric shock delivered through electrodes attached to the second and third fingers of the right hand. The subjects had previously selected a shock intensity they found "highly annoying but not painful" [36,37]. The electrodes were attached to the fingers during each phase of the study, but the US was presented only during conditioning. On day 1, subjects underwent the habituation phase in which the conditioning context and the extinction context were displayed four times while each CS was presented two to three times. In the conditioning phase, the (to later be) extinguished conditioned stimulus (CS + E) and the (to later not be extinguished) conditioned stimulus (unextinguished CS + or CS + U) were each presented eight

times with 62.5% partial reinforcement (five shocks each), while the conditioned stimulus that was never followed by a shock (CS-) was intermingled and presented 16 times. All CSs were presented in the same context. The selection of CS + and CS- colors was pseudorandom and counterbalanced across subjects. After conditioning, subjects were briefly interviewed to ensure the CS-US pattern was observed. All subjects were aware of the CS-US contingency. The extinction phase immediately followed in which the CS + E and the CS- were each shown 16 times in a new, "safe" context. On day 2, the recall phase was in the extinction context and included the presentation of the CS + U along with the CS + E and CS-.

Psychophysiological measures

During each trial, the context images were presented for nine seconds: three seconds with the light off immediately followed by six seconds in combination with the CS. The mean inter-trial interval was 15 seconds. Skin conductance responses (SCR) were calculated by subtracting the maximum response during cue presentation from the average response of the two seconds immediately preceding context onset. The SCR values were then square-root transformed to reduce heteroscedasticity. Skin conductance levels [38] were measured during the five seconds preceding the onset of each habituation session trial and then averaged across eight trials to yield a baseline SCL.

To evaluate the amount of fear during the different phases of the experiment, SCR to the CS + and SCR to the CS- were compared as follows: during conditioning,

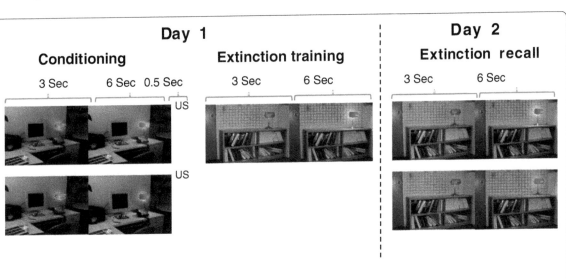

Figure 1 Illustration of the experimental fear conditioning and extinction protocol used in our experiment. Adapted from Zeidan et al., 2011. Note that the CS- (represented in a third color of light (yellow) is not shown in this figure for simplicity.

SCR to the CS + was compared to CS-; during extinction, SCR to the CS + E was compared to CS-; and during extinction recall, SCR to the CS + E was compared to CS + U. All data are reported as means ± the standard error of the mean (S.E.). A repeated-measures analysis of variance [39] was used to analyze data across experimental phases. A Student's *t*-test was used when appropriate.

Image acquisition

Image acquisition parameters were identical to previous reports [28,40,41]. A Trio 3.0-Tesla whole-body, high-speed imaging device with a 12-channel gradient head coil was used (Siemens Medical Systems, Iselin, New Jersey). An automated scout image was obtained and shimming procedures were performed followed by high-resolution, three-dimensional magnetization prepared rapid gradient echo sequences (repetition time [TR]/echo time [TE]/flip angle = 7.25 ms/3 ms/7°; 1 mm X 1 mm in plane X 1.3 mm), which were collected for spatial normalization and positioning the subsequent scans. Registration of individual functional scans was based on T1 (TR/TE/flip angle = 8 sec/39 msec/90°) and T2 (TR/TE/flip angle = 10 sec/48 msec/120°) sequences. fMRI images were acquired with gradient–echo T2*-weighted sequences (TR/TE/flip angle = 3 sec/30 msec/90°). The T1, T2, and gradient-echo functional images were all collected in the same plane (45 coronal oblique slices parallel to the anterior-posterior commissure line, tilted 30° anterior) with the same slice thickness (3 mm X 3 mm X 3 mm) except for the T1 (1 mm X 1 mm X 1 mm).

Functional MRI data analysis

Each subject's functional time series was first examined for global-signal artifacts (e.g., artifact caused by head movement) using the Artifact Detection Tool (ART) software package (http://web.mit.edu/swg/art/art.pdf) in order to control for this artifact during first-level statistical analyses. "Outlier" volumes were flagged if the average global-signal intensity of the image (i.e., average signal intensity across all voxels) was more than 3.0 standard deviations from the overall mean for all images (ART z-threshold = 3.0), the scan-to-scan translation movement was more than 0.6 mm or the scan-to-scan rotation movement was more than 0.004 radians. Once flagged, outlier volumes were modeled as regressors of no interest in the first-level general linear model (GLM) following standard fMRI pre-processing procedures using SPM8 software (http://www.fil.ion.ucl.ac.uk/spm/software/spm8).

For this pre-processing procedure, images from each functional run were first slice-timing corrected and realigned to the first image of the run. This procedure generated realignment parameters for each run that were also used as covariates of no interest in the first-level

GLM, as well as a mean image for each run. These mean images and the MPRAGE were then co-registered to the mean image of the first imaging run to facilitate later transformation of the series into MNI space. Next, the MPRAGE was segmented and spatially normalized to the T1 MNI305 template included in SPM8 (Montreal Neurological Institute, MNI). The resulting spatial-transformation parameters were applied to the EPI time series to transform them to the common anatomical coordinate space (MNI305), and voxels were re-sliced to a dimension of 2 mm isotropic. Finally, to mitigate the effects of residual spatial-transformation noise, the normalized functional images were smoothed using an 8 mm full-width-at-half-maximum Gaussian kernel.

For the first level GLM, we used an epoch model and modeled context and CS as three-second and six-second events, respectively. During conditioning, we modeled the US as a 0.5-second event. Experimental regressors were convolved with the SPM canonical hemodynamic response function (HRF), but the regressors of no interest (i.e. outliers and motion parameters) were not convolved. The time series was subjected to a 128-second high-pass filter to correct for low-frequency signal drift.

First-level statistical parametric maps were calculated using the general linear model for the contrast of interest across the time window [23]. The Stimulus Factor contrasted all 16 CS + trials vs. all 16 CS- trials in the conditioning phase (CS+ > CS-), the last 4 CS + E trials vs. the last 4 CS- trials in the extinction learning phase (CS + E > CS-), and the first 4 CS + E versus the first 4 CS + U trials in the extinction recall phase (CS + E > CS + U). The first four trials were used for extinction recall because we wanted to minimize any confound introduced by additional extinction learning during this phase, and electrophysiological data from rodents indicates that the vmPFC only signals extinction recall during the beginning of extinction recall [42].

First-level SPM contrasts were then grouped during second-level independent-groups t-tests that compared men and women using age and years of education as covariates. For this analysis, we used an uncorrected voxel-level statistical threshold of p < 0.005, and we report only peak-voxels from clusters of activation within our primary anatomical regions of interest (ROIs; vmPFC, insula, dACC, amygdala, and hippocampus). This statistical threshold was used given our focus on specific anatomical ROIs based on prior studies' findings and *a priori* hypotheses about where sex differences in brain activation should be found. Following this analysis focusing on previously identified fear conditioning circuitry regions, we conducted a stringent functional-ROI analysis of sex differences in stress-response circuitry regions during fear conditioning.

Functional ROI construction

Given our hypothesis that the brain's stress-response circuitry and fear conditioning circuitry partly overlap, sex differences found in previous fMRI studies of the stress-response circuitry should also be apparent during fear conditioning. We identified *a priori* anatomical ROIs using Goldstein and colleagues findings [4,26] of functional sex differences in the following regions during an emotional arousal task that activates the stress-response circuitry: orbitofrontal cortex (OFC), anterior cingulate cortex (ACC), the periaqueductal gray brain stem area [43], hippocampus (HIPP), anterior hypothalamus (HYP), and amygdala (AMG). However, shared functional sex differences within a broad anatomical area (particularly OFC and ACC) do not necessarily suggest any similar function for these regions in both paradigms. Therefore, we further limited our search within these anatomical regions to functional ROIs (spheres) around Goldstein's (2010) exact coordinates (Table 2). To do this, we created either 8 mm (cortical rois) or 4 mm (subcortical ROIs) spheres using the WFU Pickatlas tool for SPM8. We then examined sex differences in these spheres with an initial uncorrected voxel-level threshold of $p < .05$, which was corrected to a FWE p-value of $p < .05$ using small-volume correction. To characterize activation magnitude differences in both anatomical and functional ROIs, we calculated the average GLM beta value for each ROI by averaging across the beta value for all voxels within an ROI.

Results

Psychophysiology during conditioning, extinction, and extinction recall

Men and women showed differential conditioning. An ANOVA conducted on the SCR data revealed a significant Stimulus main effect ($F_{(1,22)} = 30.2$, $p < 0.001$) with greater responses to the CS+ than to CS- (first 4 trials of each type during conditioning) in women and men, indicating that both were able to learn the CS-US association. No significant main effects of Group ($F_{(1,22)} = 2.9$, $p = 0.11$) or Group X Stimulus interaction ($F_{(1,22)} = 0.57$, $p = 0.81$) were observed, indicating no significant sex differences in SCR during conditioning, even though males showed higher SCR than females but not significantly so (see group effect above, at $p = .11$) (see Figure 2A).

During extinction training on day 1, an ANOVA for the late extinction SCR data (last 4 CS+E vs. last 4 CS- trials) revealed no significant main effect of Stimulus ($F_{(1,21)} = 0.21$, $p = 0.65$) or Group ($F_{(1,21)} = 2.23$, $p = 0.09$) and no significant Group X Stimulus interaction ($F_{(1,21)} = 0.14$, $p = 0.71$), suggesting that comparable extinction learning had been achieved in both groups (data not shown). An ANOVA for the early extinction recall SCR data (first 4 CS+E vs. first 4 CS+U trials) also revealed no significant main effects of Stimulus ($F_{(1,22)} = 3.19$, $p = 0.09$),

Table 2 Coordinates from Goldstein et al. (2010) used in the anatomical ROI analysis

Region	X	Y	Z
Dorsal ACG			
R. BA 32	12	34	28
R. BA 32	14	16	26
R. BA 24	4	18	20
L. BA 32	−2	18	20
L. BA 32	−2	22	28
Medial PFC			
R. BA 10	20	66	10
R. BA 10	34	58	−4
L. BA 10	−4	64	20
Ventral mPFC			
R. BA 10	4	54	−8
L. BA 10	−4	42	−20
OFC - BA 1			
	2	40	−22
Amygdala			
Right	18	−2	−14
Left	−18	−4	−14
Hippocampus			
Right	30	−24	−8
Left*	−30	−24	−8
Hypothalamus			
Right*	4	2	−6
Left	−4	2	−26
Periaqueductal Gray			
	0	−30	−2

*Goldstein et al. (2010) did not report significant bi-lateral activation in these regions. Given the role of laterality in fear conditioning in these regions, we created ROIs in the contralateral hemisphere of Goldstein and colleague's significant findings.

Group ($F_{(1,22)} = 2.33$, $p = 0.14$) or Group X Stimulus Interaction ($F_{(1,22)} = 0.37$, $p = 0.55$) (Figure 3A). Analyses of the extinction retention index, which controls for the level of fear acquired during the conditioning phase [23], revealed no significant group differences in extinction retention confirming that no significant differences between groups during extinction recall (data not shown). Collectively, we did not observe any statistically significant differences between men and women in our psychophysiological measures during any experimental phase. It is important to note that several statistical sex difference trends were observed with men tending to show higher SCR to the CSs throughout conditioning and extinction even though the differences were not statistically significant.

Blood-oxygen-level dependent (BOLD) responses in anatomical ROIs

During fear conditioning, females responded to the conditioned stimulus with significantly greater activation,

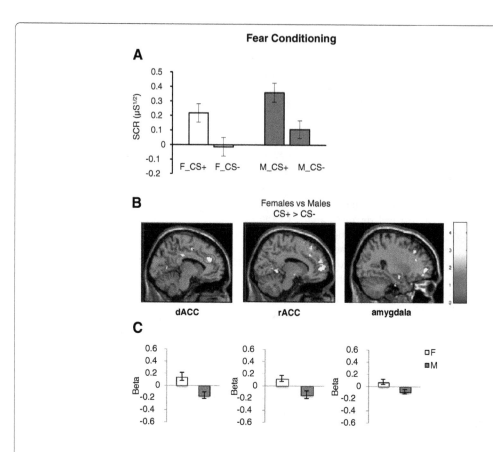

Figure 2 Differences between men and women in psychophysiological and BOLD measures during fear acquisition. **A.** Skin conductance responses (SCR) averaged across the first 4 conditioning trials for the conditioned stimulus that was reinforced, i.e. paired with the shock (CS+) and for the conditioned stimulus not paired with the shock (CS-). **B.** BOLD activation to the CS + vs. CS- contrasting Females vs. Males during fear conditioning is shown. **C.** Mean beta weights extracted from the dorsal anterior cingulate cortex (dACC), rostral anterior cingulate (rACC), and amygdala are shown, to illustrate the direction of activation within group. The threshold display for the maps in B is p < 0.01, uncorrected. M = males; F = females.

relative to males, in the following *a priori* anatomical regions of interest: the dACC, rACC, and the amygdala (see Table 3 for coordinates and statistical results and figure 2B). The average beta values for these ROIs (extracted from the between-group activation maps) show that these sex differences were present in dACC, mPFC and amygdala activation in females and deactivation in males (see Figure 2C).

We did not observe any significant sex differences in our anatomical ROIs during the extinction learning phase. During extinction recall, greater activation in the rostral region of the left rostral ACC (rACC) was observed in males relative to females. A trend in the same direction was also observed in the right rACC, which corresponds to a similar trend in right vmPFC [(6, 34, 0); z = 2.76, p = 0.006]. Additionally, greater insula activation was observed in females relative to males (see Figure 3B, Table 3). The average beta values from rACC

showed that males were activating the rACC while females were deactivating this region. In contrast, females were activating insula, while males were deactivating this region (see Figure 3C).

BOLD responses from functional ROI analysis

We extended our ROI analyses based on the anatomy of the fear-conditioning circuitry by conducting an analysis based on previously reported [4] functional sex differences in the stress-response circuitry, such as the anterior hypothalamus. These data are summarized in Table 3. Although we found sex differences in the fear conditioning circuitry in our anatomical ROIs, no significant sex differences were observed in functional stress-response ROIs (data not shown). Conversely, Table 3 shows that during extinction learning (when no sex differences in fear circuitry were found), males showed significantly greater activation in right hypothalamus, and

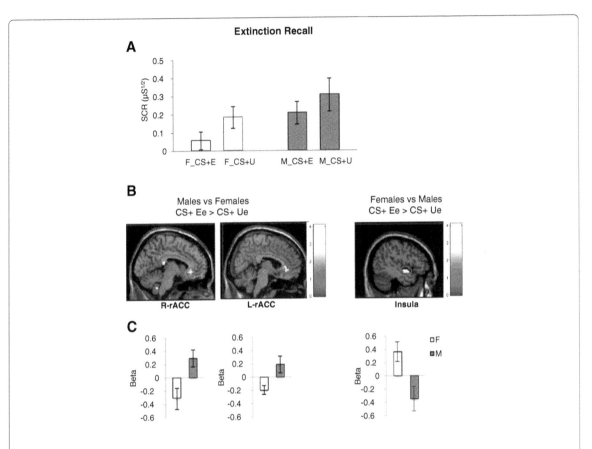

Figure 3 Differences between men and women in psychophysiological and BOLD measures during extinction memory recall.
A. Skin conductance responses (SCR) averaged across the first 4 extinction recall trials for the extinguished stimulus (CS + E) compared to the unextinguished stimulus (CS + U). **B.** BOLD activation to the CS + E vs. CS + U contrasting Females vs. Males during extinction recall are shown. **C.** Mean beta weights extracted from the left and right rostral ACC and insula are shown, to illustrate the direction of activation within group. The threshold for the maps in B is p < 0.01, uncorrected. M = males; F = females.

females showed greater activation in left hypothalamus, dACC, and mPFC. Lastly, extinction recall showed sex differences in fear and stress-response circuitry, as males exhibited significantly higher signal changes relative to females in our functional ROIs (Table 3).

Discussion

In this study, we used fMRI to investigate sex differences in BOLD-signal changes of healthy subjects exposed to a fear conditioning and fear extinction paradigm. No statistically significant sex differences in SCRs were observed during any experimental phase. However, we note that men exhibited a trend towards generally elevated SCRs during acquisition of conditioned fear responses and the extinction recall test. Regarding the BOLD responses, we observed significant sex differences in several brain regions during fear conditioning and extinction recall. Specifically, during fear conditioning,

women showed greater activation in dACC, rACC and amygdala relative to men. During extinction recall, women showed greater activation in the insula cortex relative to men, while men showed greater activation in the rACC region of the mPFC relative to women. Moreover, we found that regions where sex differences were previously identified in response to stress [4] also exhibited sex differences during fear conditioning and extinction, including the anterior hypothalamus.

Sex differences at the behavioral level have been reported in humans and rodents across a number of paradigms such as fear conditioning, active avoidance, conditioned taste aversion and eye blink conditioning [14]. Some studies report increased conditioned responding in males rats during fear learning [21], which is consistent with our findings of sex differences in SCR, whereas others found no significant sex differences in fear acquisition [20]. We previously reported that men show elevated conditioned

Table 3 BOLD responses from both our anatomical ROI analyses and our functional ROI analyses comparing males and women during the different phases of the study

Bold responses from anatomical ROI analyses

Phase	condition	regions	coordinates	z	P(≤)
conditioning	F > M	L-dACC	−8,38,26	3.54	0.001
		R-rACC	12,58,4	3.44	0.001
		Amyg	28,-6,-16	3.08	0.001
	M > F	non			
Ext learning	F > M	non			
	M > F	non			
Ext Recall	F > M	L-insula	−46,-2,-10	3.15	0.002
	M > F	L-rACC	−6,32,-4	2.79	0.005

BOLD responses from functional ROI analyses

Conditioning	F > M	non			
	M > F	non			
Ext Learning	F > M	dACC	8,12,18	3.62	0.001
		dACC	10,14,20	3.27	0.001
		mPFC	28,54,-4	3.33	0.001
		L-hypotha	−8,2,-6	2.25	0.024
	M < F	hypothalamus	6,4,-6	2.44	0.015
Ext Recall	F > M	non			
	M > F	L-rACC	−6,42,-16	3.16	0.001

ROIs are based on sexually dimorphic areas of the stress response circuitry identified by Goldstein and colleagues (2010).

fear responses relative to women [17,23]. While not statistically significant in this study, men exhibited a trend towards elevated conditioned fear responses. The lack of a statistically significant different sex difference may be due to variability of endocrine status or use of contraceptives among the women in our sample. That is, we recently demonstrated that estradiol significantly enhances fear extinction recall and its neural correlates during fear extinction [33], and others have reported that contraceptives can impact learning and memory [44]. Moreover, it has been shown that estradiol facilitated contextual fear extinction via estradiol's effect on hippocampal long-term potentiation in rats [45]. One important caveat is that in our data, men also showed a trend towards increased skin conductance responses to the CS- compared with the women. This would suggest enhanced general skin conductance reactivity in men relative to women that may not be specific to fear learning or extinction per se given that they are higher across conditions. Future studies will need to further investigate the role of sex-steroid hormones in understanding variability due to gender during conditioning and the neural responses of the fear extinction network.

Using an anatomical ROI analysis approach, we observed sex differences in fear circuitry activation. Women exhibited greater amygdala, mPFC and dACC

activation during fear acquisition and greater insula activation during extinction recall. In contrast, men showed significantly greater activation within the rACC, which is in close proximity to the locus we previously reported showing increased activation during fear extinction [35,46,47]. The mPFC and dACC have been implicated in pain processing, conflict monitoring and error processing, fear expression, and appraisal of emotionally salient stimuli [41,48-50]. The amygdala is also well known for signaling novelty and mediating emotional learning such as fear conditioning [51]. The vmPFC has been implicated in emotion regulation and fear extinction recall [2,52]. The increased mPFC activation in men during extinction recall predicted facilitated fear extinction recall in men and fear responses in women, and the increased amygdala and dACC activation in women during fear conditioning again predicted facilitated fear responses in women during this phase. The behavioral data showed lack of sex differences in fear responses. Thus brain activity *differences* in neural responses may be contributing to producing *similar* behavioral responses suggesting that men and women use different neural strategies to produce homeostasis in the brain in response to fear. This was similar to Goldstein's previous findings of sex differences in neural responses to stress to maintain homeostasis in the brain in response to stress, which was dependent on menstrual cycle phase in the women [4]. Further studies are needed to explore whether men and women use different neural networks to acquire and control fear to a similar degree.

In fact, the functional ROI analyses revealed overlap between sex differences in stress-arousal circuitry activation and sex differences in fear-arousal circuitry reported here. For example, Goldstein and colleagues [4] reported that men, compared with women in the late follicular menstrual cycle phase, exhibited significantly greater BOLD-signal changes in response to negative versus neutral stimuli in ACC, OFC, mPFC, anterior hypothalamus, hippocampus and periaqueductal gray. Although the regions of activation overlap, data from the present study indicated that women exhibited significantly greater BOLD-signal changes, compared to men, during fear conditioning in a number of these brain regions. However, no women in the current study were scanned during the mid-cycle menstrual phase, as distinct from all women in the Goldstein study who contributed to the sex difference effect were scanned during this phase. Men in both studies showed hyperactivation in vmPFC, other orbitofrontal regions, and right hypothalamus. In our study, hyperactivation was observed during extinction recall even without controlling for menstrual cycle phase. The differences between our findings and those reported by Goldstein and colleagues may be due to differences in levels of sex hormones, particularly estradiol and/or progesterone [33], but this hypothesis needs further investigation. Nevertheless, the approach underscores the importance of analyzing sex differences in shared brain circuitry across behavioral domains for understanding psychiatric disorders.

Conclusions

In summary, we present data showing sex differences in the functional responses of the fear-response circuitry during fear conditioning and extinction recall that overlap in location with previously reported sex differences in the functional response of the stress-response circuitry during arousal. Although sex differences at the neural level (i.e., BOLD-signal change) were robust, differences at the psychophysiological level (i.e., SCR) were less reliable or non-existent. Future studies examining the influence of sex hormones such as estradiol, progesterone and testosterone on sex differences are needed to further advance this line of research.

List of Abbreviations

mPFC, medial prefrontal cortex; fMRI, functional magnetic resonance imaging; SCR, skin conductance responses; BOLD, blood-oxygenated-level-dependent; SPM8, Statistical Parametric Mapping 8; ACC, anterior cingulate cortex; rACC, rostral anterior cingulated cortex; OFC, orbitofrontal cortex; vmPFC, ventral medial prefrontal cortex; CS, conditioned stimulus; US, unconditioned stimulus; CS + E, extinguished conditioned stimulus; CS + U, unextinguished conditioned stimulus; CS, conditioned stimulus that was never paired with US; SCL, skin conductance levels; ANOVA, repeated-measures analyses of variance; 3 T, 3 tesla; GLM, general linear model; ROIs, regions of interest; PAG, periaqueductal gray; HIPP, hippocampus; HYP, anterior hypothalamus; AMG, amygdala; dACC, dorsal anterior cingulate cortex.

Competing interest

Dr. Mohammed R Milad received consulting fees from Microtranspondor for a project unrelated to the one described in this manuscript. The remaining authors declare no conflicts of interest.

Acknowledgements

Dr. Kelimer Milad's time for this study was originally supported by NIMH RO1 MH56956 (JMG, PI parent grant), Administrative Supplement (for KM postdoctoral fellowship, 2008–2010). Data collection was supported by NIMH K01MH080346 to M.R.M. Dr. Goldstein's time was supported by ORWH-NIMH P50 MH082679 (JMG, P.I.). Data collection was also supported by 1UL1 RR025758-01, Harvard Clinical and Translational Science Center from NIH NCRR.

Author details

[1]Department of Psychiatry, Harvard Medical School & Massachusetts General Hospital, 149 13th St, Charlestown, MA, 02129, USA. [2]Departments of Psychiatry and Medicine, Harvard Medical School, Connors Center for Women's Health and Gender Biology, Brigham and Women's Hospital, 75 Francis St., Boston, MA, 02120, USA. [3]P.A.I.N. Group, Department of Anesthesia, Children's Hospital, Boston, MA, , USA. [4]Department of Psychiatry, Centre Hospitalier Universitaire Vaudois and University of Lausanne, 7 rue Saint-Martin1003, Lausanne, Switzerland.

Authors' contributions

All authors have made substantive intellectual contributions to the study. All authors contributed to: 1) the conception and design of the study, or acquisition of data, or analyses and interpretations of data; 2) drafting the manuscript or revising it critically for important intellectual content, and 3) final approval of the version to be publish.

References

1. Shin LM, Whalen PJ, Pitman RK, Bush G, Macklin ML, Lasko NB, Orr SP, McInerney SC, Rauch SL: An fMRI study of anterior cingulate function in posttraumatic stress disorder. BiolPsychiatry 2001, 50:932–942.
2. Graham BM, Milad MR: The Study of Fear Extinction: Implications for Anxiety Disorders. Am J Psychiatry 2011, 168:1255–1265.
3. Hettema JM, Kettenmann B, Ahluwalia V, McCarthy C, Kates WR, Schmitt JE, Silberg JL, Neale MC, Kendler KS, Fatouros P: Pilot multimodal twin imaging study of generalized anxiety disorder. Depress Anxiety 2011 (Epub ahead if print).
4. Goldstein JM, Jerram M, Abbs B, Whitfield-Gabrieli S, Makris N: Sex differences in stress response circuitry activation dependent on female hormonal cycle. J Neurosci 2010, 30:431–438.
5. Goldstein JM, Seidman LJ, Horton NJ, Makris N, Kennedy DN, Caviness VS Jr, Faraone SV, Tsuang MT: Normal sexual dimorphism of the adult human brain assessed by in vivo magnetic resonance imaging. CerebCortex 2001, 11:490–497.
6. Mong JA, Glaser E, McCarthy MM: Gonadal steroids promote glial differentiation and alter neuronal morphology in the developing hypothalamus in a regionally specific manner. J Neurosci 1999, 19:1464–1472.
7. Arnold AP, Gorski RA: Gonadal steroid induction of structural sex differences in the central nervous system. Annu Rev Neurosci 1984, 7:413–442.
8. Cahill L, Uncapher M, Kilpatrick L, Alkire MT, Turner J: Sex-related hemispheric lateralization of amygdala function in emotionally influenced memory: an FMRI investigation. LearnMem 2004, 11:261–266.
9. Canli T, Gabrieli JD: Imaging gender differences in sexual arousal. NatNeurosci 2004, 7:325–326.
10. Goldstein JM, Jerram M, Poldrack R, Anagnoson R, Breiter HC, Makris N, Goodman JM, Tsuang MT, Seidman LJ: Sex differences in prefrontal cortical brain activity during fMRI of auditory verbal working memory. Neuropsychology 2005, 19:509–519.
11. Baran SE, Armstrong CE, Niren DC, Hanna JJ, Conrad CD: Chronic stress and sex differences on the recall of fear conditioning and extinction. NeurobiolLearnMem 2009, 91:323–332.
12. Milad MR, Igoe SA, Lebron-Milad K, Novales JE: Estrous cycle phase and gonadal hormones influence conditioned fear extinction. Neuroscience 2009, 164:887–895.
13. Gupta RR, Sen S, Diepenhorst LL, Rudick CN, Maren S: Estrogen modulates sexually dimorphic contextual fear conditioning and hippocampal long-term potentiation (LTP) in rats(1). Brain Res 2001, 888:356–365.
14. Dalla C, Shors TJ: Sex differences in learning processes of classical and operant conditioning. Physiol Behav 2009, 97:229–238.
15. Ribeiro AM, Barbosa FF, Godinho MR, Fernandes VS, Munguba H, Melo TG, Barbosa MT, Eufrasio RA, Cabral A, Izidio GS, Silva RH: Sex differences in aversive memory in rats: possible role of extinction and reactive emotional factors. Brain Cogn 2010, 74:145–151.
16. Merz CJ, Tabbert K, Schweckendiek J, Klucken T, Vaitl D, Stark R, Wolf OT: Investigating the impact of sex and cortisol on implicit fear conditioning with fMRI. Psychoneuroendocrinology 2010, 35:33–46.
17. Milad MR, Goldstein JM, Orr SP, Wedig MM, Klibanski A, Pitman RK, Rauch SL: Fear conditioning and extinction: influence of sex and menstrual cycle in healthy humans. BehavNeurosci 2006, 120:1196–1203.
18. Felmingham K, Williams LM, Kemp AH, Liddell B, Falconer E, Peduto A, Bryant R: Neural responses to masked fear faces: sex differences and trauma exposure in posttraumatic stress disorder. J Abnorm Psychol 2010, 119:241–247.
19. Wiltgen BJ, Sanders MJ, Ferguson C, Homanics GE, Fanselow MS: Trace fear conditioning is enhanced in mice lacking the delta subunit of the GABAA receptor. LearnMem 2005, 12:327–333.
20. Zorawski M, Cook CA, Kuhn CM, LaBar KS: Sex, stress, and fear: individual differences in conditioned learning. Cogn Affect Behav Neurosci 2005, 5:191–201.
21. Maren S, De Oca B, Fanselow MS: Sex differences in hippocampal long-term potentiation (LTP) and Pavlovian fear conditioning in rats: positive correlation between LTP and contextual learning. Brain Res 1994, 661:25–34.
22. Aguilar R, Gil L, Gray JA, Driscoll P, Flint J, Dawson GR, Gimenez-Llort L, Escorihuela RM, Fernandez-Teruel A, Tobena A: Fearfulness and sex in F2 Roman rats: males display more fear though both sexes share the same fearfulness traits. Physiol Behav 2003, 78:723–732.

23. Milad MR, Zeidan MA, Contero A, Pitman RK, Klibanski A, Rauch SL, Goldstein JM: The influence of gonadal hormones on conditioned fear extinction in healthy humans. *Neuroscience* 2010, 168:652–658.

24. Milad MR, Igoe SA, Lebron-Milad K, Novales JE: Estrous cycle phase and gonadal hormones influence conditioned fear extinction. *Neuroscience* 2009, 164:887–895.

25. Rosenbaum JF, Biederman J, Hirshfeld DR, Bolduc EA, Faraone SV, Kagan J, Snidman N, Reznick JS: Further evidence of an association between behavioral inhibition and anxiety disorders: results from a family study of children from a non-clinical sample. *JPsychiatrRes* 1991, 25:49–65.

26. Goldstein JM, Jerram M, Poldrack R, Ahern T, Kennedy DN, Seidman LJ, Makris N: Hormonal cycle modulates arousal circuitry in women using functional magnetic resonance imaging. *JNeurosci* 2005, 25:9309–9316.

27. Protopopescu X, Pan H, Altemus M, Tuescher O, Polanecsky M, McEwen B, Silbersweig D, Stern E: Orbitofrontal cortex activity related to emotional processing changes across the menstrual cycle. *Proc Natl Acad Sci USA* 2005, 102:16060–16065.

28. Milad MR, Wright CI, Orr SP, Pitman RK, Quirk GJ, Rauch SL: Recall of fear extinction in humans activates the ventromedial prefrontal cortex and hippocampus in concert. *BiolPsychiatry* 2007, 62:446–454.

29. Uejima A, Amano T, Nomura N, Noro M, Yasue T, Shiroishi T, Ohta K, Yokoyama H, Tamura K: Anterior shift in gene expression precedes anteriormost digit formation in amniote limbs. *Dev Growth Differ* 2010, 52:223–234.

30. Foa EB, Rothbaum BO, Riggs DS, Murdock TB: Treatment of posttraumatic stress disorder in rape victims: a comparison between cognitive-behavioral procedures and counseling. *JConsult ClinPsychol* 1991, 59:715–723.

31. Insel T, Cuthbert B, Garvey M, Heinssen R, Pine DS, Quinn K, Sanislow C, Wang P: Research domain criteria (RDoC): toward a new classification framework for research on mental disorders. *Am J Psychiatry* 2010, 167:748–751.

32. Milad MR, Pitman RK, Ellis CB, Gold AL, Shin LM, Lasko NB, Zeidan MA, Handwerger K, Orr SP, Rauch SL: Neurobiological basis of failure to recall extinction memory in posttraumatic stress disorder. *BiolPsychiatry* 2009, 66:1075–1082.

33. Zeidan MA, Igoe SA, Linnman C, Vitalo A, Levine JB, Klibanski A, Goldstein JM, Milad MR: Estradiol Modulates Medial Prefrontal Cortex and Amygdala Activity During Fear Extinction in Women and Female Rats. *Biol Psychiatry* 2011, 70:920–927.

34. First MB, Spitzer RL, Gibbon M, Williams JBW: *Structured Clinical Interview for DSM-IV-TR Axis I Disorders, Research Version, Patient Edition.* New York: Biometrics Research, New York State Psychiatric Institute; 2002.

35. Milad MR, Pitman RK, Ellis CB, Gold AB, Shin LM, Lasko NB, Handwerger K, Orr SP, Rauch SL: Neurobiological basis for failure to recall extinction memory in Posttraumatic Stress Disorder. *BiolPsychiatry* 2009, 66:1075–1082.

36. Milad MR, Orr SP, Pitman RK, Rauch SL: Context modulation of memory for fear extinction in humans. *Psychophysiology* 2005, 42:456–464.

37. Orr SP, Metzger LJ, Lasko NB, Macklin ML, Peri T, Pitman RK: De novo conditioning in trauma-exposed individuals with and without posttraumatic stress disorder. *JAbnormPsychol* 2000, 109:290–298.

38. Esclassan F, Coutureau E, Di Scala G, Marchand AR: A cholinergic-dependent role for the entorhinal cortex in trace fear conditioning. *J Neurosci* 2009, 29:8087–8093.

39. Stefanova N, Ovtscharoff W: Sexual dimorphism of the bed nucleus of the stria terminalis and the amygdala. *Adv Anat Embryol Cell Biol* 2000, 158:(III-X) 1–78.

40. Rougemont-Bucking A, Linnman C, Zeffiro TA, Zeidan MA, Lebron-Milad K, Rodriguez-Romaguera J, Rauch SL, Pitman RK, Milad MR: Altered processing of contextual information during fear extinction in PTSD: an fMRI study. *CNS Neurosci Ther* 2011, 17:227–236.

41. Linnman C, Rougemont-Bucking A, Beucke JC, Zeffiro TA, Milad MR: Unconditioned responses and functional fear networks in human classical conditioning. *Behav Brain Res* 2011, 221:237–245.

42. Milad MR, Quirk GJ: Neurons in medial prefrontal cortex signal memory for fear extinction. *Nature* 2002, 420:70–74.

43. Curley JP, Jordan ER, Swaney WT, Izraelit A, Kammel S, Champagne FA: The meaning of weaning: influence of the weaning period on behavioral development in mice. *Dev Neurosci* 2009, 31:318–331.

44. Nielsen SE, Ertman N, Lakhani YS, Cahill L: Hormonal contraception usage is associated with altered memory for an emotional story. *Neurobiol Learn Mem* 2011, 96:378–384.

45. Chang YJ, Yang CH, Liang YC, Yeh CM, Huang CC, Hsu KS: Estrogen modulates sexually dimorphic contextual fear extinction in rats through estrogen receptor beta. *Hippocampus* 2009, 19:1142–1150.

46. Milad MR, Quirk GJ, Pitman RK, Orr SP, Fischl B, Rauch SL: A role for the human dorsal anterior cingulate cortex in fear expression. *Biol Psychiatry* 2007, 62:1191–1194.

47. Linnman C, Zeidan MA, Furtak SC, Pitman RK, Quirk GJ, Milad MR: Resting Amygdala and Medial Prefrontal Metabolism Predicts Functional Activation of the Fear Extinction Circuit. *Am J Psychiatry* 2012 (Epub ahead of print).

48. Etkin A, Egner T, Kalisch R: Emotional processing in anterior cingulate and medial prefrontal cortex. *Trends Cogn Sci* 2011, 15:85–93.

49. Milad MR, Quirk GJ, Pitman RK, Orr SP, Fischl B, Rauch SL: A role for the human dorsal anterior cingulate cortex in fear expression. *BiolPsychiatry* 2007, 62:1191–1194.

50. Mobbs D, Marchant JL, Hassabis D, Seymour B, Tan G, Gray M, Petrovic P, Dolan RJ, Frith CD: From threat to fear: the neural organization of defensive fear systems in humans. *J Neurosci* 2009, 29:12236–12243.

51. Davis M, Whalen PJ: The amygdala: vigilance and emotion. *MolPsychiatry* 2001, 6:13–34.

52. Quirk GJ, Mueller D: Neural mechanisms of extinction learning and retrieval. *Neuropsychopharmacology* 2008, 33:56–72.

Event-related potential studies of post-traumatic stress disorder

Arash Javanbakht[1,2]*, Israel Liberzon[1], Alireza Amirsadri[2], Klevest Gjini[2] and Nash N Boutros[2]

Abstract

Despite the sparseness of the currently available data, there is accumulating evidence of information processing impairment in post-traumatic stress disorder (PTSD). Studies of event-related potentials (ERPs) are the main tool in real time examination of information processing. In this paper, we sought to critically review the ERP evidence of information processing abnormalities in patients with PTSD. We also examined the evidence supporting the existence of a relationship between ERP abnormalities and symptom profiles or severity in PTSD patients. An extensive Medline search was performed. Keywords included PTSD or post-traumatic stress disorder, electrophysiology or EEG, electrophysiology, P50, P100, N100, P2, P200, P3, P300, sensory gating, CNV (contingent negative variation) and MMN (mismatch negativity). We limited the review to ERP adult human studies with control groups which were reported in the English language. After applying our inclusion-exclusion review criteria, 36 studies were included. Subjects exposed to wide ranges of military and civilian traumas were studied in these reports. Presented stimuli were both auditory and visual. The most widely studied components included P300, P50 gating, N100 and P200. Most of the studies reported increased P300 response to trauma-related stimuli in PTSD patients. A smaller group of studies reported dampening of responses or no change in responses to trauma-related and/or unrelated stimuli. P50 studies were strongly suggestive of impaired gating in patients with PTSD. In conclusion, the majority of reports support evidence of information processing abnormalities in patients with PTSD diagnosis. The predominance of evidence suggests presence of mid-latency and late ERP components differences in PTSD patients in comparison to healthy controls. Heterogeneity of assessment methods used contributes to difficulties in reaching firm conclusions regarding the nature of these differences. We suggest that future ERP-PTSD studies utilize standardized assessment scales that provide detailed information regarding the symptom clusters and the degree of symptom severity. This would allow assessment of electrophysiological indices-clinical symptoms relationships. Based on the available data, we suggest that ERP abnormalities in PTSD are possibly affected by the level of illness severity. If supported by future research, ERP studies may be used for both initial assessment and treatment follow-up.

Introduction

Although post-traumatic stress disorder (PTSD) is classified as an 'anxiety disorder', evidence of cognitive and information processing (IP) abnormalities in PTSD has been accumulating [1]. While many studies on emotional processing abnormalities in PTSD exist, event-related potentials (ERPs) studies focusing on early stages of IP abnormalities in PTSD are limited in number. The aim of this review was to summarize ERP findings in PTSD and determine whether there are consistent patterns of IP

deviations reported in this disorder. We also sought to gain possible insight into clinical correlates of these differences. Another aim of this review was to assess if we could present suggestions for future research methods.

Event-related brain potentials and components

Brain ERPs are the main tools available for clinical investigators to probe IP in real time, as they can assess different phases of IP in the human brain [2]. Abnormality of the initial phase of IP (the 0 to 20 ms following auditory or visual stimulation), where information is conducted through subcortical structures on its way to the cerebral cortex, is usually linked to brain stem abnormalities [3]. Abnormalities at this stage of IP are rarely reported in

* Correspondence: ajavanb@med.umich.edu
[1]Department of Psychiatry, University of Michigan, Ann Arbor, 1500 East Medical Center Drive, Ann Arbor, MI 48109, USA
Full list of author information is available at the end of the article

psychiatric patients [4]. Due to the extremely small number of ERP studies examining this stage of IP in association with PTSD, this IP stage is not further discussed in this report.

The midlatency range of information processing (following the early stage and spanning 20 to 200 ms following stimulation), when signal registration and filtering out (gating) of redundant information takes place [5], has been shown to be abnormal in a large number of psychiatric and neuropsychiatric conditions [6]. Auditory midlatency range is represented by three major event-related response components: the P50 (40 to 80 ms), N100 (75 to 150 ms) and the P200 (150 to 250 ms) [7]. Two variables are routinely examined in association with all ERPs: amplitude (how large the response is) and latency (how long after the stimulus the response is maximally seen). Amplitudes and latencies are examined using trains of identical stimuli and averaging the resulting responses [8]. Midlatency ERP responses are also widely used to examine habituation (or sensory gating) in the brain [9]. A standard paired-stimulus paradigm (S1-S2) is used for the purpose of examining habituation or gating of the P50/N100/P200 components with stimulus repetition. Habituation or gating is routinely assessed as the ratio of the responses to S2 stimuli as compared to responses to S1 stimuli (S2/S1 × 100). Higher ratios reflect decreased gating ability [10]. All three midlatency auditory event-related response (MLAER) components are demonstrated to have decreased gating in association with psychosis [5].

The later stage of IP is when higher cognitive manipulations occur [11]. The P300 ERP component is a large positive electroencephalography (EEG) deflection elicited approximately 300 ms after an individual detects a deviant stimulus imbedded among ongoing repeating stimuli [11]. The amplitude of the P300 has been linked to the amount of attentional resources allocated to the experimental task. P300 latency has been linked to the speed of IP. P500 is a positive deflection which appears between 300 and 900 ms after stimulus presentation and is believed to be involved in updating working memory representations of a specified stimulus [12]. Abnormalities of these ERP, especially the P300 (250 to 350 ms), are common in psychiatric populations.

Methods

A detailed Medline search was performed. Keywords included PTSD or post-traumatic stress disorder and EEG, electrophysiology, P50, P100, N100, P2, P200, P3, P300, sensory gating, CNV (contingent negative variation), and MMN (mismatch negativity). The search was limited to human studies reported in the English language. Because of the very small number of electrophysiological studies in children with mental illnesses in general, three of the manuscripts which reported children

studies were not included in this review. Papers which were solely EEG or sleep studies in PTSD without inclusion of ERPs were also not included. We considered only studies which included a healthy control group, enabling extraction of the differences between ERP responses in patients with PTSD and those of healthy participants. We then reviewed full texts of the selected manuscripts and summarized ERP responses from these studies in separate tables (Tables 1, 2, 3 and 4). We also extracted reported clinical correlates of the ERP results and summarized them in Table 5. This table shows the rating scales which were used in each study and the correlation of the scores of these tests with the ERP data.

Results

Initial search yielded 57 papers of which 16 were solely EEG studies, another did not include a healthy control group, and three were children or adolescents studies, which were excluded from the current work. We excluded studies in children because of the small number of reports and a lack of homogeneity in ERP procedures used. Only a single study assessed CNV differences in PTSD patients [13] and thus it was not included in this review. After exclusion of these papers, 36 manuscripts had undergone comprehensive review. All of the presented data regarding the populations, their clinical characteristics (such as rating scales and scores when provided), and the utilized event-related response measures were collected from these 36 reports. Given the fact that most of the studies did not report possible comorbidities and medication regimens, these factors are not assessed or discussed in this review.

Of the 36 studies, 15 included veterans and/or military personnel with combat/war trauma and 17 included subjects exposed to civilian traumas such as motor vehicle accidents, rape and assault. Subjects of four studies were exposed to traumas of mixed etiology. All of the considered studies included healthy control subjects and most of them (especially combat related studies) included a third group of people who were exposed to trauma but did not develop PTSD based on the Diagnostic and Statistical Manual of Mental Disorders (DSM) III or IV diagnostic criteria.

A number of rating scales were used to assess PTSD symptomatology and comorbidities (Table 5). The most widely used scale was the Clinician-Administered PTSD Scale (CAPS), utilized in 10 of the 14 studies that evaluated clinical correlates. The CAPS is a well validated 'gold standard' 30-item structured interview that corresponds to the DSM-IV criteria for PTSD [14,15]. CAPS subscores include re-experience (intrusiveness), avoidance and arousal. Other assessment instruments included the Mississippi scale for PTSD [16] (one study), a PTSD questionnaire [17] (one study), State-Trait Anxiety Inventory (STAI) [18] (three studies), brief symptom inventory [19,20] (one

Table 1 Studies examining the P50 and sensory gating

Study	Subjects	Paradigm	Results
[51]	46 prisoners of war 36 healthy controls	Checkerboard reversal (visual)	Significantly greater P50 amplitude and latency
[52]	10 inpatient combat PTSD 5 inpatient alcohol-dependents 5 combat-exposed and 5 combat-non-exposed healthy subjects	Paired click	Diminished P50 habituation in PTSD
[25]	13 female with sexual assault PTSD 16 healthy controls	Auditory oddball	No difference in P50 peak amplitude and latency
[53]	15 combat veterans 12 healthy control	Paired click	P50 amplitude in response to the conditioning stimulus did not differ. P50 T/C ratio was increased in PTSD subjects.
[54]	10 male veteran PTSD + 9 female rape victims matched control groups	Paired click	Decreased P50 gating
[32]	29 PTSD nurse veterans 38 non-PTSD	Paired click	Reduced P50 suppression associated with increased severity of general psychopathology, but not with PTSD.
[27]	12 urban violence PTSD/24 healthy subjects/12 schizophrenics	Paired click	Higher P50 ratios in subjects with PTSD
[55]	27 civilian with mixed types of trauma and 24 control subjects	Paired click	Impaired P50 suppression in PTSD subjects
[26]	Seven combat veterans with PTSD and 11 matched controls	Paired click	Impaired M50 gating in the right hemisphere in PTSD subjects. Thinner right STG (Superior Temporal Gyrus) cortical thickness was associated with worse right sensory gating in the PTSD group. The right S1 P50 source strength and gating ratio were correlated with PTSD symptomatology.

Table 2 Summary of the studies which included N100 component

Study	Subjects	Paradigm	Results
[31]	12 combat PTSD veterans 6 normal controls	Four tones intensity paradigm	No difference in N1 amplitude
[17]	20 Israeli combat veterans with PTSD 20 without PTSD	Visual oddball, trauma related non-related neutral stimuli	Combat-related pictures elicited enhanced N1 amplitude in PTSD group. Prolonged N1 latencies and reaction times to target stimuli in PTSD patients.
[56]	16 medicated, 9 un-medicated PTSD 10 healthy veterans	Auditory three-tone oddball	Longer N100 latencies in un-medicated PTSD patients compared to the medicated PTSD and healthy controls.
[51]	11 prisoners of war	Checkerboard reversal	Larger N75 amplitudes
[39]	11 PTSD survivors of a ship fire 9 psychiatric controls from the same ship	Auditory word and non-word oddball	Increased N1 latency to standard tones; Larger amplitude to emotionally meaningful words.
[25]	13 females with sexual assault PTSD 16 healthy controls	Auditory oddball	No difference in N100 amplitude and latency
[28]	17 civil PTSD 17 healthy controls	Auditory oddball	No difference in N100 amplitude or latency
[30]	36 civil PTSD 20 healthy 10 depressed 8 alcoholics	2000-Hz tone presented in increasing intensities	Increased N100 amplitudes
[38]	15 civil PTSD 15 controls	Visual presentation of angry alternating with neutral faces	Larger N110 to the angry compared to the neutral faces in the control group. Smaller and later N100 in PTSD subjects.
[35]	10 civil PTSD 10 controls	Auditory oddball	Larger N100 amplitude
[42]	19 PTSD 99 Alcohol dependence 16 personality disorder 25 anxiety or mood disorder	Visual presentation of happy, sad, and neutral faces	Larger N1 amplitudes to sad stimuli in frontotemporal leads in PTSD patients.
[57]	16 civil PTSD 16 schizophrenia 16 control subjects	Auditory Oddball	No difference in N1 amplitude and latency
[36]	14 PTSD [mixed etiologies] 12 controls	Auditory Oddball	No difference in N100 amplitude

Table 3 Summary of the studies which included P200 component

Study	Study Groups	Paradigm	Findings
[31]	12 combat PTSD veterans 6 normal controls	Four tones intensity paradigm	Reduced P2 amplitude intensity slope in PTSD subjects
[25]	13 female with sexual assault PTSD 16 healthy controls	Auditory oddball	Reduced amplitude and latency in response to deviant stimuli
[28]	17 civil PTSD 17 healthy controls	Auditory oddball	Smaller P200 to target and common tones. Earlier response to common but not target tones.
[30]	36 civil PTSD 20 healthy 10 depressed 8 alcoholics.	2000-Hz tone presented in intensity blocks of 65, 72.5, 80, 87.5, and 95 dB (SPL)	In normal subjects, depressed, and alcoholics, there was linear relationship between the tone intensity and P200 amplitude, which was not the case in combat related PTSD subjects.
[32]	29 PTSD nurse veterans 38 non-PTSD	Four-tone stimulus-intensity modulation paradigm	Increased P2 amplitude/intensity slope
[35]	10 civil PTSD 10 controls	Auditory oddball	No difference in P2 amplitude or latency
[29]	7 PTSD motor vehicle accident (MVA) 7 non-PTSD with MVA	Visual presentation of trauma related/unrelated/neutral pictures	Smaller P200 amplitude Larger response to trauma-related images in non-PTSD and healthy controls
[36]	14 PTSD [mixed etiologies] 12 controls	Auditory oddball	No difference in P200 amplitude
[33]	12 combat exposed veterans with PTSD and 33 without PTSD and their twins	Four-tone stimulus-intensity modulation paradigm	Increased P2 amplitude intensity slope in PTSD veterans. P2 amplitude intensity slopes were related to higher combat exposure, CAPS Total, and re-experience symptoms severity scores in the combat-exposed veterans but not to the remaining PTSD symptom cluster scores or the SCL-90-R (Symptom Checklist 90 Revised) general psychopathology, anxiety, or depression subscale scores. Higher combat-exposure scores, but not CAPS Total or subscale scores, were also related to increased P2 amplitude.
[34]	12 PTSD and 12 control survivors of earthquake	Subliminal visual presentation of earthquake-related/unrelated words	Increased P2 amplitude in the PTSD group in response to the trauma-related stimuli

study), Beck depression inventory [21] (two studies), Impact of Events Scale-Revised [22] (IES-R) (four studies), PTSD Check List-Military (PCL-M) [23] (one study), and Profile of Mood States (POMS) [24] (one study).

Standard tone sounds were used for the auditory oddball and gating studies. For the visual event-related potential paradigms, mostly three sets of images were presented to the subjects. These included neutral images such as nature scenes, trauma-specific aversive images and non-trauma-specific aversive pictures. Auditory stimuli were used in 22 studies, 13 used visual stimuli, and one study included both auditory and visual stimuli in their paradigms.

Most of the studies focused on the ERP component P300 (26 studies). P50, N100 and P200 components were also assessed by a fair number of studies (9 studies P50; 13 studies N100; and 10 studies P200). P100 (visual), N200 and the MMN were the least studied ERP components. Many studies probed more than one ERP component; this explains why the sum of the number of entries in tables 1, 2, 3 and 4 is larger than the total number of papers reviewed. The ERP components that were considered by at least four studies are summarized in the tables.

We first grouped all the studies together for each ERP component and counted the number of studies which reported differences in the amplitudes in each direction. We then separated studies in auditory/visual modalities and amplitudes reported in response to the trauma related (TR) and trauma nonrelated (TNR) stimuli when applicable.

P50 amplitude and gating (Table 1)

Nine papers examined the P50 auditory event-related response. Two papers only examined the amplitude and latencies of the P50 components (in other words, not using paired stimuli) of which one showed an exaggerated response to the tone and one did not [25]. Seven papers utilized the standard paired-stimulus paradigm to examine sensory gating. Six papers examining habituation showed significantly elevated gating ratios (in other words, the decreased ability to inhibit or suppress repeating (redundant) incoming sensory input) in PTSD patients as compared to controls. One study found impaired P50 gating only in the right hemisphere in PTSD patients as compared to the control group [26]. In regards to S1, four of the seven papers did not reveal a

Table 4 Summary of the studies which included P300 component

Study	Study Groups	Paradigm	Findings
[17]	20 Israeli combat veterans with PTSD 20 without PTSD	Modified target detection visual oddball paradigm, trauma related non-related neutral stimuli	Accentuated P300 amplitudes to target stimuli in both controls and PTSD patients Enhanced P300 amplitude in response to non-target combat related pictures in PTSD group Prolonged P300 latencies and reaction times to target stimuli were prolonged in PTSD subjects Increased latency in response to trauma-related stimuli in PTSD subjects
[50]	20 Israeli veterans with PTSD 20 without PTSD	Modified target detection visual oddball paradigm, trauma related, unrelated, neutral pictures	Smaller response to non-target images in the control, but equal responses to both target and non-target stimuli in the PTSD group No group difference for the target stimuli, but larger response to the non-target in the PTSD group. P300 could correctly classify 90% of PTSD and 90% of non-PTSD subjects. Increased latency of P300 response to combat-related images in relation with the severity of intrusive symptoms. This relation was negative between the P300 latency and severity of avoidance.
[58]	20 PTSD combat veterans 20 non-PTSD combat veterans	Target detection oddball, traumatic/neutral stimuli	Larger P300 amplitude in the PTSD group No difference in P300 amplitude between the target and non-target in the PTSD group; higher amplitude in response to the target stimuli in the control group. Earlier and 5 times greater P300 response to combat related pictures in PTSD patients. Repeated combat related pictures resulted in a rapid P300 amplitude reduction and latency prolongation. This effect was not observed for the target stimuli.
[59]	19 civil PTSD 17 subjects with numerous life events 18 without life events	Auditory oddball	Longer reaction times and lower amplitude P300 response
[60]	8 PTSD 8 non-PTSD combat veterans	Visual presentation of a sequence of trauma related and unrelated words	Newly identified P300tr component was suppressed to all stimuli in PTSD subjects
[43]	34 PTSD [25 male veterans/9 female victims of rape] 18 non-PTSD [10/8 from the same groups]	Auditory three-tone oddball	Smaller P300 response to the target tone. For women group, it was also smaller in response to the distracter tones.
[41]	9 PTSD [assault, rape, MVA, combat] 10 healthy controls	Modified stroop paradigm, visual presentation of neutral, positive and negative words	Smaller P300 amplitude to neutral, positive, and negative words in PTSD patients. Smaller response to neutral words as compared to positive and negative words.
[56]	16 medicated PTSD 9 un-medicated PTSD 10 healthy veterans	Auditory three-tone oddball	Significant decrease in P300 at Pz electrode in un-medicated PTSD group compared to the medicated PTSD and healthy subjects. Subjects with co-morbid panic disorder had the largest P300 amplitudes.
[39]	11 survivors of a ship fire with PTSD or near PTSD 9 controls with other psychiatric illnesses from the same ship	Auditory word and non-word oddball	Reduced P300 amplitude to non-words and negative words
[61]	25 combat veterans with PTSD/14 without PTSD	Auditory three-tone oddball	Reduced P300 amplitude to the target stimuli. Significant P300 amplitude enhancements at frontal sites to distracting stimuli during the novelty but not during the three-tone oddball tasks.
[62]	10 Vietnam war veterans with PTSD 10 without PTSD	Two oddball tasks of visual trauma-relevant and trauma-irrelevant threat (combat, social-threat, household, and neutral words)	Attenuated P300 response to neutral target stimuli Increased P300 amplitude in response to trauma-relevant combat stimuli but not to trauma-irrelevant social-threat stimuli at frontal electrode sites.
[28]	17 civil PTSD 17 healthy controls	Auditory oddball	Smaller P300 in PTSD, later at Pz

Table 4 Summary of the studies which included P300 component *(Continued)*

[32]	29 PTSD nurse veterans 38 non-PTSD	Three-tone oddball	Larger target P300 amplitudes in PTSD subjects
[38]	15 civil PTSD 15 controls	20 angry and 20 neutral faces	Slower P270 in the PTSD at occipital electrodes
[63]	25 combat PTSD 15 combat-exposed healthy controls	Three conditioned novelty visual and auditory oddball	No significant differences in P300 amplitude or latency regardless of stimulus type (target, novel) or modality (auditory, visual).
[35]	10 civil PTSD 10 controls	Auditory oddball	Same P3a amplitude in both groups, but there was a significant post-treatment attenuation of P3a in the PTSD group.
[64]	8 PTSD victims of Tokyo sarin attack 13 healthy controls	Auditory oddball	No difference in P300 latency. Significantly smaller P300 amplitudes in subjects with PTSD.
[65]	33 civil PTSD 33 matched controls	Auditory standard two-tone oddball	Delayed reduced P300 target amplitude, coupled with slower and less accurate target detection
[12]	10 male police/veteran PTSD 10 healthy controls	Auditory oddball	Smaller P550; More false negatives and positives; The higher the anxiety and depression level, the lower the amplitude; Reverse relationship between the P550 amplitude and intrusions.
[42]	19 PTSD 99 Alcohol dependence 16 personality disorder 25 anxiety or mood disorder	Visual presentation of happy, sad, and neutral faces	Longer P300 latency to happy stimuli in midline, central, and right frontal leads; Reduced P300 amplitude in response to neutral faces.
[40]	16 civil PTSD 15 trauma-exposed without PTSD 16 healthy controls	Modified auditory S1-S2 paradigm	Increased P300 and late positive complex amplitudes to trauma-specific questions; Only the PTSD group showed a differentiation between trauma-specific and neutral questions with respect to P300.
[66]	14 PTSD survivors of an air show disaster 15 trauma-exposed subjects without PTSD 15 healthy controls	Visual differential conditioning paradigm with traumatic/neutral pictures	Trauma-exposed subjects with and without PTSD showed successful differential conditioning to the trauma-relevant cue indicative of second-order conditioning
[57]	16 civil PTSD 16 schizophrenia 16 control subjects	Auditory oddball	Reduced amplitude of target and non-target P300 responses. Larger reduction in target P300 amplitude in left posterior parietal leads in PTSD group.
[49]	37 combat exposed veterans with PTSD and 47 without PTSD and their twins	Auditory oddball	No difference in P300 amplitude; When assessed the un- medicated nonsmoker group separately, P300 amplitude was smaller in the PTSD group
[1]	20 un-medicated and 14 medicated PTSD [mixed etiology] 136 controls	1-back working memory task	Reduced P300 working memory amplitude and delayed target P300 in PTSD. Amplitude reduction and delay of target P300 in medicated PTSD subjects. Little difference between the non-medicated PTSD subgroup and the controls.
[34]	12 PTSD and 12 control survivors of earthquake	Subliminal visual presentation of earthquake- related/unrelated words	Increased P2 and P3 amplitude in the PTSD group in response to the trauma-related stimuli

difference in the amplitude of response to S1 while one found a reduced response to S1 paired with an exaggerated response to S2 in PTSD subject [27]. Hunter and colleague's study [26] found reduced S1 strength only in the right hemisphere of patients with PTSD. To summarize, a small number of studies evaluated the P50 component in PTSD and among these, the majority reported impaired gating of the repetitive stimuli.

N100 (Table 2)
Thirteen studies assessed the N100 midlatency auditory event-related response. Six studies reported increased N100 amplitude in subjects with PTSD, two reported a reduction in N100 amplitude in this population, and four did not find a difference. One study did not report the N100 amplitudes. Of the nine studies reporting latencies, four found increased N100 latencies in PTSD

Table 5 Summary of studies with clinical correlates

Study	Clinical scales	Clinical correlates
[17]	IES, PTSD questionnaire	Positive correlation between P300 latency at Pz and Cz and the judged severity of intrusiveness measured by IES (Impact of Event Scale). Same applies to the level of intrusiveness measured by PTSD questionnaire. Negative correlation between P300 latency at Cz and severity of avoidance.
[52]	CAPS	P50 gating correlated negatively and significantly with PTSD subjects' CAPS re-experiencing intensity scores.
[56]	STAI	Measures of state anxiety (STAI) were significantly related to P300 amplitude at Pz; higher levels of self-reported state anxiety were associated with smaller P300 amplitudes.
[39]	CAPS	P300 amplitudes to emotionally meaningful words were significantly related to Clinician-Administered PTSD Scale subscales, in particular avoidance and arousal.
[25]	Mississippi score, STAI	Significant correlation between the magnitude of the MMN at Fz and the Mississippi PTSD Symptom Scale for civilian trauma.
[53]	CAPS, IES-R	No significant correlations were found between P50 gating and IES-R or CAPS total or subscale scores.
[28]	CAPS	Significant correlation between the intensity of numbing symptoms (reduced interest, social withdrawal, and emotional numbing) and P300 amplitude at parietal sites.
[30]	BDI, CAPS	PTSD subjects who showed N100 augmentation and P200 reduction were more depressed than PTSD patients with other patterns. Significant correlations between P200 slope and Clinician-Administered PTSD Scale total score, the Mississippi scale score, and the Hamilton depression score
[32]	Comorbidity CAPS, PCL-M	P2 slope was positively correlated with PCL-M, CAPS Total, and each of the CAPS subscale scores, indicating that a higher P2 slope was associated with more severe PTSD symptomatology P50 gating was negatively correlated with SCL-90-R Global Severity Index (GSI) score, indicating that worse gating is associated with more severe general psychopathology.
[63]	CAPS, IES-R, BDI, Mood State (POMS)	P300 amplitude to novel auditory stimuli increased as tension score in POMS increased.
[64]	CAPS, IES-R	Significantly negative correlation between present score of the cluster C of the CAPS (numbness/avoidance) and P300 amplitude at Pz.
[12]	STAI, BDI (Beck Depression Inventory), CAPS	Negative relationship between P550 amplitude and trait anxiety. Negative relationship between P550 amplitude and depression CAPS scores; negative relationship between P550 amplitude and intrusions.
[36]	Brief Symptom Inventory (BSI),	MMN was significantly correlated with the total PTSD score.
[1]	CAPS	Neither P300 nor behavioral measures were related to CAPS symptom severity measures.

patients and five did not find a difference in latency between the PTSD subjects and healthy controls. From seven auditory oddball studies, one did not report the amplitudes, four reported no differences, and two reported increased amplitude in the N100 component in the PTSD patients. Two studies presented emotional faces in the visual modality, one of which reported increased amplitude and the other reported reduced amplitude to sad faces. In summary, N100 ERP component findings are overall inconsistent in existing PTSD studies.

P200 (Table 3)

Ten studies examined the P200 MLAER component. Three studies found decreased P200 amplitude in PTSD patients [25,28,29]. In two studies, a linear relationship was found between the tone intensity and P200 amplitude in the control group, which was not detected in combat PTSD patients [30,31]. In other words, in contrast to the control subjects, PTSD patients failed to show increased P200 amplitude in response to increased tone intensity. In contrast, Metzger and colleagues reported increased P200

amplitude and intensity slope in PTSD patients [32,33]. In one of these studies, the slope was correlated with re-experience symptoms cluster but not the other symptom cluster scores. Yun and colleagues [34] found increased P2 amplitude in response to subliminal visual presentation of TR stimuli in PTSD patients. Two studies failed to detect a difference between the PTSD patients and healthy controls in P200 amplitudes or latencies [35,36]. Wessa and colleagues [29] reported reduced P200 amplitude with lack of differentiation between the TR and TNR visual stimuli in the PTSD patients.

To sum, from ten studies that compared P200 amplitudes between PTSD patients and controls, one reported increased amplitude in PTSD patients (in response to subliminal presentation of the stimuli), three reported reduced amplitude and two reported increased amplitude/slope intensity. Two studies failed to show increased P200 amplitude in response to increased intensity in PTSD patients, and two did not detect any difference between the PTSD and control groups. Given the close proximity of the N100 and P200 components, we examined the difference in the amplitudes of these two components in

PTSD studies. Among 13 studies reporting N100 amplitudes, six reported an increase while none of the five P200 studies which reported the amplitude of this component found increased amplitudes. Utilizing Fisher's exact test of 2 × 2 contingency tables, a trend towards difference in the behavior of the two components was detected (P (2-tails) = 0.102, power (2-tails) = 0.503) [37].

P300 (Table 4)

Most of the studies examining event-related responses in PTSD populations (26 studies) assessed P300 component in either an auditory or a visual oddball design.

Auditory studies

Seventeen studies assessed the P300 component in an auditory modality, 15 of which were standard oddballs. One of these 15 studies did not report the P300 amplitude [38]. Eleven studies reported reduced response amplitude to the target stimuli, one reported increased amplitude, and two failed to detect any difference between the PTSD and the control subjects. One of these studies [39] reported reduced amplitude to non-word stimuli (reversed waveforms of the digitized words) and increased amplitude to positive words in PTSD patients. Although Metzger and colleagues [33] did not find a difference in P300 amplitude, when they evaluated a subgroup of nonmedicated, nonsmoker subjects, again they reported decreased P300 amplitude in PTSD subjects. Wessa and colleagues [40] showed increased response amplitude to TR questions.

Visual studies

Eight studies reported P300 responses to TR versus aversive TNR or neutral stimuli. One study [34] reported an increased P300 response to the subliminal presentation of the TR stimuli in PTSD patients. Due to different methodology, this study is not included in the following analysis. Five studies reported increased amplitude to the TR stimuli in PTSD patients compared to the controls and one study reported increased response to all stimuli in PTSD patients. Although Metzger and colleagues [41] reported smaller P300 amplitude to all the stimuli in the PTSD patients, they found a smaller response to the neutral words as compared to the positive and negative words. Ehlers and colleagues [42] reported reduced amplitude to neutral faces in the PTSD patients and Veltmeyer and colleagues [1] in an N-back working memory task found reduced P300 amplitude in the PTSD group.

We also reviewed P300 responses to TR/aversive stimuli and neutral stimuli separately irrespective of the modality of stimulus presentation (auditory or visual). From the 17 reports on the P300 amplitudes in response to the visual or auditory TNR/neutral stimuli, 13 studies reported reduced amplitude in PTSD patients, two reported increased amplitude, and two studies failed to detect any difference between the PTSD subjects and the control group.

Eight studies reported P300 responses to TR/aversive stimuli. Seven studies found increased P300 amplitude in the PTSD patients and one study reported reduced response in the PTSD patients as compared to the control group [43]. In this last study, within group comparison showed a smaller response to the neutral words as compared to the positive and negative words in PTSD patients. On aggregate (studies pooled across visual or auditory modalities), seven out of eight studies reporting P300 responses to TR reported increased amplitudes while only two of sixteen studies examining responses to TNR stimuli reported increased P300 amplitudes (Fisher's exact test of 2 × 2 contingency tables, P (2-tailed) < 0.001, power (2-tailed) = 0.986). Conversely, while 13 of 17 papers reported decreased P300 amplitudes to TNR stimuli, only one of eight papers reported decreased amplitudes to TR stimuli (Fisher's exact test of 2 × 2 contingency tables P (2-tailed) < 0.008, power (2-tailed) = 0.889).

In summary, the majority of studies on P300 component reported sensitization of the P300 response to TR stimuli and dampening of this response to the neutral stimuli.

Other event-related responses

A host of studies examined other event-related responses including visual P100, N200 (a negativity generated with stimulus deviation), MMN (also a negativity detected with stimulus deviation) and the late positive auditory complexes. Wessa et al. [29] reported a later positivity (P550) and skin conductance to be negatively correlated with the severity of avoidance symptoms. None of these smaller bodies of literature included more than three published, full length papers and none has shown a consistent pattern. We concluded that these smaller bodies of literature were not yet at a stage that would significantly contribute to our understanding of PTSD and did not include them in this analysis.

Of all the studies reviewed, 14 examined the correlations between the assessed ERP measures and PTSD symptomatology. While 17 significant correlations were reported (see Table 5), a large number of trend level or non-significant correlations are also reported. Due to different methods and clinical rating scales used among the studies, we could not make a conclusion about the clinical correlates of the reported ERP components.

Discussion

In this manuscript, we reviewed reports that assessed ERP components in subjects with PTSD and healthy subjects. The early stage of IP was not examined due to a paucity of studies. Most of the studies presented evidence for a difference in IP between patients with PTSD and control patients during the entire midlatency range and extending into the later stages of IP.

The earlier part of the midlatency range is almost entirely pre-attentive and reflects the automatic processes of stimulus registration (reflected by response amplitudes) and filtering processes (reflected by sensory gating measures). Processes occurring at this stage are likely substantially bottom-up in nature and might be clinically correlated with 'intrusiveness' and 'hyperarousal', as these symptoms are likely to be automatic and, to a degree, pre-attentive. On the other hand, the attentive top-down level of IP is usually probed by examining the later occurring ERPs like the P300 or P550. This level of information processing could be clinically related with volitional 'avoidance' symptoms.

Results of reviewed P50 gating studies show some evidence of impaired pre-attentive habituation in PTSD patients. Whether gating deficit results from exposure to stress or represents a pre-existing vulnerability to developing PTSD can only be determined through the conduct of careful longitudinal studies. Current literature shows that decreased gating is not uncommon in seemingly healthy individuals [44,45]. On the other hand, studies also show that laboratory-induced stress (which, by definition, cannot be severe or chronic) can decrease gating in healthy individuals with normal baseline gating [46]. It is thus quite plausible to postulate that severe or chronic stress can be detrimental to the sensory gating function and possibly individuals with premorbid deficient sensory gating function are more susceptible to developing PTSD when subjected to this form of stress.

The noted possibility that the N100 and P200 components may be affected differently in association with PTSD is worthy of further investigation as the P200 along with the N100 form the vertex complex and are considered closely related. While experimentally dissociable, the two components share similar neural sources and topographical distributions [47]. A significant variance in the effects of stimulation on these two components would indeed be an interesting finding worthy of further exploration, as it could yield clues to the nature and timing of IP difficulties in this patient population. In fact, despite the small number of studies, a trend suggesting that the two components behave differently in association with PTSD is seen.

The most widely examined ERP component is the P300, which reflects task allocation of cognitive resources [3]. In a first glance at the reports that evaluated the P300 component, it is difficult to draw a conclusion as the results are contradictory. When divided into two groups of studies with presentation of visual and auditory stimuli, a higher number of auditory studies show reduced P300 amplitude while a larger number of visual studies show increased P300 amplitude in the PTSD patients. This could be due to the fact that most of the auditory studies are standard oddballs with presentation of neutral stimuli while a larger number of studies in the visual modality presented TR/aversive images as non-target stimuli. In other words, when results are examined in terms of relevance of the stimuli to the trauma, they appear to be more meaningful. Among 18 studies that reported P300 amplitude in response to the TNR/neutral stimuli in auditory/visual modalities, the majority - 13 studies - showed reduced amplitude while only two of the studies showed increased amplitude. Furthermore, among the eight studies which evaluated P300 responses to the TR/aversive stimuli, seven studies found increased P300 amplitude in patients with PTSD when compared to the control group. Of interest, the one study which showed reduced P300 amplitude in PTSD patients, in within group comparison, showed a smaller response to the neutral words as compared to the positive and negative words in PTSD patients. These findings suggest the existence of two possible P300-related abnormalities: a significant decrease in responses to TNR stimuli and a significant increase in TR stimuli. Whether these two abnormalities occur simultaneously or sequentially and whether these two abnormalities reflect different aspects of the PTSD syndrome are currently open questions. Based on the above, there might be an increased attentional resource allocation in subjects with PTSD to the cues of trauma at the expense of the neutral stimuli. In other words, subjects with PTSD show sensitization and impaired habituation to the stimuli which represent the traumatic stimuli. Considering the limited attentional resources (which might be even more limited in patients with PTSD due to causes such as traumatic brain injury), this shift in allocation of these resources (sensitization) takes place at the expense of reduced response to and processing of neutral stimuli. In a clinical language, this attentional phenomenon may be translated into hyperarousal to any reminder of the traumatic event at expense of the neutral and nonaversive stimuli. In a further speculative step, this sensitization to the TR cues/stimuli, may be extended to the top-down filtering of the TR memories and assumed to be responsible for impaired inhibition of internal TR stimuli/memories which present in the form of re-experiences, intrusive memories and flash backs.

Whether ERP findings in individuals with PTSD are the result of trauma, or are present in patients who are more susceptible to PTSD when subjected to a traumatic experience remains an open question. Hypersensitivity to aversive stimuli and lack of habituation to them could be a premorbid difference in people who are more susceptible to developing PTSD after a traumatic experience. This possibility becomes more important in light of the fact that most ERP components are heavily genetically influenced [48]. Whether the ERP findings are characteristic of people susceptible to PTSD or are results of the trauma needs to be further assessed in longitudinal cohort studies (for example, pre- and postdeployment studies in veterans). Twin studies may be utilized in assessing whether the different findings in subjects are inborn genetic characteristics or a result of traumatic experience. This review found only two twin studies, both of which reported differences in P200 and P300 components between the PTSD subjects and their non-PTSD identical twin [49,33]. Although these results suggest that the information processing differences are acquired, more studies are needed to support these findings.

Tables 1, 2, 3 and 4 show that, although the amplitudes of the ERP components are examined in most of the reviewed studies, literature is very sparse in terms of the latency of these components. A negative correlation between the latency of the P300 and severity of avoidance has been found [50], in other words, the stronger the avoidance, the shorter the P300 latency. As latency of a component reflects the number of synaptic links leading to the development of the response [3], this observation might suggest that an altered process might be engaged in some patients with PTSD. Furthermore, the same study presents a positive correlation between latency and severity of the intrusiveness symptoms. Increased latency might thus suggest altered IP pathways in PTSD and support the need for close examination of latencies in ERP-PTSD studies. Differences in the direction of correlation between avoidance and latency, and intrusiveness and latency in the same patient population may point at different pathways being involved in the formation of different symptom clusters in PTSD. While highly speculative (based on a single report) these findings are of significant interest and deserve further exploration.

Given the large number of ERP variables examined as well as the large number of PTSD symptoms (and the varied PTSD assessment methods) no clear trends can be discerned (Table 5). If ERP components indeed reflect specific symptom type or severity, this can potentially be useful in both diagnostic evaluation and treatment monitoring. However, in those studies in which clinical correlations were assessed, comparable rating scales were not utilized. As a result, for the purpose of future ERP-PTSD studies, scales providing detailed accounts of symptom severity would be most suitable to examine any clinical-electrophysiological correlations. More importantly, it will be vital to analyze and include symptom-cluster information in the reports given the current debate over the make-up of symptom composition of the PTSD clusters. Whether ERP methodologies and measures can be used to guide the development of new or revised, empirically-based symptom clusters might also be a fruitful consideration in future studies.

Conclusions

In summary, our review points to a potential relationship between ERP measures and PTSD. The most consistent findings include diminished habituation to repetitive stimuli as evidenced by reduced P50 gating, and sensitization of the P300 response to TR stimuli. The P300 response to neutral stimuli, on the other hand, is diminished in PTSD patients, suggesting a potential 'trade off' between processing traumatic versus neutral stimuli. These differences in IP are consistent with the findings in emotional processing studies in PTSD, which reveal increased emotional response to the cues of trauma. Corresponding differences in IP and emotion responses can help in a more comprehensive understanding of PTSD. Although emotion regulation and processing is more extensively addressed in research, early cognitive processing of the information needs further exploration for a better understanding of the whole picture. The findings of this review may also translate to better understanding of the mechanisms involved in clinical symptoms development. Results on the N100 and P200 components are not as conclusive and other components are not addressed in the majority of the studies.

The inconsistency in the results of different studies can stem from differences in methodologies and patient populations or differences in illness-related variables. Other contributing factors can be physiological or external factors such as patients' personality traits, pre-existing factors (such as comorbid illnesses, presence of alcohol or drugs and tiredness) or contributing conditions (availability or lack of support, use of medications such as morphine, beta blockers, and benzodiazepines) prior to or immediately after the traumatic experience. Unfortunately, many of the reviewed literature failed to assess or report comorbid illnesses or medication regimens. Prospective investigations with more uniform methodologies, unified patient populations, and pre- and post-trauma approaches are necessary to further explore such relationships.

Author details
[1]Department of Psychiatry, University of Michigan, Ann Arbor, 1500 East Medical Center Drive, Ann Arbor, MI 48109, USA. [2]Department of Psychiatry and Behavioral Neurosciences, Wayne State University, 540 E Canfield, Detroit, MI 48201-1998, USA.

Authors' contributions
AJ participated in design of the study, data collection and analysis; interpretation of the results and conceptualization of the findings; and preparation of the manuscript. IL participated in data analysis; interpretation of the results and conceptualization of the findings; and preparation of the manuscript. AA participated in design of the study; interpretation of the results and conceptualization of the findings; and preparation of the

manuscript. KG participated in data analysis, and preparation of the manuscript.

NNB participated in design of the study; data analysis, interpretation of the results and conceptualization of the findings; and preparation of the manuscript. All authors read and approved the final manuscript.

Competing interests

The authors declare that they have no competing interests.

References

1. Veltmeyer MD, Clark CR, McFarlane AC, Moores KA, Bryant RA, Gordon E: Working memory function in post-traumatic stress disorder: an event-related potential study. Clin Neurophysiol 2009, 120(6):1096-1106.
2. Lijffijt M, Lane SD, Meier SL, Boutros NN, Burroughs S, Steinberg JL, Gerard Moeller F, Swann AC: P50, N100, and P200 sensory gating: relationships with behavioral inhibition, attention, and working memory. Psychophysiology 2009, 46(5):1059-68.
3. Misulis KE, Head TC: Brainstem Auditory Evoked Potentials. In Essentials of Clinical Neurophysiology.. 3 edition. Edited by: Misulis KE, Head TC. Burlington, MA: Butterworth-Heinemann; 2003:211-220.
4. Boutros NN, Iacono WG, Galderisi S: Applied Electrophysiology. In Kaplan and Sadock's Comprehensive Textbook of Psychiatry.. Ninth edition. Edited by: Kaplan BJ, Sadock VA, Ruiz P. Philadelphia: Lippincott Williams 2009:211-248.
5. Boutros NN, Korzyukov O, Jansen B, Feingold A, Bell M: Sensory-gating deficits during the mid-latency phase of information processing in medicated schizophrenia patients. Psychiatry Research 2004, 126:203-215.
6. Cromwell HC, Mears RP, Wan L, Boutros NN: Sensory gating: a translational effort from basic to clinical science. Clin EEG Neurosci 2008, 39(2):69-72.
7. Buchsbaum MS: The middle evoked response components and schizophrenia. Schizophr Bull 1977, 3:93-104.
8. Regan D: Human Brain Electrophysiology New York: Elsevier; 1989.
9. Adler LE, Pachtman E, Franks RD, Pecevich M, Waldo MC, Freedman R: Neurophysiological evidence for a defect in neuronal mechanisms involved in sensory gating in schizophrenia. Biol Psychiatry 1982, 17:639-654.
10. Nagamoto HT, Adler LE, Waldo MC, Freedman R: Sensory gating in schizophrenia and healthy control: effects of changing stimulus interval. Biol Psychiatry 1989, 25:549-561.
11. Polich J, Kok A: Cognitive and biological determinants of P300: an integrative review. Biological Psychology 1995, 41:103-146.
12. Weber DL, Clark CR, McFarlane AC, Moores KA, Morris P, Egan GF: Abnormal frontal and parietal activity during working memory updating in post-traumatic stress disorder. Psychiatry Res 2005, 140(1):27-44.
13. Kimble M, Ruddy K, Deldin P, Kaufman M: A CNV-distraction paradigm in combat veterans with posttraumatic stress disorder. J Neuropsychiatry Clin Neurosci 2004, 16(1):102-108.
14. Blake DD, Weathers FW, Nagy LM, Kaloupek DG, Gusman FD, Charney DS, Keane TM: The development of a clinician-administered PTSD scale. J Trauma Stress 1995, 8:75-90.
15. Weathers FW, Keane TM, Davidson JR: Clinician-Administered PTSD Scale: A review of the first ten years of research. Depress Anxiety 2001, 13(3):132-156.
16. Keane TM, Caddell JM, Taylor KL: Mississippi Scale for Combat-Related Posttraumatic Stress Disorder: three studies in reliability and validity. J Consult Clin Psychol 1988, 56:85-90.
17. Attias J, Bleich A, Furman V, Zinger Y: Event-related potentials in disorder of combat origin. Biol Psychiatry 1996, 40(5):373-381.
18. Spielberger CD: State-trait Anxiety Inventory: a comprehensive bibliography Palo Alto, CA: Consultant Psychologists Press; 1984.
19. Derogatis LR, Melisaratos N: The Brief Symptom Inventory: an introductory report. Psychol Med 1983, 13:595-605.
20. Geisheim C, Hahlweg K, Fiegenbaum W, Frank M, Schroeder B, von-Witzleben I: German version of the Brief Symptom Inventory (BSI) as a tool for quality assurance in psychotherapy. Diagnostica 2002, 48:28-36.
21. Beck AT, Steer RA: Manual for the Beck Depression Inventory San Antonio, TX: Psychological Corporation; 1993.

22. Weiss DS, Marmar CR: The Impact of Event Scale - Revised. In Assessing psychological trauma and PTSD. Edited by: Wilson J, Keane TM. New York: Guilford; 1996:399-411.
23. Weathers F, Litz B, Herman D, Huska J, Keane T: The PTSD Checklist (PCL): Reliability, Validity, and Diagnostic Utility. Paper presented at the Annual Convention of the International Society for Traumatic Stress Studies San Antonio, TX; 1993.
24. Pollock V, Cho DW, Reker D, Volavka J: Profile of mood states: the factors and their physiological correlates. J Nerv Ment Dis 1979, 167(10):612-614.
25. Morgan CA, Grillon C: Abnormal mismatch negativity in women with sexual assault-related posttraumatic stress disorder. Biol Psychiatry 1999, 45(7):827-832.
26. Hunter M, Villarreal G, McHaffie GR, Jimenez B, Smith AK, Calais LA, Hanlon F, Thoma RJ, Cañive JM: Lateralized abnormalities in auditory M50 sensory gating and cortical thickness of the superior temporal gyrus in post-traumatic stress disorder: preliminary results. Psychiatry Res 2011, 191(2):138-144.
27. Ghisolfi ES, Margis R, Becker J, Zanardo AP, Strimitzer IM, Lara DR: Impaired P50 sensory gating in post-traumatic stress disorder secondary to urban violence. Int J Psychophysiol 2004, 51(3):209-214.
28. Felmingham KL, Bryant RA, Kendall C, Gordon E: Event-related potential dysfunction in posttraumatic stress disorder: the role of numbing. Psychiatry Res 2002, 109(2):171-179.
29. Wessa M, Karl A, Flor H: Central and peripheral psychophysiological responses to trauma-related cues in subclinical posttraumatic stress disorder: a pilot study. Exp Brain Res 2005, 167(1):56-65.
30. Lewine JD, Thoma RJ, Provencal SL, Edgar C, Miller GA, Canive JM: Abnormal stimulus-response intensity functions in posttraumatic stress disorder: an electrophysiological investigation. Am J Psychiatry 2002, 159(10):1689-1695.
31. Paige SR, Reid GM, Allen MG, Newton JE: Psychophysiological correlates of posttraumatic stress disorder in Vietnam veterans. Biol Psychiatry 1990, 27(4):419-430.
32. Metzger LJ, Carson MA, Paulus LA, Lasko NB, Paige SR, Pitman RK, Orr SP: Event-related potentials to auditory stimuli in female Vietnam nurse veterans with posttraumatic stress disorder. Psychophysiology 2002, 39(1):49-63.
33. Metzger LJ, Pitman RK, Miller GA, Paige SR, Orr SP: Intensity dependence of auditory P2 in monozygotic twins discordant for Vietnam combat: associations with posttraumatic stress disorder. J Rehabil Res Dev 2008, 45(3):437-449.
34. Yun X, Li W, Qiu J, Jou J, Wei D, Tu S, Zhang Q: Neural mechanisms of subliminal priming for traumatic episodic memory: An ERP study. Neurosci Lett 2011, 498(1):10-14.
35. Lamprecht F, Köhnke C, Lempa W, Sack M, Matzke M, Münte TF: Event-related potentials and EMDR treatment of post-traumatic stress disorder. Neurosci Res 2004, 49(2):267-272.
36. Menning H, Renz A, Seifert J, Maercker A: Reduced mismatch negativity in posttraumatic stress disorder: a compensatory mechanism for chronic hyperarousal? Int J Psychophysiol 2008, 68(1):27-34.
37. Cardillo G: MyFisher22.[http://www.mathworks.com/matlabcentral/fileexchange/15434-myfisher22].
38. Felmingham KL, Bryant RA, Gordon E: Processing angry and neutral faces in post-traumatic stress disorder: an event-related potentials study. Neuroreport 2003, 14(5):777-780.
39. Blomhoff S, Reinvang I, Malt UF: Event-related potentials to stimuli with emotional impact in posttraumatic stress patients. Biol Psychiatry 1998, 44(10):1045-1053.
40. Wessa M, Jatzko A, Flor H: Retrieval and emotional processing of traumatic memories in posttraumatic stress disorder: peripheral and central correlates. Neuropsychologia 2006, 44(10):1683-1696.
41. Metzger LJ, Orr SP, Lasko NB, McNally RJ, Pitman RK: Seeking the source of emotional Stroop interference effects in PTSD: a study of P3s to traumatic words. Integr Physiol Behav Sci 1997, 32(1):43-51.
42. Ehlers CL, Hurst S, Phillips E, Gilder DA, Dixon M, Gross A, Lau P, Yehuda R: Electrophysiological responses to affective stimuli in American Indians experiencing trauma with and without PTSD. Ann N Y Acad Sci 2006, 1071:125-136.
43. Metzger LJ, Orr SP, Lasko NB, Berry NJ, Pitman RK: Evidence for diminished P3 amplitudes in PTSD. Ann N Y Acad Sci 1997, 821:499-503.

44. Smith D, Boutros NN, Schwarzkopf SB: **Reliability of P50 auditory event-related potential indices of SG.** *Psychophysiology* 1994, **31**:495-502.

45. Fuerst DR, Gallinat J, Boutros NN: **Range of SG values and test-retest reliability in normal subjects.** *Psychophysiology* 2007, **44**:620-626.

46. Kurayama T, Nakazawa K, Matsuzawa D, Yoshida S, Nanbu M, Suto C, Shimizu E: **Alterations of auditory P50 suppression in human fear conditioning and extinction.** *Biol Psychiatry* 2009, **65**(6):495-502.

47. Boutros NN, Korzyukov O, Oliwa G, Feingold A, Campbell D, McClain-Furmanski D, Struve F, Jansen BH: **Morphological and latency abnormalities of the mid-latency auditory evoked responses in schizophrenia: a preliminary report.** *Schizophr Res* 2004, **70**(2-3):303-313.

48. Anokhin AP, Vedeniapin AB, Heath AC, Korxyukov O, Boutros NN: **Genetic and environmental influences on sensory gating of mid-latency auditory evoked responses: a twin study.** *Schizophr Res* 2007, **89**(1-3):312-319.

49. Metzger LJ, Clark CR, McFarlane AC, Veltmeyer MD, Lasko NB, Paige SR, Pitman RK, Orr SP: **Event-related potentials to auditory stimuli in monozygotic twins discordant for combat: association with PTSD.** *Psychophysiology* 2009, **46**(1):172-178.

50. Attias J, Bleich A, Gilat S: **Classification of veterans with post-traumatic stress disorder using visual brain evoked P3s to traumatic stimuli.** *Br J Psychiatry* 1996, **168**(1):110-115.

51. Vrca A, Bozikov V, Malinar M: **The use of visual evoked potentials to follow-up prisoners of war after release from detention camps.** *Coll Antropol* 1997, **21**(1):229-233.

52. Gillette GM, Skinner RD, Rasco LM, Fielstein EM, Davis DH, Pawelak JE, Freeman TW, Karson CN, Boop FA, Garcia-Rill E: **Combat veterans with posttraumatic stress disorder exhibit decreased habituation of the P1 midlatency auditory evoked potential.** *Life Sci* 1997, **61**(14):1421-1434.

53. Neylan TC, Fletcher DJ, Lenoci M, McCallin K, Weiss DS, Schoenfeld FB, Marmar CR, Fein G: **Sensory gating in chronic posttraumatic stress disorder: reduced auditory P50 suppression in combat veterans.** *Biol Psychiatry* 1999, **46**(12):1656-1664.

54. Skinner RD, Rasco LM, Fitzgerald J, Karson CN, Matthew M, Williams DK, Garcia-Rill E: **Reduced sensory gating of the P1 potential in rape victims and combat veterans with posttraumatic stress disorder.** *Depress Anxiety* 1999, **9**(3):122-130.

55. Holstein DH, Vollenweider FX, Jäncke L, Schopper C, Csomor PA: **P50 suppression, prepulse inhibition, and startle reactivity in the same patient cohort suffering from posttraumatic stress disorder.** *J Affect Disord* 2010, **126**(1-2):188-197.

56. Metzger LJ, Orr SP, Lasko NB, Pitman RK: **Auditory event-related potentials to tone stimuli in combat-related posttraumatic stress disorder.** *Biol Psychiatry* 1997, **42**(11):1006-1015.

57. Galletly CA, McFarlane AC, Clark R: **Differentiating cortical patterns of cognitive dysfunction in schizophrenia and posttraumatic stress disorder.** *Psychiatry Res* 2008, **159**(1-2):196-206.

58. Bleich AV, Attias J, Furman V: **Effect of repeated visual traumatic stimuli on the event related P3 brain potential in post-traumatic stress disorder.** *Int J Neurosci* 1996, **85**(1-2):45-55.

59. Boudarene M, Timsit-Berthier M: **Interest of events-related potentials in assessment of posttraumatic stress disorder.** *Ann N Y Acad Sci* 1997, **821**:494-498.

60. Kounios J, Litz B, Kaloupek D, Riggs D, Knight J, Weathers F, Anderson JE, Keane T: **Electrophysiology of combat-related PTSD.** *Ann N Y Acad Sci* 1997, **821**:504-507.

61. Kimble M, Kaloupek D, Kaufman M, Deldin P: **Stimulus novelty differentially affects attentional allocation in PTSD.** *Biol Psychiatry* 200, **47**(10):880-890.

62. Stanford MS, Vasterling JJ, Mathias CW, Constans JI, Houston RJ: **Impact of threat relevance on P3 event-related potentials in combat-related post-traumatic stress disorder.** *Psychiatry Res* 2001, **102**(2):125-137.

63. Neylan TC, Jasiukaitis PA, Lenoci M, Scott JC, Metzler TJ, Weiss DS, Schoenfeld FB, Marmar CR: **Temporal instability of auditory and visual event-related potentials in posttraumatic stress disorder.** *Biol Psychiatry* 2003, **53**(3):216-225.

64. Araki T, Kasai K, Yamasue H, Kato N, Kudo N, Ohtani T, Nakagome K, Kirihara K, Yamada H, Abe O, Iwanami A: **Association between lower P300 amplitude and smaller anterior cingulate cortex volume in patients with posttraumatic stress disorder: a study of victims of Tokyo subway sarin attack.** *Neuroimage* 2005, **25**(1):43-50.

65. Veltmeyer MD, McFarlane AC, Bryant RA, Mayo T, Gordon E, Clark CR: **Integrative assessment of brain function in PTSD: brain stability and working memory.** *J Integr Neurosci* 2005, **5**(1):123-138.

66. Wessa M, Flor H: **Failure of extinction of fear responses in posttraumatic stress disorder: evidence from second-order conditioning.** *Am J Psychiatry* 2007, **164**(11):1684-1692.

Reduced hippocampal and medial prefrontal gray matter mediate the association between reported childhood maltreatment and trait anxiety in adulthood and predict sensitivity to future life stress

Adam X Gorka[1*], Jamie L Hanson[1,2], Spenser R Radtke[1] and Ahmad R Hariri[1]

Abstract

Background: The experience of early life stress is a consistently identified risk factor for the development of mood and anxiety disorders. Preclinical research employing animal models of early life stress has made inroads in understanding this association and suggests that the negative sequelae of early life stress may be mediated by developmental disruption of corticolimbic structures supporting stress responsiveness. Work in humans has corroborated this idea, as childhood adversity has been associated with alterations in gray matter volumes of the hippocampus, amygdala, and medial prefrontal cortex. Yet, missing from this body of research is a full understanding of how these neurobiological vulnerabilities may mechanistically contribute to the reported link between adverse childhood experiences and later affective psychopathology.

Results: Analyses revealed that self-reported childhood maltreatment was associated with reduced gray matter volumes within the medial prefrontal cortex and left hippocampus. Furthermore, reduced left hippocampal and medial prefrontal gray matter volume mediated the relationship between childhood maltreatment and trait anxiety. Additionally, individual differences in corticolimbic gray matter volume within these same structures predicted the anxious symptoms as a function of life stress 1 year after initial assessment.

Conclusions: Collectively, these findings provide novel evidence that reductions in corticolimbic gray matter, particularly within the hippocampus and medial prefrontal cortex, are associated with reported childhood maltreatment and individual differences in adult trait anxiety. Furthermore, our results suggest that these structural alterations contribute to increased affective sensitivity to stress later in life in those that have experienced early adversity. More broadly, the findings contribute to an emerging literature highlighting the critical importance of early stress on the development of corticolimbic structures supporting adaptive functioning later in life.

Keywords: Stress, Hippocampus, Gray matter, Anxiety, MRI, Childhood maltreatment, Medial prefrontal cortex

* Correspondence: axgorka@gmail.com
[1]Laboratory of NeuroGenetics, Department of Psychology and Neuroscience, Duke University, 417 Chapel Drive, Durham, NC 27708, USA
Full list of author information is available at the end of the article

Background

Stress early in life is associated with increased rates of mood and anxiety disorders in adulthood [1] with a recent meta-analysis showing a 62% increase in the risk for anxiety disorders in individuals who have suffered early trauma [2]. With over one in eight children in the US experiencing early adversity such as child maltreatment [3], this represents a major public health problem. Though well-studied and well-replicated in psychological and epidemiological research, little is known regarding the mechanisms mediating the association between adverse childhood experiences and later affective psychopathology, particularly anxiety disorders.

Preclinical research has begun to uncover potential neurobiological mechanisms underlying these relationships, as a multitude of animal models of early life stress (e.g., maternal deprivation, maternal abuse), result in an increase in anxiety-like behavioral phenotypes and also structural alterations in corticolimbic regions such as the hippocampus, amygdala, and prefrontal cortex [4,5]. Similar alterations have been noted in human samples exposed to childhood maltreatment, with reduced gray matter volume within the hippocampus and alterations in an interconnected network of corticolimbic structures, including the amygdala, orbitofrontal cortex, and anterior cingulate cortex as a function of stressors experienced during childhood [6-10]. Such results have important implications for the vulnerability to affective psychopathology. Reduced gray matter within these brain structures has also been associated with higher trait anxiety as well as mood and anxiety disorders in adults [11-17].

Missing from this body of research, however, are strong links to behavior, as many of the past studies have simply noted brain differences between groups. Rao and colleagues [18] took an important initial step to close this gap, finding decreased hippocampal gray matter mediated the relationship between adversity during childhood and increased risk for major depression. While these investigators importantly connected alterations in neurobiology and behavior, it is still unclear how differences in the brain are associated with higher rates of affective dysregulation after early stress. Further studies are needed to drill down to understand how neurobiological vulnerabilities may mechanistically contribute to the reported link between adverse childhood experiences and later affective psychopathology.

Related to this idea, a growing body of psychological research has found that environmental stressors often play a precipitating role in the onset of mood and anxiety disorders and that the experience of stress early in life confers risk for psychopathology by sensitizing organisms to stress in adulthood [19,20]. Tellingly, childhood maltreatment is further associated with increased trait anxiety, alterations in hypothalamic-pituitary-adrenal (HPA) axis stress reactivity, and greater potentiated startle to threat [1,21,22]. These collective findings suggest that early adversity may create a dispositional sensitivity to perceived threat and may be associated with elevated risk for mood and anxiety disorders following stressful life events in adulthood [23-25]. No study to date, however, has formally linked individual differences in the intermediate risk phenotype of trait anxiety with the experience of childhood maltreatment, particularly in relation to later stress, and associated changes in corticolimbic morphology. It is likely that alterations in corticolimbic gray matter associated with childhood maltreatment interact with experiences of stress in the future and these neural phenotypes associated with early adversity may aid researchers in prospectively predicting relative risk and resilience in the context of environmental challenge.

In the current study, we examined if the association between self-reported childhood maltreatment and the expression of trait anxiety in adulthood is mediated by differences in corticolimbic morphology. Specifically, we tested whether childhood maltreatment was associated with trait anxiety via reductions in gray matter within neural circuits regulating stress responsiveness. To this end, structural MRI and self-reported measures of childhood maltreatment, recent life stress, and negative affect were examined in 818 participants of the ongoing Duke Neurogenetics Study (DNS). A subset of 196 participants completed additional behavioral assessments at least 1 year after the DNS. This unique longitudinal component allowed us to further determine if the structural correlates of childhood maltreatment predict subsequent vulnerability to future stressful life events. Based on prior preclinical and clinical research, we hypothesized that childhood maltreatment would be negatively correlated with corticolimbic gray matter volume with a specific focus on the hippocampus, amygdala, and medial prefrontal cortex (mPFC) including the orbitofrontal cortex (OFC) and anterior cingulate cortex (ACC). Further, we hypothesized that gray matter reductions within these structures would mediate the relationship between childhood maltreatment and adult trait anxiety. Given the importance of these corticolimbic structures in orchestrating adaptive responses to stress, we lastly hypothesized that these gray matter reductions would predict increased anxiety, following stressful life events in the future.

Methods

Participants

This study was approved by the Duke University Medical Center Institutional Review Board. Data were available from 906 participants who had successfully completed the ongoing DNS, which assesses a wide range of behavioral and biological traits among non-patient, 18–22-year-old university students. All participants provided informed consent in accordance with Duke University

Medical Center Institutional Review Board guidelines prior to participation. The participants were in good general health and free of the following study exclusions: (1) medical diagnoses of cancer, stroke, head injury with loss of consciousness, untreated migraine headaches, diabetes requiring insulin treatment, chronic kidney or liver disease, or lifetime history of psychotic symptoms; (2) use of psychotropic, glucocorticoid, or hypolipidemic medication; and (3) conditions affecting cerebral blood flow and metabolism (e.g., hypertension). As diagnoses of mood disorders are associated with gray matter volume and trait anxiety, we excluded participants based on a diagnosis of any past or current DSM-IV axis I or select axis II (antisocial and borderline personality) disorders as identified through clinical interviews using the electronic MINI [26]. The participants were administered a neuropsychological battery that included the Wechsler Abbreviated Scale of Intelligence (WASI) [27].

Analyses testing primary hypotheses were limited to 818 participants (469 females, mean age =19.62 ± 1.24 SD) with overlapping structural MRI and self-report data surviving our stringent, multilevel quality control procedures described below. All successful DNS participants are contacted every 3 months after initial study completion and asked to complete a brief online assessment of recent life events, mood, and affect in the past week. Secondary longitudinal analyses were restricted to a subset of 196 participants (123 females, mean age =19.49 ± 1.17 SD) that completed these follow-up measures at least 1 year after their structural scan (mean time since scan = 466.98 days ±131.66 at the time of follow-up). See Table 1 for descriptive statistics of the full sample and longitudinal subsample.

Self-report measures

The State-Trait Anxiety Inventory - Trait (STAI-T) version was used to assess the general tendency with which individuals perceive encountered situations to be threatening and to respond to such situations with subjective feelings of apprehension and tension [28].

The Childhood Trauma Questionnaire (CTQ) was used to assess exposure to childhood maltreatment in five categories: emotional, physical and sexual abuse, and emotional and physical neglect [29]. Each of the

instrument's subscales has robust internal consistency and convergent validity with a clinician-rated interview of childhood abuse and therapists' ratings of abuse [30]. As each type of stressor would contribute to allostatic load which is thought to impact the hippocampus, we conducted analyses using total scores, summed from all subscales, which have previously been demonstrated to predict gray matter reductions within the brain [6,31].

We used a modified version of the Life Events Scale for Students (LESS) [32] to assess the occurrence and self-reported subjective impact of common stressful life events within the past 12 months (see Additional file 1 for details on items). As the experience of each life event would contribute to allostatic load, which is thought to impact corticolimbic circuitry, we conducted analyses using cumulative impact scores (i.e., the sum of self-reported impact from all stressful life events reported within the last 12 months).

Recent negative affect was assessed using the Mood and Anxiety Symptom Questionnaire (MASQ) [33]. The MASQ is a well-validated measure yielding four subscales assessing symptoms experienced within the last 7 days specific to Anxious Arousal (MASQ-AA) or Anhedonic Depression (MASQ-AD) as well as General Distress Anxiety (MASQ-GDA) and General Distress Depression (MASQ-GDD). Previous research has demonstrated that MASQ-AA, which represents items assessing physiological arousal, has higher discriminant validity than MASQ-GDA, which represents items assessing general and nonspecific distress [33,34]. Here, we utilize MASQ-AA as it best represents a state measure related to our measure of trait anxiety.

Acquisition of structural MRI data

Each participant was scanned on one of two identical research-dedicated GE MR750 3T scanners at the Duke-UNC Brain Imaging and Analysis Center. Each identical scanner was equipped with high-power high-duty cycle 50-mT/m gradients at 200 T/m/s slew rate and an eight-channel head coil for parallel imaging at high bandwidth up to 1 MHz. For optimized voxel-based morphometry (VBM), T1-weighted images were obtained using a 3D Ax FSPGR BRAVO sequence with the following parameters: TR =8.148 s; TE =3.22 ms; 162 sagittal slices;

Table 1 Descriptive statistics of all participants

	Age	Gender	Childhood maltreatment (CTQ)	Recent life stress (LESS)	Trait anxiety (STAI-T)	IQ score[a] (WASI)	State anxiety (MASQ-AA)	Days since MRI scan
Full sample (N =818)	19.6 ± 1.24	349 male, 469 female	33.2 ± 8.12	4.2 ± 2.95	37.2 ± 5.65	121.62 ± 8.57		
Longitudinal sample (N =196)	19.5 ± 1.17	73 male, 123 female	32.5 ± 7.26	2.2 ± 2.37	37.0 ± 9.0		20.9 ± 5.75	477.0 ± 131.66

Full sample: all participants who completed the structural MRI, trait anxiety assessment (STAI-T), and inventories of life stress (CTQ, LESS) and were free of current or past mood and anxiety disorders. Longitudinal sample: subset of those participants who completed a follow-up assessment at least 1 year after their MRI scan. [a]WASI IQ scores were not collected for one participants (N =817).

flip angle, 12°; FOV, 240 mm; matrix =256 × 256; slice thickness =1 mm with no gap; and total scan time =4 min and 13 s.

Optimized voxel-based morphometry

Regional gray matter volumes from T1-weighted images were determined using the VBM8 toolbox (version 369 http://dbm.neuro.uni-jena.de/vbm/) within SPM8. The toolbox is an extension of the unified segmentation model [35]. Using this approach, individual T1-weighted images were segmented into gray, white, and CSF images using an adaptive maximum a posterior technique, partial volume estimation, an optimized block-wise nonlocal means denoising filter and spatial constraints based on a classical Markov random field model. Resulting gray matter images were normalized to a gray matter template in Montreal Neurological Institute (MNI) space using affine transformations. Subsequently, gray matter voxel values were scaled using the Jacobian matrix parameters from normalization to adjust for volume changes during the affine transformation. In line with the methodology of Good et al. [36], normalized gray matter images were then smoothed with a 12-mm FWHM kernel [36].

Hypothesis testing

Associations between CTQ total scores and local gray matter volume were assessed by entering the resulting processed whole brain gray matter images into a second-level multiple regression analysis within SPM8. To ensure that results were unique to CTQ scores, we controlled for recent life stress (LESS cumulative impact) in addition to age and gender. We corrected against type I error in these analyses resulting from multiple comparisons by applying a p <0.05 family wise error (FWE)-corrected threshold on a voxel level across bilateral medial temporal lobe and medial PFC regions of interest, which were defined using a medial frontal gyrus regions of interest (ROI) selected from the Talairach Daemon - Labels toolbox and a medial temporal lobe ROI, comprised of bilateral hippocampus and amygdala masks, using the Automatic Anatomical Labeling (AAL) toolbox within SPM8. Gray matter volumes from a 5-mm sphere surrounding the max voxel of resulting clusters showing significant associations with CTQ scores were then extracted and entered into SPSS v21 for mediation and moderation analyses using the PROCESS macro [37].

Our mediation analyses assessed the indirect effect (the a path multiplied by the b path) of self-reported childhood maltreatment on trait anxiety via variability in gray matter volume. Previous research has demonstrated that the indirect effect, in contrast with the variables used to calculate it, is only normally distributed in special cases

which can lead to unbalanced confidence limits [38]. Consequently, we determined significance using confidence intervals obtained using bias-corrected bootstrapping which previous research suggests is the best resampling method for testing indirect effects [38]. Reported regression coefficients reflect standardized betas.

Results
Demographic data

The observed means and distributions of our self-report measures were broadly in line with previous reports. For the CTQ total scores, the mean was 33.03 for men and 33.33 for women with a range of 25–75 (score of 25 was the minimum possible value with participants selecting a "1 = Never True" for all items). Previous CTQ total scores derived from young adults in a community sample was 32.96 for men and 30.27 for women [39]. Although ranges were not reported for this community sample, the 90th percentile had a mean of 41.00 for men and 41.49 for women, while the 90th percentile in our sample has a mean of 49.15 for men and 52.46 for women. Previous assessments of cumulative impact for all 36 LESS items in undergraduate samples report means of 248.32 with a range of 0–1,009 (with impact for each event scored on a scale of 0–100) [40]. The version of the LESS collected in this study assessed 45 items (see Additional file 1 for all items) with impact scored on a scale of 1–4 for each event. Although we collect data on a broader number of negative life events, using a truncated Likert scale for impact rating, our results (mean =9.26, range: 0–52) are broadly in line with previous reports after scaling adjustments (mean =231.57, range: 0–1,300). STAI-T scores from our sample (mean =37.21, range: 20–71) are similar to those reported from other samples of young adults (mean =32.68 for men and 36.85 for women) [41].

Our MASQ-AA scores (mean =20.9, range: 17–52) included values that were larger than those observed in previous reports from undergraduate samples (mean =18.63, range: 17–23; and mean =18.70, range: 17–26) [42] (see Table 1 for additional demographic information).

Primary analyses (full sample)
Childhood maltreatment and corticolimbic gray matter volume

CTQ total scores were negatively correlated with gray matter volume within the left hippocampus after controlling for recent life stress cumulative impact scores, gender, and age ($x = -18$, $y = -21$, $z = -18$; $T =4.46$; p <0.05, FWE-corrected; 334 voxels; Figure 1A). No significant correlations were observed between CTQ total scores and gray matter volume within the right hippocampus or bilateral amygdala. CTQ total scores were, however, negatively correlated with gray matter volume within

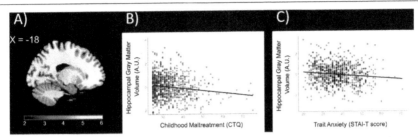

Figure 1 Relationships between hippocampal gray matter volume, childhood maltreatment, and trait anxiety (N = 818). (A) Statistical parametric map from medial temporal lobe ROI analyses illustrating voxels exhibiting a significant negative correlation with CTQ total scores within the left hippocampus while controlling for age, gender, and recent life stress (LESS) ($x = -18$). **(B)** Scatterplot depicting hippocampal gray matter volume from a 5-mm sphere surrounding max voxel ($x = -18$, $y = -21$, $z = -18$) as a function of CTQ total scores. **(C)** Trait anxiety plotted against gray matter volumes from 5-mm sphere. Scatterplots reflect partial correlations between variables after controlling for gender, age, and recent life stress (LESS). Y axes reflect standardized residuals. (AU = arbitrary units).

the mPFC ($x = -3$, $y = 57$, $z = 16$; $T = 3.88$; $p < 0.05$, FWE-corrected; 19 voxels; Figure 2A).

Correlations with trait anxiety

CTQ total scores were positively correlated with trait anxiety as assessed by the STAI-T ($\beta = 0.366$, $p < 0.001$). Individual differences in gray matter volumes from 5-mm spheres surrounding the max voxels within the left hippocampus and mPFC identified from the regression analyses with CTQ total scores reported above were correlated with trait anxiety (left hippocampus: $\beta = -0.126$, $p < 0.001$; mPFC: $\beta = -0.116$, $p < 0.001$; Figures 1C and 2C). Mediation analyses revealed that left hippocampal gray matter volume significantly mediated the relationship between CTQ total scores and STAI-T scores ($\beta = 0.011$, lower limit confidence interval (LLCI) $= 0.0006$, upper limit confidence interval (ULCI) $= 0.0246$; Figure 3). Mediation analyses further demonstrated that mPFC gray matter volume significantly mediates the relationship between CTQ total scores and STAI-T scores ($\beta = 0.009$,

LLCI $= 0.0007$, ULCI $= 0.0230$; Figure 4). These significant relationships were all robust to inclusion of LESS cumulative impact scores, gender, and age as covariates.

Secondary analyses (longitudinal sample)
Corticolimbic morphology and responsiveness to stress
There was a significant positive correlation between LESS cumulative impact scores in the year following initial assessment and MASQ-AA scores at follow-up ($\beta = 0.204$, $p = 0.008$) after controlling for age, gender, and number of days between MRI scan and follow-up assessment. This correlation was significantly moderated by the same left hippocampal gray matter volumes described above ($\beta = -0.181$, $p = 0.038$) (Figure 5) while controlling for covariates. The participants with relatively less hippocampal gray matter volume exhibited stronger correlations between LESS and MASQ-AA than those with average or relatively more gray matter volumes (simple slopes: -1 SD: $\beta = 0.345$, $p = 0.001$; mean: $\beta = 0.164$, $p = 0.033$, $+1$ SD: $\beta = -0.017$, $p = 0.893$; Figure 4). Gray

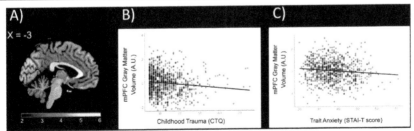

Figure 2 Relationships between mPFC gray matter volume, childhood maltreatment, and trait anxiety (N = 818). (A) Statistical parametric map from frontal gyrus ROI analyses illustrating voxels exhibiting a significant negative correlation with CTQ total scores within the mPFC while controlling for age, gender, and recent life stress (LESS) ($x = -3$). **(B)** Scatterplot depicting mPFC gray matter volume from a 5-mm sphere surrounding max voxel ($x = -3$, $y = 57$, $z = 16$) as a function of CTQ total scores. **(C)** Trait anxiety plotted against mPFC gray matter volumes from 5-mm sphere. Scatterplots reflect partial correlations between variables after controlling for gender, age, and recent life stress (LESS). Y axes reflect standardized residuals. (AU = arbitrary units).

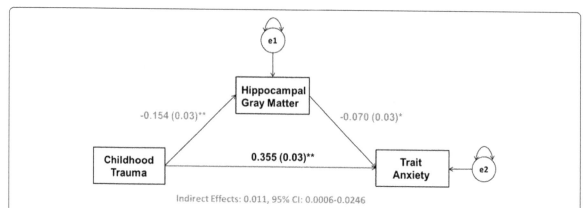

Figure 3 Hippocampal gray matter volume mediates the relationship between childhood maltreatment and trait anxiety in adulthood. Results from a path analysis testing a model wherein left hippocampal gray matter volume mediates the relationship between childhood maltreatment and trait anxiety in adulthood. Values represent standardized parameter estimates with standard errors presented in parentheses after controlling for age, gender, and recent life stress (LESS). The circles labeled e1 and e2 denote the variance in left hippocampal gray matter volume and trait anxiety scores unaccounted for by the model. *p <0.05, **p <0.005.

matter within the medial prefrontal cortex similarly moderated the relationship between LESS cumulative impact scores and MASQ-AA (interaction term: $\beta = -0.178$, $p = 0.008$; simple slopes: -1 SD: $\beta = 0.378$, $p = 0.002$; mean: $\beta = 0.200$, $p = 0.008$, $+1$ SD: $\beta = 0.023$, $p = 0.823$; Figure 6) while controlling for covariates.

Discussion

Here, fitting with past research, we find that self-reported childhood maltreatment was associated with reduced gray matter volumes within the medial prefrontal cortex and left hippocampus. We also for the first time to date, formally demonstrate that gray matter volume reductions within the hippocampus and mPFC mediate the association

between the self-reported childhood maltreatment and the increased expression of trait anxiety in adulthood. Our results expand on prior preclinical and clinical research and begin to fill in important gaps in the understanding of the sequelae of early life stress including associated variance in neurobiology. Unique to our work, we then attempted to link these neurobiological phenotypes to susceptibility to environmental challenge in the future by focusing on the relationship between stress later in life and state anxiety as a function of individual differences in corticolimbic morphology. Consistent with our hypotheses, our secondary analyses demonstrate this intermediate behavioral phenotype is related to reduced hippocampal and mPFC gray matter volume. As such, gray matter within these structures

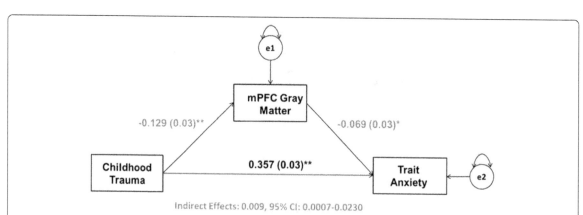

Figure 4 mPFC gray matter volume mediates the relationship between childhood maltreatment and trait anxiety in adulthood. Results from a path analysis testing a model wherein mPFC gray matter volume mediates the relationship between childhood maltreatment and trait anxiety in adulthood. Values represent standardized parameter estimates with standard errors presented in parentheses after controlling for age, gender, and recent life stress (LESS). The circles labeled e1 and e2 denote the variance in mPFC gray matter volume and trait anxiety scores unaccounted for by the model. *p <0.05, **p <0.005.

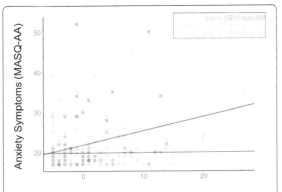

Figure 5 The relationship between recent life stress (LESS) and current anxiety symptoms (MASQ-AA). The relationship between recent life stress (LESS) and current anxiety symptoms (MASQ-AA) measured at least 1 year after initial assessment, plotted at low (−1 SD), intermediate (mean), and high (+1 SD) levels of left hippocampal gray matter volume. Scatterplots reflect partial correlations between LESS and STAI-T after controlling for gender, age, and time since MRI scan. MASQ-AA scores reflect standardized residuals.

may represent a neural embedding of early life stress through which later psychopathology emerges.

Our findings of structural alterations within the hippocampus and mPFC associated with self-reported childhood maltreatment are broadly consistent with findings from animal models showing decreased dendritic arborization, spine density, and neuronal number within these areas [43-45]. Though, care should be taken in direct translation, as the resolution of MRI precludes focusing on neural

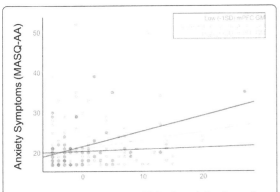

Figure 6 The relationship between recent life stress (LESS) and current anxiety symptoms (MASQ-AA). The relationship between recent life stress (LESS) and current anxiety symptoms (MASQ-AA) measured at least 1 year after initial assessment, plotted at low (−1 SD), intermediate (mean), and high (+1 SD) levels of mPFC gray matter volume. Scatterplots reflect partial correlations between LESS and STAI-T after controlling for gender, age, and time since MRI scan. MASQ-AA scores reflect standardized residuals.

architecture at that level and our data is correlative in nature. Thinking about what these neural alterations may mean for behavior, the hippocampus is critical in shaping emotional responses to environmental challenge through its regulation of the HPA axis and encoding of contextual memory for emotional experiences as exemplified by fear learning [40,41]. The mPFC is essential for the process of fear extinction and functions to regulate behavioral and neuroendocrine responses to controllable stressors [46,47]. The hippocampus and mPFC both support multiple processes that likely contribute to trait anxiety; however, it is currently unclear which exact processes are being affected by gray matter reductions in these regions.

Of note, our study contained both (primary) cross-sectional and (secondary) longitudinal assessments. The deployment of longitudinal designs is especially important when considering how stress affects brain structure across development and how early adversity shapes future responses to stress. Although much research has addressed the relationship between childhood maltreatment and gray matter volume in adulthood, certain studies provide unique insight into the complexity of these relationships. Meta-analyses demonstrate that childhood maltreatment is associated with reduced hippocampal gray matter in adulthood, but not during childhood [34] suggesting that the impact of adversity on neural morphology is not immediate but develops over time. A better understanding of how childhood maltreatment is associated with gray matter in neural structures that generate and regulate responses to stress may facilitate our understanding of how early adversity impacts risk in the context of stress over the lifespan and may implicate specific developmental windows during which treatment and prevention strategies are most effective. It is possible that intervention strategies immediately following childhood maltreatment may prevent the emergence of hippocampal deficits, which are associated with risk for mood and anxiety disorders. Preventing these morphological changes via intervention during childhood may be more effective than treating the negative sequelae that emerge in adulthood.

Our work is not without limitations. First, our measures of self-reported childhood maltreatment, trait anxiety, and gray matter morphology were assessed concurrently, and as such are correlative in nature and cannot establish temporal order. For example, it is possible that persons who are high in trait anxiety, in addition to having reduced gray matter volume, are also more likely to retrospectively remember or report maltreatment during childhood. It is thus possible that hippocampal and mPFC gray matter volume mediates the impact of trait anxiety on self-reported childhood maltreatment, rather than vice versa. However, our finding that individual differences in gray matter volume within these structures prospectively predicts anxious arousal and subsequent to the experience of stressful life events supports the importance of gray matter deficits within the hippocampus and mPFC associated with childhood maltreatment as a mechanism through which sensitivity to stressful life events emerges. Developmental longitudinal studies in high-risk populations (e.g., individuals with positive family history for disorder) could advance the relevance of this potential mechanism for understanding etiology and pathophysiology of anxiety disorders.

Additionally, we observed decreased gray matter within the left hippocampus as a function of self-reported childhood maltreatment, but no effect of early life stress was significant within the right hemisphere. We did not hypothesize a lateralized effect, and it is possible that results in the right hemisphere are simply less robust. A recent meta-analysis found evidence for bilateral reductions in hippocampal gray matter in participants with PTSD related to childhood trauma [34]. We observe only a weak effect of childhood maltreatment on gray matter volume within the right hippocampus and only at more liberal statistical threshold (p <0.005 uncorrected, 21 voxels). Future research will be needed to determine whether gray matter reductions in the right hippocampus are linked to vulnerability to stress similarly to the results reported here.

Lastly, the effect sizes observed in our analyses are relatively small. Further, our sample consists of undergraduate students who report experiencing childhood maltreatment yet are free of past or current mood and anxiety disorders. As such, this sample may represent a relatively resilient population, and it is not immediately clear if our results have direct parallels to clinical outcomes. Nonetheless, previous research has demonstrated that reduced gray matter within the hippocampus mediates the association between early life adversity and vulnerability to major depression [42], which parallels the results reported here. Additionally, the age of our participants (18–22 years of age) is relatively young compared to the average onset of mood and anxiety disorders [48,49], and it is possible that some of our participants will go on to develop psychopathology within their lifetime. Future research will be needed to determine whether gray matter reductions within healthy participants exist on a continuum with clinical samples, and whether gray matter morphology is associated with responses to stress later in life in a manner that is clinically meaningful.

These limitations notwithstanding, our results suggest that structural variance in hippocampal and mPFC gray matter volume represent mechanisms through which childhood maltreatment may shape not only the expression of trait anxiety but also the responsiveness to stress. By specifically modeling the effects of childhood maltreatment onto behavioral processes indirectly through variability in neural phenotypes, our work can serve as a springboard

for future research. A wealth of preclinical and clinical evidence suggests that the experience of stress early in life and higher levels of trait anxiety are risk factors for the development of mood and anxiety disorders. Our results suggest that structural changes within the hippocampus and mPFC may represent the neural embedding of early life stress, which shapes risk for subsequent psychopathology by affecting how we respond to challenges in the environment.

Conclusions

Our findings suggest that reduced corticolimbic gray matter, particularly within the hippocampus and medial prefrontal cortex, mediates the relationship between reported childhood maltreatment and individual differences in adult trait anxiety. Further, our results suggest that these structural alterations contribute to increased affective sensitivity to stress later in life. These findings contribute to the literature addressing how early stress may affect the development of corticolimbic structures supporting adaptive functioning later in life.

Additional file

Additional file 1: Modified Life Events Scale for Students (LESS). This supplementary file contains the items used in our modified version of the Life Events Scale for Students.

Abbreviations
AAL: Automatic anatomical labeling; ACC: Anterior cingulate cortex; AU: Arbitrary units; CTQ: Childhood trauma questionnaire; DNS: Duke neurogenetics study; FWE: Family wise error; HPA: Hypothalamic-pituitary-adrenal; LESS: Life events scale for students; LLCI: Lower limit confidence interval; MASQ-AA: Mood and anxiety symptom questionnaire - anxious arousal; MASQ-GDA: Mood and anxiety symptom questionnaire - general distress anxiety; MNI: Montreal neurological institute; mPFC: Medial prefrontal cortex; OFC: Orbitofrontal cortex; ROI: Region of interest; STAI-T: State-trait anxiety inventory - trait version; ULCI: Upper limit confidence interval; VBM: Voxel-based morphometry; WASI: Wechsler abbreviated scale of intelligence.

Competing interests
The authors declare that they have no competing interests.

Authors' contributions
AXG performed the statistical analyses, participated in the study design and data collection, and helped draft the manuscript. JLH helped draft the manuscript and aided with the statistical analyses. SRR helped draft the manuscript and participated in the data collection. ARH conceived of the study, participated in the study design, and helped draft the manuscript. All authors read and approved the final manuscript.

Acknowledgements
We thank Bartholomew Brigidi, Kelly Faig, Annchen Knodt, and Yuliya Nikolova for their assistance in the DNS data collection and analysis. This work was supported by the research grants from Duke University and also the National Institute on Drug Abuse (R01-DA033369 and R01-DA031579 to ARH; P30-DA023026 to JLH), as well as a postdoctoral fellowship provided by the National Institute of Child Health and Human Development (T32-HD07376-25) through the Center for Developmental Science, University of North Carolina at Chapel Hill, to JLH.

Author details
[1]Laboratory of NeuroGenetics, Department of Psychology and Neuroscience, Duke University, 417 Chapel Drive, Durham, NC 27708, USA. [2]Center for Developmental Science, University of North Carolina at Chapel Hill, 100 East Franklin Street, Suite 200 CB#8115, Chapel Hill, NC 27599, USA.

References

1. Heim C, Nemeroff CB: The role of childhood trauma in the neurobiology of mood and anxiety disorders: preclinical and clinical studies. *Biol Psychiatry* 2001, 49:1023–1039.

2. Norman RE, Byambaa M, De R, Butchart A, Scott J, Vos T: The long-term health consequences of child physical abuse, emotional abuse, and neglect: a systematic review and meta-analysis. *PLoS Med* 2012, 9:e1001349.

3. Wildeman C, Emanuel N, Leventhal JM, Putnam-Hornstein E, Waldfogel J, Lee H: The prevalence of confirmed maltreatment among US children, 2004 to 2011. *JAMA Pediatr* 2014, 168(8):706–713.

4. Lupien SJ, McEwen BS, Gunnar MR, Heim C: Effects of stress throughout the lifespan on the brain, behaviour and cognition. *Nat Rev Neurosci* 2009, 10:434–445.

5. McEwen BS, Eiland L, Hunter RG, Miller MM: Stress and anxiety: structural plasticity and epigenetic regulation as a consequence of stress. *Neuropharmacology* 2012, 62:3–12 [Anxiety and Depression].

6. Dannlowski U, Stuhrmann A, Beutelmann V, Zwanzger P, Lenzen T, Grotegerd D, Domschke K, Hohoff C, Ohrmann P, Bauer J, Lindner C, Postert C, Konrad C, Arolt V, Heindel W, Suslow T, Kugel H: Limbic scars: long-term consequences of childhood maltreatment revealed by functional and structural magnetic resonance imaging. *Biol Psychiatry* 2012, 71:286–293 [Mechanisms of Compromised Stress Resilience During Development and Aging].

7. Mehta MA, Golembo NI, Nosarti C, Colvert E, Mota A, Williams SCR, Rutter M, Sonuga-Barke EJS: Amygdala, hippocampal and corpus callosum size following severe early institutional deprivation: the English and Romanian Adoptees Study Pilot. *J Child Psychol Psychiatry* 2009, 50:943–951.

8. Teicher MH, Anderson CM, Polcari A: Childhood maltreatment is associated with reduced volume in the hippocampal subfields CA3, dentate gyrus, and subiculum. *Proc Natl Acad Sci* 2012, 109:E563–E572.

9. Tottenham N, Sheridan MA: A review of adversity, the amygdala and the hippocampus: a consideration of developmental timing. *Front Hum Neurosci* 2010, 3:68.

10. Woon FL, Hedges DW: Hippocampal and amygdala volumes in children and adults with childhood maltreatment-related posttraumatic stress disorder: a meta-analysis. *Hippocampus* 2008, 18:729–736.

11. Bremner JD, Vythilingam M, Vermetten E, Nazeer A, Adil J, Khan S, Staib LH, Charney DS: Reduced volume of orbitofrontal cortex in major depression. *Biol Psychiatry* 2002, 51:273–279.

12. Campbell S, Marriott M, Nahmias C, MacQueen GM: Lower hippocampal volume in patients suffering from depression: a meta-analysis. *Am J Psychiatry* 2004, 161:598–607.

13. DeYoung CG, Hirsh JB, Shane MS, Papademetris X, Rajeevan N, Gray JR: Testing predictions from personality neuroscience brain structure and the big five. *Psychol Sci* 2010, 21:820–828.

14. Gardini S, Cloninger CR, Venneri A: Individual differences in personality traits reflect structural variance in specific brain regions. *Brain Res Bull* 2009, 79:265–270.

15. Karl A, Schaefer M, Malta LS, Dörfel D, Rohleder N, Werner A: A meta-analysis of structural brain abnormalities in PTSD. *Neurosci Biobehav Rev* 2006, 30:1004–1031.

16. Spampinato M, Wood J, De Simone V, Grafman J: Neural correlates of anxiety in healthy volunteers: a voxel-based morphometry study. *J Neuropsychiatry Clin Neurosci* 2009, 21:199–205.

17. Treadway MT, Grant MM, Ding Z, Hollon SD, Gore JC, Shelton RC: Early adverse events, HPA activity and rostral anterior cingulate volume in MDD. *PLoS ONE* 2009, 4:e4887.

18. Rao U, Chen L-A, Bidesi AS, Shad MU, Thomas MA, Hammen CL: Hippocampal changes associated with early-life adversity and vulnerability to depression. *Biol Psychiatry* 2010, 67:357–364 [Posttraumatic Stress Disorder: Translational Neuroscience Perspectives on Gene-Environment Interactions].

19. Finlay-Jones R, Brown GW: Types of stressful life event and the onset of anxiety and depressive disorders. *Psychol Med* 1981, 11:803–815.

20. Kendler KS, Karkowski LM, Prescott CA: Causal relationship between stressful life events and the onset of major depression. *Am J Psychiatry* 1999, 156:837–841.

21. Jovanovic T, Blanding NQ, Norrholm SD, Duncan E, Bradley B, Ressler KJ: Childhood abuse is associated with increased startle reactivity in adulthood. *Depress Anxiety* 2009, 26:1018–1026.

22. Pole N, Neylan TC, Otte C, Metzler TJ, Best SR, Henn-Haase C, Marmar CR: Associations between childhood trauma and emotion-modulated psychophysiological responses to startling sounds: a study of police cadets. *J Abnorm Psychol* 2007, 116:352–361.

23. Gross C, Hen R: The developmental origins of anxiety. *Nat Rev Neurosci* 2004, 5:545–552.

24. Kendler KS, Kuhn J, Prescott CA: The interrelationship of neuroticism, sex, and stressful life events in the prediction of episodes of major depression. *Am J Psychiatry* 2004, 161:631–636.

25. Sandi C, Richter-Levin G: From high anxiety trait to depression: a neurocognitive hypothesis. *Trends Neurosci* 2009, 32:312–320.

26. Sheehan DV, Lecrubier Y, Sheehan KH, Amorim P, Janavs J, Weiller E, Hergueta T, Baker R, Dunbar GC: The Mini-International Neuropsychiatric Interview (MINI): the development and validation of a structured diagnostic psychiatric interview for DSM-IV and ICD-10. *J Clin Psychiatry* 1998, 59:22–33.

27. Axelrod BN: Validity of the Wechsler abbreviated scale of intelligence and other very short forms of estimating intellectual functioning. *Assessment* 2002, 9:17–23.

28. Spielberger CD, Sydeman SJ, Owen AE, Marsh BJ: Measuring Anxiety and Anger with the State-Trait Anxiety Inventory (STAI) and the State-Trait Anger Expression Inventory (STAXI). In *Use Psychol Test Treat Plan Outcomes Assess*. 2nd edition. Mahwah, NJ, US: Lawrence Erlbaum Associates Publishers; 1999:993–1021.

29. Bernstein DP, Stein JA, Newcomb MD, Walker E, Pogge D, Ahluvalia T, Stokes J, Handelsman L, Medrano M, Desmond D, Zule W: Development and validation of a brief screening version of the Childhood Trauma Questionnaire. *Child Abuse Negl* 2003, 27:169–190.

30. Fink LA, Bernstein D, Handelsman L, Foote J, Lovejoy M: Initial reliability and validity of the childhood trauma interview: a new multidimensional measure of childhood interpersonal trauma. *Am J Psychiatry* 1995, 152:1329–1335.

31. McEwen BS: Sex, stress and the hippocampus: allostasis, allostatic load and the aging process. *Neurobiol Aging* 2002, 23:921–939 [Brain Aging: Identifying the Brakes and Accelerators].

32. Clements K, Turpin G: The life events scale for students: validation for use with British samples. *Personal Individ Differ* 1996, 20:747–751.

33. Watson D, Weber K, Assenheimer JS, Clark LA, Strauss ME, McCormick RA: Testing a tripartite model: I. Evaluating the convergent and discriminant validity of anxiety and depression symptom scales. *J Abnorm Psychol* 1995, 104:3–14.

34. Reidy J, Keogh E: Testing the discriminant and convergent validity of the mood and anxiety symptoms questionnaire using a British sample. *Personal Individ Differ* 1997, 23:337–344.

35. Ashburner J, Friston KJ: Unified segmentation. *NeuroImage* 2005, 26:839–851.

36. Good CD, Johnsrude I, Ashburner J, Henson RNA, Friston KJ, Frackowiak RSJ: Cerebral asymmetry and the effects of sex and handedness on brain structure: a voxel-based morphometric analysis of 465 normal adult human brains. *NeuroImage* 2001, 14:685–700.

37. Hayes AF: PROCESS: a versatile computational tool for observed variable mediation, moderation, and conditional process modeling. [White paper]. Retrieved from http://www.afhayes.com/public/process2012.pdf.

38. MacKinnon DP, Lockwood CM, Williams J: Confidence limits for the indirect effect: distribution of the product and resampling methods. *Multivar Behav Res* 2004, 39:99.

39. Scher CD, Stein MB, Asmundson GJG, McCreary DR, Forde DR: The childhood trauma questionnaire in a community sample: psychometric properties and normative data. *J Trauma Stress* 2001, 14:843–857.

40. Lightsey OR Jr, Hulsey CD: Impulsivity, coping, stress, and problem gambling among university students. *J Couns Psychol* 2002, 49:202.

41. Knight RG, Waal-Manning HJ, Spears GF: Some norms and reliability data for the state-trait anxiety inventory and the zung self-rating depression scale. *Br J Clin Psychol* 1983, 22:245–249.

42. Bogdan R, Perlis RH, Fagerness J, Pizzagalli DA: The impact of
     mineralocorticoid receptor ISO/VAL genotype (rs5522) and stress on
     reward learning. *Genes Brain Behav* 2010, **9**:658–667.
43. Cook SC, Wellman CL: Chronic stress alters dendritic morphology in rat
     medial prefrontal cortex. *J Neurobiol* 2004, **60**:236–248.
44. Fabricius K, Wörtwein G, Pakkenberg B: The impact of maternal separation
     on adult mouse behaviour and on the total neuron number in the
     mouse hippocampus. *Brain Struct Funct* 2008, **212**:403–416.
45. Monroy E, Hernández-Torres E, Flores G: Maternal separation disrupts
     dendritic morphology of neurons in prefrontal cortex, hippocampus, and
     nucleus accumbens in male rat offspring. *J Chem Neuroanat* 2010,
     40:93–101.
46. Sotres-Bayon F, Cain CK, LeDoux JE: Brain mechanisms of fear extinction:
     historical perspectives on the contribution of prefrontal cortex.
     Biol Psychiatry 2006, **60**:329–336.
47. Maier SF, Ryan SM, Barksdale CM, Kalin NH: Stressor controllability and the
     pituitary-adrenal system. *Behav Neurosci* 1986, **100**:669–674.
48. Kessler RC, Berglund P, Demler O, Jin R, Merikangas KR, Walters EE: Lifetime
     prevalence and age-of-onset distributions of DSM-iv disorders in the
     National Comorbidity Survey Replication. *Arch Gen Psychiatry* 2005,
     62:593–602.
49. Burke K, Burke JD Jr, Regier DA, Rae DS: Age at onset of selected mental
     disorders in five community populations. *Arch Gen Psychiatry* 1990,
     47:511–518.

13

Quantitative meta-analysis of neural activity in posttraumatic stress disorder

Jasmeet P Hayes[1,2,3*], Scott M Hayes[2,3,4] and Amanda M Mikedis[1,2]

Abstract

Background: In recent years, neuroimaging techniques such as functional magnetic resonance imaging (fMRI) and positron emission tomography (PET) have played a significant role in elucidating the neural underpinnings of posttraumatic stress disorder (PTSD). However, a detailed understanding of the neural regions implicated in the disorder remains incomplete because of considerable variability in findings across studies. The aim of this meta-analysis was to identify consistent patterns of neural activity across neuroimaging study designs in PTSD to improve understanding of the neurocircuitry of PTSD.

Methods: We conducted a literature search for PET and fMRI studies of PTSD that were published before February 2011. The article search resulted in 79 functional neuroimaging PTSD studies. Data from 26 PTSD peer-reviewed neuroimaging articles reporting results from 342 adult patients and 342 adult controls were included. Peak activation coordinates from selected articles were used to generate activation likelihood estimate maps separately for symptom provocation and cognitive-emotional studies of PTSD. A separate meta-analysis examined the coupling between ventromedial prefrontal cortex and amygdala activity in patients.

Results: Results demonstrated that the regions most consistently hyperactivated in PTSD patients included mid- and dorsal anterior cingulate cortex, and when ROI studies were included, bilateral amygdala. By contrast, widespread hypoactivity was observed in PTSD including the ventromedial prefrontal cortex and the inferior frontal gyrus. Furthermore, decreased ventromedial prefrontal cortex activity was associated with increased amygdala activity.

Conclusions: These results provide evidence for a neurocircuitry model of PTSD that emphasizes alteration in neural networks important for salience detection and emotion regulation.

Keywords: Activation likelihood estimation, fMRI, PET, Amygdala, Anterior cingulate cortex, Ventromedial prefrontal cortex, Salience network, Fear conditioning

Background

In the aftermath of highly distressing and shocking events such as combat, genocide, and rape, a subset of individuals develop posttraumatic stress disorder (PTSD), which is characterized by distressing memories of the event, physiological hyperarousal, and impairment in daily functioning. With the growing interest in PTSD due in part to its high prevalence among veterans of the Iraq and Afghanistan wars, there is an urgency to understand the neural pathogenesis of the disorder. Neuroimaging studies have been conducted to examine brain regions involved in PTSD [1-26]. Based on these findings and the non-human animal literature, the prevailing neurocircuitry model of PTSD suggests that PTSD can be understood in terms of circuits involved in fear conditioning in the brain. Specifically, this model suggests that heightened amygdala activity gives privileged status to feared and threatening stimuli. Whereas the ventromedial prefrontal cortex would normally temper amygdala activity, abnormal function of this region reduces regulation of amygdala output [27]. Furthermore, altered hippocampal function may result in impaired ability to discern safe from dangerous contexts.

The aforementioned brain regions, which play a key role in nonhuman animal fear conditioning [28], likely

* Correspondence: jphayes@bu.edu
[1]National Center for PTSD, VA Boston Healthcare System, Boston, MA, USA
[2]Neuroimaging Research Center, VA Boston Healthcare System, Boston, MA, USA
Full list of author information is available at the end of the article

play an important role in PTSD. PTSD is more likely to develop following highly fear-provoking and life-threatening events than less intense events [29]. Influential psychological theories of PTSD have emphasized the role of fear structures and fear conditioning in the development and maintenance of the disorder [30,31]. Furthermore, exposure therapy, which involves the principles of extinction learning [30], is one of the most effective therapeutic interventions for PTSD.

However, fear conditioning models are limited in their ability to explain the full range of human experience and emotion. Fear conditioning can occur outside of conscious awareness, yet conscious processes such as voluntary and effortful avoidance of thoughts and memories of the trauma play a vital role in the development and maintenance of the disorder [32]. This has led to growing supposition that fear-circuitry models are unable to fully account for the heterogeneity of symptoms following a traumatic event [33] and that anxiety and fear may not be the central components in explaining PTSD symptomatology as previously believed [34]. Accordingly, the proposed revision of the Diagnostic and Statistical Manual (DSM-V) may now recognize negative cognitions and persistent negative mood states as key symptoms of the diagnosis [35], suggesting that other emotions such as dysphoria are important in the development and maintenance of the disorder in addition to fear. Therefore, a primary goal of the present study was to examine patterns of brain activation in neuroimaging studies of PTSD that may provide a more complete understanding of the neural circuitry of PTSD.

In the present study, we performed a quantitative meta-analysis of neuroimaging studies in PTSD using activation likelihood estimation (ALE). This method calculates the probability that a given voxel is activated consistently across studies rather than a single study [36] and therefore provides a more objective measure of brain activity in PTSD than qualitative reviews. Although there have been two prior functional neuroimaging meta-analyses in PTSD [37,38], the present study includes more recent studies, focuses solely on adult PTSD, and considers separately the effects of study type (symptom provocation versus cognitive-emotional) and neuroimaging analysis type (whole-brain voxel-wise analysis versus region-of-interest [ROI] analysis). Symptom provocation studies are designed to elicit trauma-related symptoms whereas cognitive-emotional studies include emotional stimuli (e.g., fearful face) but do not explicitly cue the patient to their traumatic event. In contrast to previous meta-analyses in PTSD, the current study separates symptom provocation and cognitive-emotional studies to examine the neural correlates of two primary characteristics of PTSD: specific recall of a traumatic event (symptom provocation) and emotional response

generalization (cognitive-emotional studies). Furthermore, examining results from whole-brain voxel-wise analyses separately from ROI analyses may provide greater insight whether the regions typically targeted in ROI studies (e.g., the amygdala) are also robustly active when taking into account all voxels in the brain. ROI analyses restrict statistical analysis to the small number of a priori defined voxels, reducing the need for more stringent correction for multiple comparisons; thus, ROI studies are not entirely comparable to studies employing whole-brain voxel-wise statistics. In the present study, we examined the results from ROI studies as they comprise a significant proportion of imaging studies in PTSD, with the recognition that whole brain voxel-wise analyses represent a less biased statistical approach. Finally, we performed a separate meta-analysis to test the fear-model hypothesis that hypoactivity in the ventromedial prefrontal cortex is associated with hyperactivity in the amygdala, reflecting insufficient inhibition of prefrontal cortex over the amygdala.

Methods
Article selection
Using keywords "PTSD," "neuroimaging," "fMRI," and "PET," a literature search in PubMed and Published International Literature on Traumatic Stress (PILOTS) was conducted for PET and fMRI studies of adult PTSD that were published before February 2011. The article search resulted in 79 functional neuroimaging studies. Included studies contrasted a traumatic or negative emotional condition with a resting baseline, positive condition, or neutral condition, conducted between-group analyses using subtraction methodology, and reported between-group peak activation coordinates in standard space. For relevant articles that did not report whole-brain results, the authors were contacted to request activation coordinates [6,10]. Case studies were excluded [39,40] as well as studies examining PTSD and co-morbidity with other disorders, although an exception was made for major depressive disorder (MDD) because of its high co-morbidity with PTSD [13]. Based on these inclusion and exclusion criteria, 26 adult PTSD neuroimaging studies reporting results from 342 patients and 342 controls remained in the analyses (see Table 1).

Inclusion/exclusion criteria for activation foci
For each of the articles listed in Table 1, significant peak activation coordinates were extracted for negative > other (baseline, positive, or neutral) between-group contrasts (PTSD > Controls; Controls > PTSD). When coordinates for more than one type of negative > other contrast were reported in the same study, only one contrast was included to avoid using foci from the same participants twice [4,9,16,25]. In these cases, the selected contrast

Table 1 Functional neuroimaging studies included in meta-analysis

Study	PTSD	TC*	NTC**	Type of trauma	Contrast used in meta-analysis	Scanning task	Imaging method	Design
Symptom Provocation Whole Brain Analyses (10)								
Bremner et al. 1999a	10	10		Combat	Combat vs. neutral pictures and sounds	View and listen	PET	Block
Bremner et al. 1999b	10	12		SA[+]	Childhood abuse vs. neutral scripts	Image and remember event	PET	Block
Britton et al. 2005	16	15		Combat	Combat vs. neutral scripts	Listen and maintain evoked emotional state	PET	Block
Hou et al. 2007	10	7		Mining accident	Mining accident vs. neutral pictures	View	fMRI	Block
Lanius et al. 2001	9	9		Mixed	Trauma scripts vs. baseline	Listen and remember event	fMRI	Block
Lanius et al. 2002	7	10		SA (1 MVA) [+]	Trauma scripts vs. baseline	Listen and remember event	fMRI	Block
Lanius et al. 2003	10	10		Mixed	Trauma scripts vs. baseline	Listen and remember event	fMRI	Block
Lanius et al. 2007	26	16		MVA[+]	Trauma vs. neutral scripts	Listen and remember event	fMRI	Block
Shin et al. 1999	8	8		SA[+]	Sexual abuse vs. neutral scripts	Recall and imagine contents of script	PET	Block
Shin et al. 2004	17	19		Combat	Combat vs. neutral scripts	Recall and imagine contents of script	PET	Block
Symptom Provocation ROI Analyses (2)								
Frewen et al. 2008	25	16		MVA[+]	Trauma vs. neutral scripts	Listen to and image script	fMRI	Block
Protopopescu et al. 2005	9	14		SA, PA[+]	PTSD vs. neutral words	Read word	fMRI	Block
Cognitive-Emotional Whole Brain Analyses (12)								
Bremner et al. 2003	10		11	SA[+]	Negative emotional vs. neutral word pairs	Declarative memory task	PET	Block
Bremner et al. 2004	12	9		SA[+]	Negative emotional vs. neutral words	Stroop task	PET	Block
Brunetti et al. 2010	10		10	Assault	Negative emotional vs. neutral IAPS pictures	Visuo-attentional task	fMRI	Block
Felmingham et al. 2010	23	21		Mixed	Fearful vs. neutral faces	Backward masking task	fMRI	Block
Fonzo et al. 2010	12		12	IPV[+]	Fearful vs. happy faces	Emotional face matching task	fMRI	Block
Kim et al. 2008	12		12	Fire	Fearful vs. neutral faces	Same-different judgment task	fMRI	Event-related
Sakamoto et al. 2005	16		16	Mixed	Traumatic vs. neutral images	View stimuli below perceptual threshold	fMRI	Block
Shin et al. 2005	13	13		Combat, fire	Fearful vs. happy faces	Overt passive viewing task	fMRI	Block
Thomaes et al. 2009	9		9	SA, PA[+]	Negative words vs. baseline	Word classification task	fMRI	Event-related
Whalley et al. 2009	16	16	16	Mixed	Negative vs. neutral background pictures with neutral foreground pictures	Episodic memory retrieval task	fMRI	Event-related
Williams et al. 2006	13		13	Mixed	Fearful vs. neutral faces	Overt fear perception task	fMRI	Block
Hou et al. 2007				Same Hou et al. 2007 article as the one listed above (in addition to symptom provocation coordinates, article reported coordinates from a short-term memory recall task)				
Cognitive-Emotional ROI Analyses (6)								
Bryant et al. 2008	15		15	Mixed	Fearful vs. neutral faces	View stimuli below conscious threshold	fMRI	Block
Phan et al. 2006	16	15		Combat	Negative vs. neutral IAPS pictures	View and rate pictures	PET	Block
Rauch et al. 2000	8	8		Combat	Fearful vs. positive faces	Masked faces paradigm	fMRI	Block
Felmingham et al. 2010				Same as whole brain article above				

Table 1 Functional neuroimaging studies included in meta-analysis *(Continued)*

Fonzo et al. 2010	Same as whole brain article above
Williams et al. 2006	Same as whole brain article above

*TC: trauma exposed controls without PTSD.
**NTC: non-traumatized controls.
+ SA: sexual abuse/assault; PA: physical abuse/assault; MVA: motor vehicle accident; NSA: non sexual assault; IPV: intimate partner violence.

compared a trauma-specific or fear-inducing condition with a neutral condition. If a study conducted a whole-brain and a ROI analysis [8,9,12,26], coordinates from both analyses were included provided that the ROIs were not reported in the whole-brain results [8,9,26].

In studies that included two levels of control groups (e.g., healthy controls and trauma-exposed controls) or PTSD patients (e.g., PTSD with MDD versus PTSD without MDD), only foci from one of the between-group comparisons were used (i.e., between-group foci for PTSD vs. traumatized controls [5,8] and PTSD without co-morbidity vs. controls [13]). Following inclusion and exclusion of coordinates, 218 between-group activation foci remained (Table 2).

Meta-analyses

Coordinate-based random-effects meta-analyses were conducted using GingerALE software version 2.1 (http://brainmap.org/ale/). Coordinates reported in MNI space were converted to Talairach space using the Lancaster transform [41] as implemented in GingerALE. Coordinates from symptom provocation and cognitive-emotional tasks were first combined to examine the neural regions involved across tasks and then were analyzed separately to examine differences between the two design types. A replicate set of analyses was performed that included ROI-based studies. Differences in the whole-brain voxel-wise results with the inclusion of ROIs, when present, are noted in the tables and results.

For each analysis reported, peak activation coordinates were smoothed using a three-dimensional Gaussian filter and transformed into Gaussian probability distributions. These probability distributions were combined to generate whole-brain statistical maps of the ALE values on a voxel-wise basis. ALE statistics calculated the probability that at least one of the foci lay within each voxel and, therefore, the likelihood that each voxel was activated across all studies included in the analysis. The ALE statistic maps were compared with a null-distribution of random spatial associations between experiments (random-effects model) to assess for above chance clustering between experiments using a threshold at false discovery rate (FDR) corrected $P < 0.05$ and a cluster-extent of 100 mm^3.

To explore the hypothesis that activity in the ventro-medial prefrontal cortex and the amygdala was inversely related, we first identified whole-brain studies that reported increased ventromedial prefrontal cortex activity in controls relative to PTSD patients (which would suggest that this region was hypoactive in PTSD) and also reported regions of increased activity in PTSD relative to controls. Six studies were identified that met these criteria [1,11,12,21-23]. A meta-analysis was performed on the coordinates from these studies for the PTSD > Control contrast. Thus, we examined the regions that were hyperactive in PTSD when the ventromedial prefrontal cortex was hypoactive. Due to the small number of studies included, the analysis was thresholded at FDR corrected $P < 0.05$ and a less conservative cluster-extent of 40 mm^3 (i.e., 5 contiguous voxels) was used.

Results

Separate meta-analyses were run to examine the neural activity across and within symptom provocation and cognitive-emotional tasks in PTSD. Because of the variability in naming conventions of medial prefrontal cortex regions across different studies, activated regions are listed in the text and tables both by their structure specific name (e.g., medial frontal gyrus) and a general name signifying their contribution to a broader, less defined area (e.g., ventromedial prefrontal cortex which broadly includes the pregenual and subgenual anterior cingulate cortex, medial orbitofrontal cortex, and the ventral part of the medial prefrontal cortex).

Common activations for PTSD across tasks

The regions that were hyper- and hypoactive when studies were collapsed across task type (i.e., symptom provocation and cognitive-emotional) in PTSD relative to control subjects are reported in Table 3. We defined hyperactivity in PTSD as the results stemming from the PTSD > Control contrast and hypoactivity in PTSD as brain regions active from the Control > PTSD contrast. Patients with PTSD showed hyperactivation in the mid- and dorsal anterior cingulate (Figure 1A), left superior temporal gyrus, and left supplementary motor area. Robust bilateral amygdala and left dorsomedial prefrontal cortex activity was observed when ROI studies were included (Figure 1B).

Notably, there were several regions of hypoactivation in PTSD relative to controls including the medial frontal gyrus (ventromedial prefrontal cortex; Figure 1B), thalamus, right inferior frontal gyrus (Figure 1B), and right

Table 2 Number of activation foci included in between-group analyses

Study	P > C[+]	C > P[+]	Statistical threshold
Symptom Provocation Whole Brain Analyses			
Bremner et al. 1999a	5	5	P < .001
Bremner et al. 1999b	9	19	P < .001
Britton et al. 2005	–	1	P < .005
Hou et al. 2007	1	9	P < .005
Lanius et al. 2001	–	4	P < .001
Lanius et al. 2002	9	3	P < .001, > 10 voxels
Lanius et al. 2003	–	9	P < .001, > 10 voxels
Lanius et al. 2007	–	2	P < .05 cor., > 10 voxels
Shin et al. 1999	4	14	P < .001
Shin et al. 2004	1	3	P < .001
Symptom Provocation ROI Analyses			
Protopopescu et al. 2005	1	–	P < .01 cor.
Frewen et al. 2008	–	3	P < .05, > 10 voxels
Cognitive-Emotional Whole Brain Analyses			
Bremner et al. 2003	15	14	P < .01 cor.
Bremner et al. 2004	2	6	P < .005 cor., > 65 voxels
Brunetti et al. 2010	6	3	P < .001
Felmingham et al. 2010	1	–	P < .001, > 10 voxels
Fonzo et al. 2010	3	1	P < .05
Kim et al. 2007	7	6	P < .001
Sakamoto et al. 2005	1	4	P < .01
Shin et al. 2005	4	4	P < .001
Thomaes et al. 2009	2	–	P < .001
Whalley et al. 2009	3	1	P < .001
Williams et al. 2006	7	1	P < .001
Hou et al. 2007*	–	2	P < .005
Cognitive-Emotional ROI Analyses			
Bryant et al. 2008	4	–	P < .05, > 3 voxels
Phan et al. 2006	–	1	P < .005 cor.
Rauch et al. 2000	1	–	P < .05
Felmingham et al. 2010**	9	–	P < .001, > 10 voxels
Fonzo et al. 2010**	2	–	P < .05
Williams et al. 2006**	2	4	P < .001
Total SP foci	30	72	
Total cognitive-emotional foci	69	47	
Total number of foci	99	119	

[+] P > C: PTSD patients > Controls; C > P: Controls > PTSD patients.
*Paper also reported symptom provocation coordinates.
**Papers also reported whole brain coordinates.
cor. = corrected for multiple comparisons.

middle temporal gyrus. When ROI studies were included, the results remained consistent with additional activity observed in the pregenual anterior cingulate cortex (Table 3).

Symptom provocation studies

A meta-analysis of symptom provocation designs was conducted to reveal the regions that were involved in reliving one's traumatic event (Table 4). The regions consistently hyperactivated in PTSD were the mid- and dorsal anterior cingulate cortex. By contrast, widespread hypoactivity was observed, including the medial frontal gyrus (ventromedial prefrontal cortex), right inferior frontal gyrus, and right precuneus. These results were unchanged with the inclusion of ROI studies. Figure 2 displays brain activation separately for symptom provocation and cognitive-emotional studies.

Cognitive-emotional studies

Cognitive-emotional studies included stimuli that were negative, but not trauma-specific (e.g., fearful faces). The whole-brain voxel-wise analysis revealed hyperactivity in supplementary motor area. Bilateral amygdala and medial frontal gyrus (dorsomedial prefrontal cortex, BA 8) activity was observed when ROI studies were included (see Table 4). Regions of hypoactivity (Figure 2) included the pregenual anterior cingulate cortex (ventromedial prefrontal cortex) and medial frontal gyrus (dorsomedial prefrontal cortex, BA 9).

Ventromedial prefrontal cortex meta-analysis

We next performed a meta-analysis on regions that were hyperactive in PTSD within studies that reported decreased ventromedial prefrontal cortex activity (see Methods). The analysis showed that when the ventromedial prefrontal cortex was hypoactivated, greater amygdala activation was observed in PTSD, supporting the hypothesis that activity in the ventromedial prefrontal cortex and amygdala are inversely related. Other regions that showed increased activity included the right middle and inferior temporal gyrus, left superior temporal gyrus, bilateral precuneus, and right putamen (Table 5).

Discussion

The present study used quantitative meta-analysis to examine the pathophysiology of PTSD. The results confirmed involvement of a subset of regions implicated in fear-circuitry models of PTSD, including robust hyperactivity in the dorsal anterior cingulate cortex, hypoactivity in the ventromedial prefrontal cortex in PTSD, and an inverse relationship between activity in the ventromedial prefrontal cortex and amygdala. However, additional regions were found to be hyper- and hypoactive in PTSD, suggesting that a broader view of the neural circuitry of PTSD should be considered. Collapsing across symptom provocation and cognitive-emotional studies, the whole-brain voxel-wise analysis revealed hyperactivation of the mid/dorsal anterior cingulate

Table 3 Between-group comparison of activity across symptom provocation and cognitive-emotional studies

Region	Hemisphere	Talairach			BA	Volume (mm³)
		x	y	z		
PTSD > Controls						
Whole Brain Analysis						
Dorsal ACC	R	17.3	38.35	15.53	32	672
Mid/Dorsal ACC	R	3.49	−3.51	34.37	24	400
Superior Temporal Gyrus	L	−63.02	−47.37	18.13	22	152
Supplementary Motor Area	L	−22.02	−1.55	57.56	6	112
Whole Brain + ROI Analysis						
Amygdala	R	22.86	1.06	−13.32	−	1328
Amygdala	L	−25.95	−0.02	−17.87	−	1136
Dorsal ACC	R	17.33	38.35	15.44	32	640
Mid/Dorsal ACC	R	3.61	−3.18	34.29	24	288
Medial Frontal Gyrus (dmPFC)	R	1.08	31.44	37.87	8	216
Superior Temporal Gyrus	L	−63.15	−47.34	18.13	22	144
Controls > PTSD						
Whole Brain Analysis						
Medial Frontal Gyrus (vmPFC)	R	3.07	36.09	−6.69	11	984
Thalamus	L	−4.12	−14.12	17.89	−	480
Thalamus	R	12.06	−12.03	1.97	−	464
Inferior Frontal Gyrus	R	16.02	21.76	−12.36	47	440
Middle Occipital Gyrus	L	−31.42	−86.95	−1.35	18	392
Medial Frontal Gyrus	R	6.23	48.66	9.06	10	344
Middle Temporal Gyrus	R	45.03	−68.88	13.16	39	336
Inferior Frontal Gyrus	R	45.79	15.16	10.21	44	304
Precuneus	R	24.34	−56.37	38.59	7	280
Cerebellum	R	35.16	−82.16	−20	−	272
Medial Frontal Gyrus	R	11.89	42.19	24.43	9	272
Fusiform Gyrus	L	−51.87	−47.57	−15.78	37	256
Precuneus	R	25.76	−84.66	39.71	19	248
Superior Temporal Gyrus	L	−39.88	−23.07	5.88	13	144
Cerebellum	R	20	−47.03	−14.64	−	128
Inferior Frontal Gyrus	R	41.45	39.85	7.14	46	112
Whole Brain + ROI Analysis						
Pregenual ACC	R	5.17	44.99	14.35	32	1824
Medial Frontal Gyrus (vmPFC)	R	3.11	36.03	−6.34	11	864
Thalamus	L	−4.12	−14.11	17.88	−	480
Thalamus	R	12.01	−12.01	2	−	456
Inferior Frontal Gyrus	R	16.14	21.75	−12.28	47	424
Middle Occipital Gyrus	L	−31.35	−86.97	−1.34	18	384
Dorsal ACC	L	−6.43	9.14	25.01	24	368
Middle Temporal Gyrus	R	44.97	−68.82	13.1	39	328
Superior Frontal Gyrus	L	−23.94	50.88	8.8	10	256
Fusiform Gyrus	L	−51.75	−47.62	−15.77	37	248
Thalamus	L	−7.65	−6.83	7.93	−	248

Table 3 Between-group comparison of activity across symptom provocation and cognitive-emotional studies (Continued)

Precuneus	R	24.44	−56.35	38.82	7	248
Inferior Frontal Gyrus	R	45.69	14.86	10.31	44	240
Precuneus	R	25.73	−84.68	39.86	19	216
Cerebellum	R	35.01	−82	−20	–	208
Superior Temporal Gyrus	L	−39.98	−22.77	5.98	13	120

$P < .05$ FDR-corrected, cluster activation extent ≥ 100 mm³. ACC = anterior cingulate cortex, BA = Brodmann area, dmPFC = dorsomedial prefrontal cortex, L = left, R = right, vmPFC = ventromedial prefrontal cortex.

cortex, supplementary motor area, and superior temporal gyrus in PTSD. These regions have been previously shown to be part of a putative 'salience network' that processes autonomic, interoceptive, homeostatic, and cognitive information of personal relevance [42,43]. Ultimately, the salience network helps an organism evaluate whether stimuli in the environment should be approached or avoided. Importantly, activity in this salience network is positively correlated with anxiety [43]. We propose that in PTSD, the behavioral manifestation of increased output of the salience network may provide privileged cognitive resources to a broad range of salient stimuli leading to hypervigilance and disruption of goal-directed activity. This notion is consistent with observations

in PTSD patients of deficits in working memory for not only trauma-related negative distractors, but also neutral distractors [44], suggesting that a variety of stimuli become potentially salient for patients with PTSD. From this viewpoint, negative emotions other than fear can be associated with the disorder, as long as they are salient and associated with a stress response.

The dorsal anterior cingulate cortex is a key node in the salience network. Earlier conceptualizations of the region suggested that its role was primarily in "cold" cognitive processes, in contrast to the ventral aspects of the anterior cingulate cortex that were thought to be involved in affective processing [45]. However, more recent data have not corroborated a cognitive versus

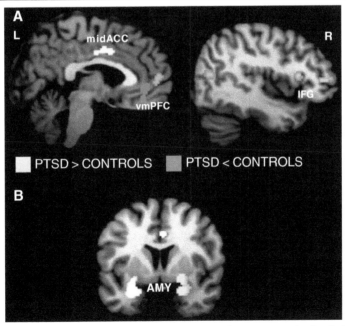

Figure 1 A. Brain regions associated with PTSD across symptom provocation and cognitive-emotional tasks in the whole-brain voxelwise analysis. B. Bilateral amygdala activity is observed after including symptom provocation and cognitive-emotional ROI studies to the whole-brain voxel-wise results. Areas of hyperactivation in PTSD (PTSD > Control) are shown in yellow and areas of hypoactivation in PTSD (Control > PTSD) are shown in blue. Amy = amygdala, IFG = inferior frontal gyrus, L = left, midACC = mid anterior cingulate cortex, R = right, vmPFC = ventromedial prefrontal cortex.

Table 4 Between-group comparison results of symptom provocation articles and cognitive-emotional articles

Region	Hemisphere	Talairach			BA	Volume (mm³)
		x	y	z		
SYMPTOM PROVOCATION						
PTSD > Controls						
Whole Brain Analysis						
Dorsal ACC	R	15.38	37.69	16.96	32	344
Mid/Dorsal ACC	R	2.65	−8.91	33.77	24	296
Mid/Dorsal ACC	R	0.3	−19.11	37.4	24	104
Whole Brain + ROI Analysis						
Dorsal ACC	R	15.38	37.69	16.96	32	344
Mid/Dorsal ACC	R	2.65	−8.91	33.77	24	296
Controls > PTSD						
Whole Brain Analysis						
Medial Frontal Gyrus (vmPFC)	R	3.32	36.07	−6.42	11	1152
Thalamus	R	12	−12	2	–	648
Thalamus	L	−4.02	−14.02	17.98	–	648
Inferior Frontal Gyrus	R	45.62	14.54	8.65	44	480
Precuneus	R	25.83	−84.66	39.57	19	296
Inferior Frontal Gyrus	R	41.77	40.46	7.18	46	216
Medial Frontal Gyrus	R	3.94	50.11	7.37	10	208
Whole Brain + ROI Analysis						
Medial Frontal Gyrus (vmPFC)	R	3.34	36.13	−6.34	11	1168
Thalamus	R	12	−12	2	–	648
Thalamus	L	−4.03	−14.01	17.97	–	648
Medial Frontal Gyrus	R	0.63	47.89	5.66	10	504
Inferior Frontal Gyrus	R	45.69	14.62	8.52	44	464
Precuneus	R	25.83	−84.66	39.57	19	296
Inferior Frontal Gyrus	R	41.77	40.46	7.18	46	216
COGNITIVE- EMOTIONAL						
PTSD > Controls						
Whole Brain Analysis						
Supplementary Motor Area	L	−22.13	−1.49	57.27	6	128
Supplementary Motor Area	L	−25.39	2.02	40.31	6	104
Whole Brain + ROI Analysis						
Amygdala	R	22.93	1.03	−13.28	–	1376
Amygdala	L	−27.21	−0.16	−17.37	–	840
Medial Frontal Gyrus (dmPFC)	R	0.98	31.46	37.87	8	224
Controls > PTSD						
Whole Brain Analysis						
Pregenual ACC (vmPFC)	L	−13.93	49.87	−2.12	32	400
Medial Frontal Gyrus (dmPFC)	R	10.63	40.6	23.03	9	272
Whole Brain + ROI Analysis						
Medial Frontal Gyrus (dmPFC)	R	11.17	41.96	21.25	9	984
Pregenual ACC (vmPFC)	L	−13.97	49.76	−2.16	32	384

$P < 0.05$ FDR-corrected, activation extent ≥ 100 mm³. *ACC* = anterior cingulate cortex, *BA* = Brodman area, *dmPFC* = dorsomedial prefrontal cortex, *L* = left, *R* = right, *vmPFC* = ventromedial prefrontal cortex.

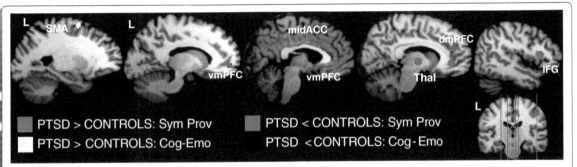

Figure 2 Overlay of brain regions associated with PTSD by task design. Warm colors indicate regions of hyperactivity in PTSD patients during symptom provocation study designs (red) and cognitive-emotional study designs (yellow). Cool colors indicate regions of hypoactivity in PTSD during symptom provocation designs (purple) and cognitive-emotional designs (blue). Cog-Emo = Cognitive-emotional, DmPFC = dorsomedial prefrontal cortex, IFG = inferior frontal gyrus, L = left, midACC = mid anterior cingulate cortex, SMA = supplementary motor area, Sym Prov = symptom provocation, Thal = thalamus, vmPFC = ventromedial prefrontal cortex.

affective dissociation. Recent reviews have called attention to the involvement of the dorsal anterior cingulate cortex in PTSD [46,47], which may subserve learned fear, fear appraisal and expression, and sympathetic activity [48]. More broadly, dorsomedial prefrontal regions (including the dorsal anterior cingulate cortex) have been associated with appraisal and evaluation whereas ventromedial prefrontal regions are associated with regulatory functions. This dissociation is consistent with the findings reported here, where more dorsal prefrontal regions, including the dorsomedial prefrontal cortex and mid/dorsal anterior cingulate cortex were active in patients with PTSD and may suggest heightened appraisals of potential threats in the environment, whereas hypoactivity in ventromedial prefrontal regions may reflect dysfunction in emotion regulation.

Interestingly, the present results highlight the contribution of the mid-cingulate in PTSD, adding to the growing evidence that this region plays an important role in this disorder [49-51] and may be important for fear conditioning [52]. The dorsal anterior cingulate spans a large area, encompassing BAs 24, 32, and 33. Whereas a more anterior portion of the dorsal anterior cingulate was activated in both PTSD patients and control subjects in the present meta-analysis, a more posterior region was hyperactivated only in PTSD. A previous study demonstrated that individuals with severe PTSD symptomatology activated the mid/dorsal anterior cingulate to a greater extent than controls during an emotional oddball task, suggesting that distracting stimuli are given attentional preference at the expense of a goal-relevant task in PTSD [49]. These findings provide converging evidence for the role of the mid/dorsal anterior cingulate cortex in salience processing. Another region in the salience network, the amygdala, was observed only when using a less stringent spatial extent in the whole-brain analysis or when considering ROI analyses. The amygdala is notoriously difficult to image due to

Table 5 Ventromedial prefrontal cortex meta-analysis results

Region	Hemisphere	Talairach			BA	Volume (mm³)
		x	y	z		
PTSD > Controls						
Middle Temporal Gyrus	R	49.54	−36.22	−12.82	20	136
Amygdala	L	−19.01	−0.97	−19.03	−	64
Precuneus	L	−12.98	−53.03	33.02	31	64
Putamen	R	19.43	1.15	−7.72	−	56
Cerebellum	R	36.64	−65.35	−37.02	−	48
Amygdala	R	19.35	0.65	−18.99	−	48
Superior Temporal Gyrus	L	−62.66	−48.01	18.66	22	48
Precuneus	R	20.65	−76.99	40.66	7	48
Supplementary Motor Area	L	−47.98	4.01	41.66	6	48
Inferior Temporal Gyrus	R	54.78	−45.22	−11.61	20	40

$P < .05$ FDR-corrected, activation extent ≥ 40 mm³. BA = Brodmann area, L = left, R = right.

vulnerability to susceptibility artifact and its relatively small volume, which could account for lack of robust findings in the whole-brain analysis. Alternatively, it is possible that the amygdala is not as central of a region in PTSD as current neurocircuitry models suggest, consistent with previous meta-analysis data showing that the amygdala is more frequently active in patients with social anxiety disorder and specific phobia than PTSD [37].

With the addition of ROI analyses, amygdala activity was observed for cognitive-emotional tasks but not symptom provocation tasks, suggesting that the type of task employed within a study influences amygdala activity in PTSD. There is emerging recognition that the amygdala may play a more general role in processing ambiguous and salient stimuli in the environment [53-55], of which fear may be one particularly potent instance. The amygdala, which is composed of several distinct but highly interconnected nuclei, is not specific to fear states but is also activated for unusual and novel stimuli [56] and unpredictability [57]. Therefore, the stimuli and study designs employed during cognitive-emotional studies of PTSD, which often present novel and ambiguous stimuli intermittently, may evoke more central involvement of the amygdala than autobiographical trauma scripts, which were often familiar and unambiguous from the start. Other explanations for the lack of amygdala activity in symptom provocation designs are less likely. Both the symptom provocation designs and the cognitive-emotional ROI studies (in which amygdala activity was observed most robustly) were block designs; therefore, the results are unlikely to be attributable to differences in neuroimaging experimental design (i.e., event-related vs. block designs). Furthermore, the majority of both symptom provocation and cognitive-emotional studies were fMRI rather than PET, suggesting that the difference is not due to imaging modality. The discrepancy in amygdala activity for cognitive-emotional and symptom provocation studies underscores the importance of considering the cognitive task when interpreting activation differences (or lack thereof) in the amygdala in PTSD and control participants.

In the present study, widespread hypoactivity in prefrontal cortex in PTSD was observed, including both medial and lateral regions. Notably, hypoactivity in the ventromedial prefrontal cortex was present in both symptom provocation and cognitive-emotional study designs. To examine the relationship between the ventromedial prefrontal cortex and amygdala, we performed a meta-analysis that identified regions of hyperactivity within a subset of studies that showed a decrease in ventromedial prefrontal cortex activity in PTSD patients. We reasoned that under conditions of diminished ventromedial prefrontal cortex activity, which may

signify reduced top-down governance of interconnected regions, we would observe greater amygdala activity. The results showed that when the ventromedial prefrontal cortex was hypoactive, the amygdala, putamen, and temporal cortex were hyperactivated. These results support the notion that a consequence of hypoactivity of the ventromedial prefrontal cortex may be greater responsivity of the amygdala in the face of negative information. Although the direction of this effect cannot be determined conclusively because the neural connections between the amygdala and ventromedial prefrontal cortex are bidirectional, there is a well-established literature showing the involvement of ventromedial prefrontal cortex in regulatory control across species [58]. It is important to note that the ventromedial prefrontal cortex is not a single entity, but rather is composed of multiple distinct regions (i.e., subgenual and pregenual anterior cingulate cortex, medial portions of orbitofrontal gyrus, and medial frontal gyrus) that subserve a variety of functions. For instance, the non-human animal literature suggests that bordering divisions within ventromedial prefrontal cortex may be responsible for both inhibition and facilitation of autonomic arousal [58]. This may help to explain why some studies of PTSD show increased activation in this region [59] and suggests that a more fine-grained analysis is required to better elucidate the various functions of the ventromedial prefrontal cortex. Nevertheless, the results of the current meta-analysis show robust hypoactivation in the ventromedial prefrontal cortex consistent across task type, underscoring its hypothesized role in regulatory control.

Importantly, additional prefrontal cortex regions such as the inferior frontal gyrus were hypoactivated in PTSD. This finding is notable as previous work has implicated the role of inferior frontal gyrus in emotion regulation, including inhibition from emotional distraction [60] and emotional thought suppression [61]. Moreover, the inferior frontal gyrus is purported to be involved in a network of lateral prefrontal cortex regions involved in changing one's negative thoughts to reduce the impact of negative feelings (i.e., cognitive reappraisal) [62]. Although speculative, it is possible that decreased activity in lateral prefrontal cortex may reflect PTSD patients' difficulty challenging negative thoughts to cope with emotional stimuli. Contemporary psychological models of PTSD highlight the role of negative appraisals and emotion regulation in the etiology and maintenance of PTSD. One of the most successful psychosocial interventions for PTSD, cognitive processing therapy, is based upon the notion that faulty cognitions and interpretation surrounding the traumatic event interferes with the natural recovery process after a trauma [63]. For example, a female rape victim who misattributes blame to herself for attending a party where the rape occurred may then mistrust her decisions in every aspect of her life, leading to experiential avoidance and withdrawal from social relationships. Research has supported the notion that negative self-appraisals are associated with PTSD symptom maintenance [64] and therefore the DSM-V may now include the presence of negative cognitions as a core feature of the disorder [35]. Cognitive processing therapy encourages the patient to adopt a more balanced view of the circumstances surrounding the traumatic event, as well as current personal events by challenging negative thoughts. Given the present results, future studies should examine whether individuals who benefitted from cognitive processing therapy recruit the inferior frontal gyrus to a greater extent compared to pre-therapy, as well as compared to individuals who did not benefit from therapy.

Limitations

A constraint of the current study is the availability of studies that met our criteria for inclusion into the analyses. Although the literature search started with 79 studies, the exclusion of studies that did not include stereotaxic coordinates likely reduced our power to detect less robust activations. Although the number of foci included in this study is more than the minimum recommended for a meta-analysis, it remains an open question whether a larger sample will reveal additional networks central to the PTSD diagnosis. For example, amygdala activity was observed in the PTSD group only when considering ROI analyses or using a less stringent spatial extent. Therefore, the limited number of studies available for the meta-analysis may have had an impact on the ability to detect amygdala activity within the whole-brain analysis. Activity in another key node within the salience network, the anterior insula, was observed in the PTSD group using a less stringent cluster threshold (FDR corrected, $P < 0.05$, cluster-extent = 24 mm^3). Future studies could isolate resting-state networks as a more powerful and robust method towards understanding the functional connections between nodes of the salience network in PTSD. Interestingly, a recent resting-state study in PTSD revealed greater connectivity between the amygdala and insula in patients with PTSD than trauma-exposed controls [65]. The results are consistent with the notion that key nodes within the salience network are highly coactive in PTSD and may underlie the hallmark symptoms of the disorder.

Although there is convincing evidence that the hippocampus becomes dysfunctional as a result of chronic stress [66] and activity in this region has shown to be negatively correlated with arousal symptoms in PTSD [67], hippocampal activity was not observed in the present meta-analysis making it unclear how this region contributes to neurocircuitry models of PTSD. Many of the tasks included in this meta-analysis were not optimal for eliciting hippocampal activity and those that do examine hippocampal function in PTSD show mixed results. There is a growing functional neuroimaging literature examining learning and memory in PTSD, which may clarify the role of hippocampus given that these types of paradigms traditionally activate the hippocampus in healthy individuals.

Finally, working with a limited sample required inclusion of studies with patients on medication and/or comorbid depression. As additional studies are published and software development continues, future meta-analyses may be able to focus exclusively on PTSD or include depression and medication status as covariates in the analyses.

Conclusions

The goal of the present meta-analysis was to examine the neurocircuitry of PTSD by considering a set of studies that were diverse in terms of functional imaging modality, study design, and PTSD trauma type. The results provide evidence for hyperactivation of regions important for vigilance and salience detection, and hypoactivation of regulatory networks engaged in regulation of autonomic arousal and cognition. The key salience network regions that appear to be important in PTSD include the dorsomedial prefrontal cortex (including mid/dorsal anterior cingulate cortex), supplementary motor area, and superior temporal gyrus.

Furthermore, regulatory control regions include two primary networks that appear to be dysfunctional in PTSD, including ventromedial prefrontal cortex control over the amygdala and lateral prefrontal regions putatively involved in modification of thought and inhibition of distracting emotions. This model is consistent with the findings that therapies designed to both extinguish fear responses and promote emotion regulation through challenging negative cognitions are helpful for the treatment of PTSD.

Competing interests

The author(s) declare that they have no competing interests.

Authors' contributions

Ms. Amanda Mikedis conducted a literature review, performed data analysis, and assisted in writing the Methods section. Dr. Jasmeet Hayes and Dr. Scott Hayes helped with the literature review and data analysis, and wrote the paper. All authors read and approved the final manuscript.

Acknowledgements

We would like to thank Drs. Marcella Brunetti and Ruth Lanius for providing unpublished activation coordinates for inclusion in the current meta-analysis, and Dr. Lisa Shin for providing insightful comments on the manuscript. This work was supported by the National Institutes of Health, National Institutes of Mental Health [grant number K23 MH084013 awarded to JPH] and the Department of Veterans Affairs, Veterans Health Administration, Rehabilitation Research & Development Service [grant number CDA E7822W awarded to SMH]. These funding sources had no further role in the study analysis, interpretation of the data, writing of the report, or approval of the paper.

Author details
[1]National Center for PTSD, VA Boston Healthcare System, Boston, MA, USA. [2]Neuroimaging Research Center, VA Boston Healthcare System, Boston, MA, USA. [3]Department of Psychiatry, Boston University School of Medicine, Boston, MA, USA. [4]Memory Disorders Research Center, VA Boston Healthcare System and Boston University School of Medicine, Boston, MA, USA.

References
1. Bremner JD, Narayan M, Staib LH, Southwick SM, McGlashan T, Charney DS: Neural correlates of memories of childhood sexual abuse in women with and without posttraumatic stress disorder. *Am J Psychiatry* 1999, **156**:1787–1795.
2. Bremner JD, Staib LH, Kaloupek D, Southwick SM, Soufer R, Charney DS: Neural correlates of exposure to traumatic pictures and sound in Vietnam combat veterans with and without posttraumatic stress disorder: A positron emission tomography study. *Biol Psychiatry* 1999, **45**:806–816.
3. Bremner JD, Vermetten E, Vythilingam M, Afzal N, Schmahl C, Elzinga B, et al: Neural correlates of the classic color and emotional Stroop in women with abuse-related posttraumatic stress disorder. *Biol Psychiatry* 2004, **55**:612–620.
4. Bremner JD, Vythilingam M, Vermetten E, Southwick SM, McGlashan T, Staib LH, et al: Neural correlates of declarative memory for emotionally valenced words in women with posttraumatic stress disorder related to early childhood sexual abuse. *Biol Psychiatry* 2003, **53**:879–889.
5. Britton JC, Phan KL, Taylor SF, Fig LM, Liberzon I: Corticolimbic blood flow in posttraumatic stress disorder during script-driven imagery. *Biol Psychiatry* 2005, **57**:832–840.
6. Brunetti M, Sepede G, Mingoia G, Catani C, Ferretti A, Merla A, et al: Elevated response of human amygdala to neutral stimuli in mild post traumatic stress disorder: Neural correlates of generalized emotional response. *Neuroscience* 2010, **168**:670–679.
7. Bryant RA, Kemp AH, Felmingham KL, Liddell B, Olivieri G, Peduto A, et al: Enhanced amygdala and medial prefrontal activation during nonconscious processing of fear in posttraumatic stress disorder: An fMRI study. *Hum Brain Mapp* 2008, **29**:517–523.
8. Felmingham K, Williams LM, Kemp AH, Liddell B, Falconer E, Peduto A, et al: Neural responses to masked fear faces: Sex differences and trauma exposure in posttraumatic stress disorder. *J Abnorm Psychol* 2010, **119**:241–247.
9. Fonzo GA, Simmons AN, Thorp SR, Norman SB, Paulus MP, Stein MB: Exaggerated and disconnected insular-amygdalar blood oxygenation level-dependent response to threat-related emotional faces in women with intimate-partner violence posttraumatic stress disorder. *Biol Psychiatry* 2010, **68**:433–441.
10. Frewen P, Lane RD, Neufeld RWJ, Densmore M, Stevens T, Lanius R: Neural correlates of levels of emotional awareness during trauma script-imagery in posttraumatic stress disorder. *Psychosom Med* 2008, **70**:27–31.
11. Hou C, Liu J, Wang K, Li L, Liang M, He Z, et al: Brain responses to symptom provocation and trauma-related short-term memory recall in coal mining accident survivors with acute severe PTSD. *Brain Res* 2007, **1144**:165–174.
12. Kim MJ, Chey J, Chung A, Bae S, Khang H, Ham B, et al: Diminished rostral anterior cingulate activity in response to threat-related events in posttraumatic stress disorder. *J Psychiatr Res* 2008, **42**:268–277.
13. Lanius RA, Frewen PA, Girotti M, Neufeld RW, Stevens TK, Densmore M: Neural correlates of trauma script-imagery in posttraumatic stress disorder with and without comorbid major depression: A functional MRI investigation. *Psychiat Res-Neuroim* 2007, **155**:45–56.
14. Lanius RA, Williamson PC, Boksman K, Densmore M, Gupta M, Neufeld RW, et al: Brain activation during script-driven imagery induced dissociative responses in PTSD: A functional magnetic resonance imaging investigation. *Biol Psychiatry* 2002, **52**:305–311.
15. Lanius RA, Williamson PC, Densmore M, Boksman K, Gupta MA, Neufeld RW, et al: Neural correlates of traumatic memories in posttraumatic stress disorder: A functional MRI investigation. *Am J Psychiatry* 2001, **158**:1920–1922.

16. Lanius RA, Williamson PC, Hopper J, Densmore M, Boksman K, Gupta MA, et al: Recall of emotional states in posttraumatic stress disorder: An fMRI investigation. *Biol Psychiatry* 2003, **53**:204–210.
17. Phan KL, Britton JC, Taylor SF, Fig LM, Liberzon I: Corticolimbic blood flow during nontraumatic emotional processing in posttraumatic stress disorder. *Arch Gen Psychiatry* 2006, **63**:184–192.
18. Protopopescu X, Pan H, Tuescher O, Cloitre M, Goldstein M, Engelien W, et al: Differential time courses and specificity of amygdala activity in posttraumatic stress disorder subjects and normal control subjects. *Biol Psychiatry* 2005, **57**:464–473.
19. Rauch SL, Whalen PJ, Shin LM, McInerney SC, Macklin ML, Lasko NB, et al: Exaggerated amygdala response to masked facial stimuli in posttraumatic stress disorder: A functional MRI study. *Biol Psychiatry* 2000, **47**:769–776.
20. Sakamoto H, Fukuda R, Okuaki T, Rogers M, Kasai K, Machida T, et al: Parahippocampal activation evoked by masked traumatic images in posttraumatic stress disorder: A functional MRI study. *Neuroimage* 2005, **26**:813–821.
21. Shin LM, McNally RJ, Kosslyn SM, Thompson WL, Rauch SL, Alpert NM, et al: Regional cerebral blood flow during script-driven imagery in childhood sexual abuse-related PTSD: A PET investigation. *Am J Psychiatry* 1999, **156**:575–584.
22. Shin LM, Orr SP, Carson MA, Rauch SL, Macklin ML, Lasko NB, et al: Regional cerebral blood flow in the amygdala and medial prefrontal cortex during traumatic imagery in male and female Vietnam veterans with PTSD. *Arch Gen Psychiatry* 2004, **61**:168–176.
23. Shin LM, Wright CI, Cannistraro PA, Wedig MM, McMullin K, Martis B, et al: A functional magnetic resonance imaging study of amygdala and medial prefrontal cortex responses to overtly presented fearful faces in posttraumatic stress disorder. *Arch Gen Psychiatry* 2005, **62**:273–281.
24. Thomaes K, Dorrepaal E, Draijer N, de Ruiter M, Elzinga B, van Balkom A, et al: Increased activation of the left hippocampus region in Complex PTSD during encoding and recognition of emotional words: A pilot study. *Psychiat Res-Neuroim* 2009, **171**:44–53.
25. Whalley MG, Rugg MD, Smith APR, Dolan RJ, Brewin CR: Incidental retrieval of emotional contexts in post-traumatic stress disorder and depression: An fMRI study. *Brain Cognition* 2009, **69**:98–107.
26. Williams LM, Kemp AH, Felmingham K, Barton M, Olivieri G, Peduto A, et al: Trauma modulates amygdala and medial prefrontal responses to consciously attended fear. *Neuroimage* 2006, **29**:347–357.
27. Rauch SL, Shin LM, Phelps EA: Neurocircuitry models of posttraumatic stress disorder and extinction: Human neuroimaging research - Past, present, and future. *Biol Psychiatry* 2006, **60**:376–382.
28. LeDoux JE: Emotion circuits in the brain. *Annu Rev Neurosci* 2000, **23**:155–184.
29. Kilpatrick DG, Resnick HS, Acierno R: Should PTSD Criterion A be retained?. *J Trauma Stress* 2009, **22**:374–383.
30. Foa EB, Kozak MJ: Emotional processing of fear: Exposure to corrective information. *Psychol Bull* 1986, **99**:20–35.
31. Keane T, Fairbank J, Caddell J, Zimering R, Bender M: A behavioral approach to assessing and treating post-traumatic stress disorder in Vietnam Veterans. In *Trauma and its Wake: The Study and Treatment of Post-traumatic Stress Disorder.* Edited by Bristol FC. PA: Brunner/Mazel; 1985:257–294.
32. Ehlers A, Mayou RA, Bryant B: Psychological predictors of chronic posttraumatic stress disorder after motor vehicle accidents. *J Abnorm Psychol* 1998, **107**:508–519.
33. Suvak MK, Barrett LF: Considering PTSD from the perspective of brain processes: A psychological construction approach. *J Trauma Stress* 2011, **24**:3–24.
34. Resick PA, Miller MW: Posttraumatic stress disorder: Anxiety or traumatic stress disorder?. *J Trauma Stress* 2009, **22**:384–390.
35. Friedman MJ, Resick PA, Bryant RA, Brewin CR: Considering PTSD for DSM 5. *Depress Anxiety* 2011, **28**:750–769.
36. Turkeltaub PE, Eden GF, Jones KM, Zeffiro TA: Meta-analysis of the functional neuroanatomy of single-word reading: Method and validation. *Neuroimage* 2002, **16**:765–780.
37. Etkin A, Wager TD: Functional neuroimaging of anxiety: A meta-analysis of emotional processing in PTSD, social anxiety disorder, and specific phobia. *Am J Psychiatry* 2007, **164**:1476–1488.
38. Simmons AN, Matthews SC: Neural circuitry of PTSD with or without mild traumatic brain injury: A meta-analysis. *Neuropharmacology* 2012, **62**:598–606.

39. Flatten G, Perlitz V, Pestinger M, Arin T, Kohl B, Kastrau F, et al: Neural processing of traumatic events in subjects suffering PTSD-a case study of two surgical patients with severe accident trauma. GMS Psycho-social Medicine 2004, 1:1–10.

40. Lanius RA, Hopper JW, Menon RS: Individual differences in a husband and wife who developed PTSD after a motor vehicle accident: A functional MRI case study. Am J Psychiatry 2003, 160:667–669.

41. Laird AR, Robinson JL, McMillan KM, Tordesillas-Gutierrez D, Moran ST, Gonzales SM, et al: Comparison of the disparity between Talairach and MNI coordinates in functional neuroimaging data: Validation of the Lancaster transform. Neuroimage 2010, 51:677–683.

42. Downar J, Crawley AP, Mikulis DJ, Davis KD: A cortical network sensitive to stimulus salience in a neutral behavioral context across multiple sensory modalities. J Neurophysiol 2002, 87:615–620.

43. Seeley WW, Menon V, Schatzberg AF, Keller J, Glover GH, Kenna H, et al: Dissociable intrinsic connectivity networks for salience processing and executive control. J Neurosci 2007, 27:2349–2356.

44. Morey R, Dolcos F, Petty C, Cooper D, Hayes J, LaBar K, et al: The role of trauma-related distractors on neural systems for working memory and emotion processing in posttraumatic stress disorder. J Psychiatr Res 2009, 43:809–817.

45. Bush G, Luu P, Posner MI: Cognitive and emotional influences in anterior cingulate cortex. Trends Cogn Sci 2000, 4:215–222.

46. Hughes KC, Shin LM: Functional neuroimaging studies of post-traumatic stress disorder. Expert Rev Neurother 2011, 11:275–285.

47. Shin LM, Handwerger K: Is posttraumatic stress disorder a stress-induced fear circuitry disorder?. J Trauma Stress 2009, 22:409–415.

48. Etkin A, Egner T, Kalisch R: Emotional processing in anterior cingulate and medial prefrontal cortex. Trends Cogn Sci 2011, 15:85–93.

49. Pannu Hayes J, LaBar K, Petty C, McCarthy G, Morey R: Alterations in the neural circuitry for emotion and attention associated with posttraumatic stress symptomatology. Psychiat Res-Neuroim 2009, 172:7–15.

50. Shin LM, Bush G, Milad MR, Lasko NB, Brohawn KH, Hughes KC, et al: Exaggerated activation of dorsal anterior cingulate cortex during cognitive interference: A monozygotic twin study of posttraumatic stress disorder. Am J Psychiatry 2011, 168:979–985.

51. Shin LM, Lasko NB, Macklin ML, Karpf RD, Milad MR, Orr SP, et al: Resting metabolic activity in the cingulate cortex and vulnerability to posttraumatic stress disorder. Arch Gen Psychiatry 2009, 66:1099–1107.

52. Milad MR, Quirk GJ, Pitman RK, Orr SP, Fischl B, Rauch SL: A role for the human dorsal anterior cingulate cortex in fear expression. Biol Psychiatry 2007, 62:1191–1194.

53. Davis M, Whalen PJ: The amygdala: Vigilance and emotion. Mol Psychiatr 2001, 6:13–34.

54. Pessoa L, Adolphs R: Emotion processing and the amygdala: From a 'low road' to 'many roads' of evaluating biological significance. Nat Rev Neurosci 2010, 11:773–783.

55. Whalen PJ: Fear, vigilance, and ambiguity: Initial neuroimaging studies of the human amygdala. Curr Dir Psychol Sci 1998, 7:177–188.

56. Blackford JU, Buckholtz JW, Avery SN, Zald DH: A unique role for the human amygdala in novelty detection. Neuroimage 2010, 50:1188–1193.

57. Sarinopoulos I, Grupe D, Mackiewicz K, Herrington J, Lor M, Steege E, et al: Uncertainty during anticipation modulates neural responses to aversion in human insula and amygdala. Cereb Cortex 2010, 20:929–940.

58. Quirk GJ, Beer JS: Prefrontal involvement in the regulation of emotion: convergence of rat and human studies. Curr Opin Neurobiol 2006, 16:723–727.

59. Morey RA, Petty CM, Cooper DA, LaBar KS, McCarthy G: Neural systems for executive and emotional processing are modulated by symptoms of posttraumatic stress disorder in Iraq War veterans. Psychiat Res-Neuroim 2008, 162:59–72.

60. Dolcos F, McCarthy G: Brain systems mediating cognitive interference by emotional distraction. J Neurosci 2006, 26:2072–2079.

61. Depue B, Curran T, Banich M: Prefrontal regions orchestrate suppression of emotional memories via a two-phase process. Science 2007, 317:215–219.

62. Ochsner KN: For better or for worse: Neural systems supporting the cognitive down- and up-regulation of emotion. Neuroimage 2004, 23:483–499.

63. Resick PA, Monson C, Chard K: Cognitive processing therapy: Veteran/military version. Washington DC: Department of Veterans' Affairs; 2008.

64. Owens G, Cox TA, Chard K: The relationship between maladaptive cognitions, anger expression, and posttraumatic stress disorder among Veterans in residential treatment. Journal of Aggression, Maltreatment & Trauma 2008, 17:439–452.

65. Rabinak CA, Angstadt M, Welsh RC, Kennedy A, Lyubkin M, Martis B, et al: Altered amygdala resting-state functional connectivity in post-traumatic stress disorder. Front. Psychiatry 2011, 2:62.

66. Ulrich-Lai YM, Herman JP: Neural regulation of endocrine and autonomic stress responses. Nat Rev Neurosci 2009, 10:397–409.

67. Hayes J, LaBar K, McCarthy G, Selgrade E, Nasser J, Dolcos F, et al: Reduced hippocampal and amygdala activity predicts memory distortions for trauma reminders in combat-related PTSD. J Psychiatr Res 2011, 45:660–669.

14

Amygdala activation to threat under attentional load in individuals with anxiety disorder

Thomas Straube*, Judith Lipka, Andreas Sauer, Martin Mothes-Lasch and Wolfgang HR Miltner

Abstract

Background: Previous studies in healthy subjects have shown that strong attentional distraction prevents the amygdala from responding to threat stimuli. Here, we investigated the effects of attentional load on amygdala activation to threat-related stimuli in individuals suffering from an anxiety disorder.

Methods: During functional magnetic resonance imaging, spider-phobicand healthy control subjects were presented with phobia-related and neutral stimuli while performing a distraction task with varying perceptual load (high vs low).

Results: Our data revealed a pattern of simultaneously increased amygdala and visual cortical activation to threat vs neutral pictures in phobic individuals, compared with controls, occurring regardless of attentional load.

Conclusions: These results suggest that, in contrast to studies in healthy subjects, amygdala activation to clinically relevant threat stimuli is more resistant to attentional load.

Background

In accordance with theories suggesting a critical function of the amygdala in the processing of threat signals and the mediation of fear responses [1,2], several studies found increased amygdala activation to threatening vs neutral stimuli in individuals with anxiety disorders [3-8] and in healthy subjects [9-14]. Furthermore, there are strong theoretical accounts proposing an automatic response of the amygdala to threat signals even when target stimuli are presented during attentional distraction [1,2,14]. Whereas some studies indeed suggest an automaticity of amygdala activation to threat-related stimuli under conditions of attentional distraction [9,13,14], several recent studies in healthy subjects, however, indicated a complete inhibition of differential activation to threat vs neutral stimuli within the amygdala, given sufficiently strong perceptual load by a main task [15-18]. Thus, it seems that, at least in healthy subjects, automatic activation of the amygdala to emotional stimuli does not occur when demanding cognitive tasks exhaust the available processing resources.

Bishop *et al.*, for example, used a perceptual load task, while subjects were exposed to fearful and neutral faces.

Perceptual load was induced by varying the number of task-relevant items [19,20] within a letter string presented along with the facial expression. When perceptual identification was easy (low load), elevated state anxiety was associated with a heightened response to threat distractors in the amygdala and superior temporal sulcus, whereas individuals scoring high in trait anxiety showed a reduced prefrontal response to these stimuli. The latter finding was interpreted as weakened recruitment of control mechanisms when confronted with salient distractors. This finding is in accordance with theories assuming an imbalance between the stimulus-driven processing of salient threat-related stimuli, associated with automatic orienting, and goal-directed attentional control (for example, [21]). This would lead to a relatively stronger role of the posterior attentional systems in the brain involved in bottom-up attention as compared to the more anterior top-down control system [22]. However, in the study of Bishop *et al.*, neither high-anxious nor low-anxious subjects showed an increased amygdala response to threat distractors when perceptual identification was more attention demanding (high perceptual load). Furthermore, high attentional load in previous studies also prevented differential activation to threat vs neutral stimuli in areas of the extrastriate visual cortex, suggesting the absence of

* Correspondence: straube@biopsy.uni-jena.de
Department of Biological and Clinical Psychology, Friedrich-Schiller-University, Jena, Germany

differential processing of threat and neutral stimuli also in areas beyond the amygdala [15,17,23].

Thus, in line with a recent model of selective attention [19,20], processing of task-unrelated stimuli is prevented when task-related demands exhaust perceptual capacity limits. Even though this model does not predict that also the processing of salient emotional stimuli is impaired by high perceptual load [24], it has been extended to the domain of threat processing [15,23]. Furthermore, based on the findings of Bishop et al., effects of subjects' anxiety on the neural processing of threat-related stimuli seem to appear only during relatively low-load tasks. Thus, high load should prevent neural responses to threat and also the attentional processing of these stimuli, that is automatic orienting [22]. This position is in contrast to cognitive models of anxiety [25] predicting a mandatory processing of threat stimuli in anxious subjects or models predicting that anxiety increases the processing of threat-related signals under high demands on the central executive [21].

Even though it has been shown that high perceptual load prevents the processing of threat stimuli in anxious healthy subjects, it is unknown whether similar findings will be observed in individuals suffering from an anxiety disorder. Automatic processing of disorder-related stimuli seems to be a main feature of anxiety disorders and this might be represented in attention-independent activation of the amygdala [1,2,8]. An example is specific phobia, which is among the most common anxiety disorders [26]. Neuroimaging research implicates the amygdala in the processing of phobia-related stimuli, specifically in the initial detection of such stimuli and perhaps in the lowering of thresholds for the induction of rapid fear responses, rather than in the sustained processing of phobia-relevant information [8,27,28]. For example, activation of the amygdala in spider-phobic subjects has been demonstrated regardless of whether attention was focused on the stimuli or distracted by an unrelated foreground task [8], supporting the hypothesis that the amygdala is automatically activated by phobogenic stimuli [1,2,29]. Furthermore, this attention independent response in the amygdala was associated with increased activation in the extrastriate visual cortex [8], which is typically coactivated with the amygdala in spider phobia in response to phobia-related stimuli (for example, [3,30-32]).

A recent study with spider-phobic subjects reported attention-dependent activation of the amygdala to spider pictures [33]. However, in this study the number of phobia-related stimuli and attention focus were confounded, making a clear interpretation of the results difficult. Thus, the findings might even be interpreted to support the hypothesis of automatic amygdala activation to task-irrelevant (background) spider pictures. To date, there has been no functional imaging study that employed a parametric variation of attentional load in individuals with specific phobia or any other anxiety disorder.

In the present study, we used event-related functional magnetic resonance imaging (fMRI) to explore the question whether amygdala activation to phobia-relevant stimuli is modulated by a parametric variation of attentional distraction in patients with specific phobia. We used a perceptual load task that has been previously shown to inhibit amygdala activation to threat-related stimuli in high-anxious healthy subjects [15]. An absence of attentional modulation of amygdala activation in the present experiment would indicate a role of the amygdala in threat processing even under high attentional load in individuals with anxiety disorder. Additionally, we examined the neural activation in the visual cortex and several brain areas proposed to be involved in the processing of threat-related stimuli.

The results show a pattern of simultaneously increased amygdala and visual cortical activation to threat vs neutral pictures in phobic individuals, compared with controls, occurring regardless of attentional load. These findings suggest that amygdala activation to clinically relevant threat stimuli is resistant to attentional load.

Methods

Subjects

A total of 17 spider-phobic (mean age = 25.2, SD = 4.9) and 16 control subjects (mean age = 26.6, SD = 9.2) participated in the study. Participants were right handed female university students with normal or corrected-to-normal vision who provided written informed consent to volunteer in the study. The ethics committee of the University of Jena approved all experimental procedures. All phobic subjects fulfilled the diagnostic criteria for spider phobia according to the *Diagnostic and Statistical Manual of Mental Disorders*, fourth edition (DSM-IV; [34]) as assessed by a structured clinical interview [35]. According to this interview, spider-phobic subjects had no additional psychopathological disorders. In addition, spider-phobic subjects, but not controls, showed high scores on a spider phobia questionnaire ([36]; mean = 23.4, SD = 2.3 vs mean = 2.8, SD = 1.6; t = 29.55, P < 0.001). There was no difference in trait or state anxiety scores between groups ([37]; trait: mean phobics = 36.94, SD = 11.02, mean controls = 41.93, SD = 7.40; t = 1.43, P > 0.05; state: mean phobics = 38.27, SD = 10.42, mean controls = 34.45, SD = 4.45; t = 1.27, P > 0.05). Further demographic and clinical characteristics are summarized in Table 1.

Stimuli and tasks

Subjects were exposed to 48 different pictures of spiders and 48 different pictures of mushrooms while performing

Table 1 Demographic and clinical characteristics

	Phobic subjects (N = 17)	Healthy controls (N = 16)
Age in years, mean (SD)	25.2 (4.9)	26.6 (9.2)
Ethnicity	Caucasian	Caucasian
Education	At least secondary high school	At least secondary high school
Prior/current medication	No	No
Psychotherapy	No	No
SPQ, mean (SD)	23.4 (2.3)	2.8 (1.6)
STAI, mean (SD)	36.94 (11.02)	34.45 (4.45)

SPQ = spider phobia questionnaire; STAI = State-Trait Anxiety Index.

a letter search task (adapted from [15]). The spider pictures represented the disorder-related stimuli. We used mushrooms as control stimuli, mainly for reasons of comparability with several previous studies (for example, [8,12,38,39]). A string of six letters written in red ink was superimposed onto the task-irrelevant spider or mushroom picture, respectively. In half of the trials (high perceptual load), the string comprised a single target letter (N or X) and five non-target letters (H, K, M, W, Z), which were arranged in random order. In the other half of the trials (low load), the letter string comprised either six Xs or six Ns. The task was to decide by button press whether the letter string contained an 'X' or an 'N'. The low-load and high-load conditions were arranged in blocks of four trials (see [15]). In total, there were 24 blocks of 4 trials each. Load was varied across blocks and picture category was varied within blocks. The stimulus onset asynchrony (SOA) was 4.5 sec allowing improved sampling of the BOLD response due to jittering between SOA relative to the repetition time (TR), thus representing an effective interval for event-related designs. The pictures were randomized across and within blocks with the restriction that two mushroom and two spider pictures were shown within each block. The stimuli (including the letter strings) were presented for 200 ms in random order with a resulting interstimulus interval of 4300 ms. Figure 1 shows an example of two trials. The overall picture size was 15 × 20° visual angle, with the stimuli subtending approximately 11.5 × 11.5°. After the fMRI session, participants rated the pictures using a nine-point Likert scale to assess valence (1 = 'very pleasant' to 9 = 'very unpleasant') and arousal (1 = 'not arousing' to 9 = 'very arousing'). Behavioral data were analyzed by repeated measures analysis of variance using SPSS (V. 17; SPSS, Chicago, IL, USA) with subsequent post hoc t tests (Bonferroni corrected). For analysis of performance data, one control subject had to be excluded due to technical problems during the registration of button presses.

fMRI data acquisition and analysis

A run of 294 volumes (40 axial slices per volume, thickness = 3 mm, in plane resolution = 3 × 3 mm) was acquired (3 T; 'Tim Trio', Siemens, Erlangen, Germany) using a T2*-weighted echo planar sequence (echo time (TE) = 30 ms, flip angle = 90°, matrix = 64 × 64, field of view (FOV) = 192 mm, TR = 2.9 s). Additionally, a T1-weighted anatomical volume was recorded (192 slices, echo time (TE) = 6 ms, matrix = 256 × 256, voxel size = 1 × 1 × 1 mm). Preprocessing and analysis of the functional data were performed using the software Brain Voyager QX (Brain Innovation, Maastricht, The Netherlands). All volumes were realigned to the first, corrected for slice time errors, and spatially (8 mm full-width half-maximum isotropic Gaussian kernel) as well as temporally (high pass filter: cut-off = 0.006 Hz) smoothed. Furthermore, data preprocessing included removal of linear trends and of the mean. Anatomical and functional images were coregistered and normalized to the Talairach space. Statistical analysis was performed by multiple linear regression of the signal time course at each voxel. The expected blood oxygen level-dependent signal change for each predictor was modeled by a hemodynamic response function (based on a two-gamma-function model, which models rise and undershoot of the BOLD response, as implemented in Brain Voyager). Predictors of non-interest were the six movement parameters. The four predictors of interest were the spider pictures/low load, spider pictures/high load, mushroom pictures/low load, and mushroom pictures/high load. Statistical comparisons were conducted using a mixed-effect analysis. In the first step, voxelwise statistical maps were generated and predictor estimates (β weights) were computed for each individual. In the second step, contrasts of predictor estimates were analyzed across subjects with repeated-measures analysis of variance (ANOVA). Statistical parametric maps resulting from the voxelwise analysis were considered significant for statistical values that survived a cluster-based correction for multiple comparisons. Voxel-level threshold was initially set to $P < 0.005$ (uncorrected) to strike a balance between type I and type II errors. Thresholded maps were then submitted to a region of interest (ROI)-specific or whole brain-specific correction criterion, which was based on the estimate of the map's spatial

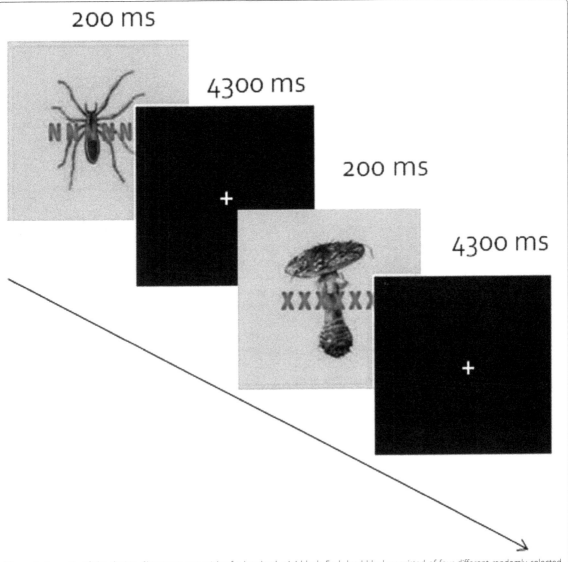

Figure 1 Example of the design. Shown are two trials of a low load mini block. Each load block consisted of four different randomly selected pictures. Load was varied across blocks and picture category was varied within blocks.

smoothness and on an iterative procedure (Monte Carlo simulation) used to estimate cluster-level false-positive rates. After 1,000 iterations, the minimum cluster size threshold that yielded a cluster-level false-positive rate of 5% was applied to the statistical maps (11 voxels for whole brain analysis). According to our previous studies [7,8,12,13,18,32], the following anatomical ROIs were defined a priori using Talairach daemon software [40,41]: amygdala, insula, anterior cingulate cortex (ACC), dorsolateral prefrontal cortex (DLPFC), dorsomedial prefrontal cortex (DMPFC), and fusiform gyrus, with the latter region consistently shown to be

involved in the visual processing of spider pictures in spider-phobic subjects (for example, [8]). Statistical data are only shown for significantly activated voxels.

Results
Performance data
For accuracy (Table 2), a main effect of load was found (F(1,30) = 70.8, P <0.0001) due to decreased accuracy during the high-load condition. For reaction times (Table 2), a main effect of load (F(1,30) = 201.6, P <0.0001), due to increased reaction times during the high-load condition, and an interaction of Task ×

Table 2 Behavioral data

	Phobics		Controls	
	Spider	Mushroom	Spider	Mushroom
Performance				
Reaction times (ms):				
High load	973.04 (166.0)	986.8 (160.98)	1047.51 (154.37)	1062.14 (152.33)
Low load	683.79 (146.9)	664.4 (108.6)	665.79 (58.75)	655.85 (61.54)
Accuracy (% correct):				
High load	68.38 (12.48)	62.38 (17.16)	67.5 (11.16)	64.31 (16.31)
Low load	87.87 (16.09)	87.13 (18.48)	88.01 (22.08)	90.0 (22.27)
Ratings				
Valence (range 1 to 9)	8.59 (0.44)	3.41 (1.79)	5.46 (1.06)	4.58 (1.05)
Arousal (range 1 to 9)	8.24 (0.69)	1.05 (0.30)	2.89 (1.87)	1.08 (0.36)

Data shown are mean (SD).

picture category ($F(1,30) = 6.5$, $P < 0.05$), due to increased reaction times to spiders vs mushrooms during low but not high load, were found.

Rating data

Post-scanning arousal and valence ratings (Table 2) showed a main effect of group ($F(1,30) = 101.3$, $P < 0.0001$; $F(1,30) = 11.3$, $P < 0.005$), picture category ($F(1,30) = 324.9$, $F(1,30) = 102.4$, both $P < 0.0001$), and an interaction of group × picture category ($F(1,30) = 116.0$, $F(1,30) = 51.6$, both $P < 0.0001$). Post hoc analysis using t tests (Bonferroni corrected) revealed that phobic subjects rated spiders, but not mushrooms, as more arousing and unpleasant than control subjects (arousal: t = 10.7, $P < 0.001$ (spiders), t = 0.3; $P > 0.05$ (mushrooms); t = 10.9, $P < 0.001$ (spiders), t = -2.0; $P > 0.05$ (mushrooms)).

fMRI analysis
Amygdala ROI

For both the right and left amygdala, there was only a main effect of load (left: (x, y, z) = -25, -8, -12; $F[1,31] = 45.09$; right: (x, y, z) = 27, -10, -11; $F[1,31] = 55.54$; both $P < 0.05$, corrected; cluster size: left: 2771 mm^3; right: 2571 mm^3) and an interaction of group × picture category (left: (x, y, z) = -27, -1, -17; $F[1,31] = 10.15$; right: (x, y, z) = 23, -1, -11; $F[1,31] = 11.54$; both $P < 0.05$, corrected; cluster size: left: 108 mm^3; right: 116 mm^3). Thus, our data did not reveal an interaction of group × picture category × load. The main effect of load resulted from decreased amygdala activation across pictures and groups under high vs low load. The interaction of group by picture category was due to increased activation to spider versus neutral pictures in phobic subjects, as compared to healthy controls. However, as also indicated in Figure 2, the increased activation to threat vs neutral pictures in phobic subjects was independent of perceptual load.

Other ROIs and whole brain analysis

As indicated in Table 3, an effect of load was also evident in several other brain regions. While regions such as the dorsal ACC and other areas in the frontal and parietal cortex implicated in dealing with task difficulty showed increased activation during high load, other areas such as the ventromedial prefrontal cortex, which is typically deactivated during demanding tasks, as well as areas in the visual cortex showed a decreased activation under high vs low load.

Furthermore, there were main effects of picture category in the superior temporal gyrus and the visual cortex due to decreased (superior temporal gyrus (STG)) and increased (visual cortex) activation to spiders vs mushrooms across subjects and tasks (see Table 3). Most importantly, there was an interaction of group × picture specifically in the left fusiform gyrus (see Table 2 and Figure 2). The interaction of group by picture category was due to increased activation to spiders versus neutral pictures in phobic subjects, as compared to healthy controls. As also indicated in Figure 3, the increased activation to threat vs neutral pictures in phobic subjects was independent of perceptual load, comparable with the profile of activation in the amygdala. There were no further significant main effects or interactions.

Discussion

The present study provides evidence for a critical involvement of the amygdala in threat processing under attentional load in subjects suffering from an anxiety disorder. Thus, amygdala activation to disorder-related vs neutral stimuli was observed regardless of attentional load. A similar finding was evident for the left fusiform gyrus.

This finding contrasts with prior studies in healthy subjects [15-18], especially with a study where the same task resulted in a strong modulation of amygdala

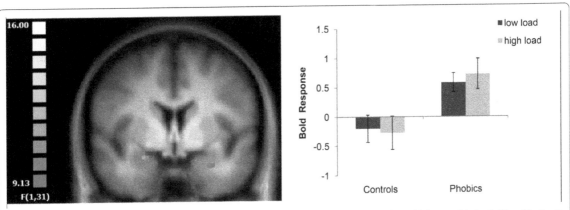

Figure 2 Amygdala responses to spider vs mushroom pictures. Increased activation in the right and left amygdala in phobic subjects was found regardless of perceptual load. Statistical parametric maps are overlaid on a T1 scan (radiological convention: left = right; y = -1). The plot shows the difference of parameter estimates (spider vs mushroom; mean and standard error) for the maximally activated voxel in the left amygdala.

activation to fearful vs neutral faces, with the differential amygdala activation completely inhibited under the high-load condition [15]. The study of Bishop *et al.* found that, during a low-load condition, when perceptual distractor identification was less demanding, elevated state anxiety was associated with a heightened response to fearful faces in the amygdala and superior temporal sulcus, whereas individuals scoring high in

Table 3 Significant brain activation

Area	Side	x	y	z	Size (mm^3)	F value	Signal change (%)
Main effect load (ROI):							
Amygdala	R	27	-10	-11	2571	55.54	0.35
	L	-25	-8	-12	2771	45.09	0.35
Insula	R	33	15	11	1674	54.72	0.43
	L	-35	15	12	1431	59.68	0.43
FG	L	-45	-55	-14	662	45.06	0.49
Dorsal ACC	R/L	-7	43	11	10652	65.54	0.70
DMPFC	R/L	-10	43	15	8391	54.61	0.45
DLPFC	R	23	23	52	1489	42.11	0.38
	L	-19	28	52	3604	57.51	0.53
Main effect load (whole brain):							
Parietal cortex	R	2	-53	21	11751	62.70	0.76
	L	-25	-66	34	17118	103.44	0.83
VMPFC	R/L	-7	43	9	4503	71.67	0.70
Visual cortex	R	3	-77	-7	373	23.06	0.37
	L	-3	-81	-8	328	27.06	0.36
Main effect picture (whole brain):							
STG	R	53	-14	-3	377	13.12	0.14
Visual cortex	R	16	-93	-5	783	20.79	0.19
	L	-18	-94	-10	513	22.57	0.21
Interaction picture by group (ROI):							
Amygdala	R	23	-1	-11	116	11.54	0.40
	L	-27	-1	-17	108	10.15	0.35
FG	L	-42	-55	-11	179	12.11	0.32

x, y, z are the Talairach coordinates of peak voxel activation threshold: $P < 0.05$, corrected. Cluster threshold whole brain: 11 voxels; other thresholds: 3 to 5 voxels; voxel threshold: $P < 0.005$.
ACC = anterior cingulate cortex; DLPFC = dorsolateral prefrontal cortex; DMPFC = dorsomedial prefrontal cortex; FG = fusiform gyrus; ROI = region of interest; STG = superior temporal gyrus; VMPFC = ventromedial prefrontal cortex.

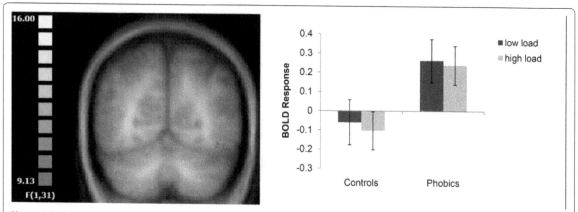

Figure 3 Activation to spider vs mushroom pictures in the extrastriate visual cortex. Increased activation in the left fusiform gyrus in phobic subjects was found regardless of perceptual load. Statistical parametric maps are overlaid on a T1 scan (radiological convention: left = right; y = -55). The plot shows the difference of parameter estimates (spider vs mushroom; mean and standard error) for the maximally activated voxel.

trait anxiety showed a reduced prefrontal response to these stimuli. The latter finding was interpreted to indicate a weakened recruitment of cortical control mechanisms in anxious individuals when confronted with threat distractors. However, neither high-anxious nor low-anxious volunteers showed an increased amygdala response to threat distractors when the perceptual identification task was more attention demanding (high perceptual load).

Thus, it seems that the findings in subjects showing high, but subclinical, levels of state and trait anxiety may not necessarily be comparable to those of a subject sample meeting the diagnostic criteria for a clinically relevant anxiety disorder such as specific phobia. This difference suggests an increased responsiveness of the amygdala to threat signals in anxiety disorder patients. This increased responsiveness might be mainly associated with differences in the threat relevance of stimuli used in the different studies. Thus, while fearful facial expressions are associated with rather low anxiety ratings, disorder-related stimuli evoke strong fear responses in subjects suffering from an anxiety disorder. Furthermore, our findings are also not associated with trait or state anxiety scores of subjects, since there was no difference between groups. Thus, the use of increased trait or state scores as analogue to clinical disorders might be often of limited relevance. Rather, it may be the disorder-related importance of the stimuli that determines differential brain responses, at least in phobias.

Our results support previous findings of amygdala activation to threat under conditions of attentional distraction in specific phobia [8,33]. However, no previous study in individuals with anxiety disorders employed a parametric manipulation of attentional load as yet. Also,

prior work may differ in that the distraction conditions might not have been very demanding [8], or that they were confounded with other factors [33]. The present results suggest that, at least in specific phobia, the salience of stimuli evokes differential amygdala activation to threat vs neutral stimuli independent of attentional load, even though the amygdala and other areas were found to be modulated by attentional load in general. Thus, high load led to decreased activation of the amygdala and several other brain areas. Conversely, regions implicated in attentional control and dealing with task difficulty showed increased activation under high as compared to low load. This general effect of load or attentional distraction is in line with prior work [15,17,23].

We did not detect any evidence for a decreased prefrontal control of threat distractors as suggested by Bishop *et al.* However, one has to keep in mind that the results in the Bishop *et al.* study are based on a correlation with trait anxiety scores and a comparable significance of the facial expressions for all subjects (high and low anxious). Here, we compared subjects with anxiety disorder to healthy controls. That is, for spider-phobic subjects the spider pictures were disorder related, while for the control group the (attentional control of these) pictures had no relevance. This prevents a meaningful comparison of differential control mechanisms between groups.

Beyond its role in the rapid induction of defense behaviors [1,2], the amygdala might also be involved in attentional functions [2,42-45], for example, through the modulation of activation in visual areas by feedback connections [46]. This influence of the amygdala might allow the enhanced perception of threat [47].

Accordingly, it has been shown that the amygdala drives the activation of areas within the inferior temporo-occipital cortex such as the fusiform gyrus [14] and increased activations to threat even under distraction conditions or perceptual unawareness have been found in visual areas [48,49]. In line with these findings, our data revealed a significant activation of the fusiform gyrus to spider vs neutral stimuli in spider-phobic subjects occurring in conjunction with the amygdala activation during both attentional conditions.

The amygdala's influence on attentional functions is not specific for anxious subjects or anxiety disorders, but can be found in healthy subjects as well (for example, [43,44,50]). Animal research also implicates the amygdala in forming a crucial part of a pervasive vigilance system subserving facilitated processing of biologically relevant information [45,51,52]. Thus, the meaning of automatic amygdala activations for phobic symptomatology might be associated with such functions. Individuals suffering from specific phobias show increased vigilance for phobia-relevant stimuli [48,53]. Under divided attention conditions, the amygdala might be activated even by crude representations of threat stimuli requiring the brain to gather more information by potentiating subsequent sensory information processing.

It should be noted that we do not suggest that these findings are necessarily specific for the processing of phobogenic stimuli. Rather, the processing of phobogenic stimuli represents a highly aversive condition and might be a specific case where personally relevant and salient aversive stimuli are processed even during high perceptual load. Generally, we suggest that activation of the amygdala and visual cortex is due to the interplay between the saliency of stimuli and available cognitive resources. Thus, other threat stimuli might be processed in non-clinical populations as well, given that the saliency and the personal importance of these stimuli are sufficiently high. Future studies should use negative and positive affective control stimuli in order to disentangle the general role of valence and arousal for amygdala responses under high perceptual load.

Furthermore, there was a remarkable reduction of the activation of the amygdala by high load regardless of group and picture category. This is in accordance with previous work (for example, [16]) and provides clear evidence that even in the absence of emotional stimuli the activation in the amygdala is affected by attentional conditions. However, in our study, the differential activation to phobia-related vs neutral pictures was stable across load conditions, indicating a dissociation between a general decrease of the amygdala responsiveness regardless of the specific stimuli and intact relative increased amygdala activation to phobia-related vs neutral stimuli during high load.

Remarkably, there were no effects on task performance in spider-phobic subjects as compared to healthy subjects. However, this finding is in accordance with previous results [8]. Furthermore, impairments in task performance are not consistently observed in subjects with phobias (for example, [7,8,54,55]). Moreover, for the kind of task used in the present study, Bishop et al. showed differential brain activation in anxious subjects that was not accompanied by indications of behavioral impairment. Thus, effects on brain activation can be dissociated from those on behavioral measures, at least when assessed through reaction times and errors. Future studies should investigate whether amygdala responses can predict other behavioral measures. Furthermore, it would be interesting to investigate whether automatic amygdala activations can be modified by successful psychotherapy and if these responses are associated with therapeutic success in the short and long term.

Conclusions

Our results indicate a hyper-responsiveness of the amygdala to disorder-related stimuli in phobic subjects that proved to be independent of attentional load when using a task which induces a high load and which has been shown to prevent amygdala activation to threat in high anxious subjects. This suggests that anxiety disorder patients are characterized by a high level of automaticity of their amygdala responsiveness. Although we did not find an effect of perceptual load on differential amygdala responses, future work might aim to investigate whether a further increase of perceptual load may result in different outcomes as revealed in this study. Thus, also in anxiety patients, the amygdala response to threat might be characterized by a relative instead of an absolute automaticity.

Acknowledgements
The study was supported by the Deutsche Forschungsgemeinschaft (STR 987/2-1; 987/2-3).

Authors' contributions
TS participated in the design and the data analysis of the study and drafted the manuscript. AS and JL carried out the experiments. AS and MML established the experimental procedures. AS performed the data preprocessing and analysis and wrote parts of the manuscript. WM participated in the development and coordination of the study. All authors read and approved the final manuscript.

Competing interests
The authors declare that they have no competing interests.

References
1.   LeDoux JE: **Fear and the brain: where have we been, and where are we going?** *Biol Psychiatry* 1998, **44**:1229-1238.

2. Öhman A, Mineka S: **Fears, phobias, and preparedness: toward an evolved module of fear and fear learning.** *Psychol Rev* 2001, **108**:483-522.

3. Dilger S, Straube T, Mentzel HJ, Fitzek C, Reichenbach JR, Hecht H, Krieschel S, Gutberlet I, Miltner WH: **Brain activation to phobia-related pictures in spider phobic humans: an event-related functional magnetic resonance imaging study.** *Neurosci Letters* 2003, **348**:29-32.

4. Liberzon I, Taylor SF, Amdur R, Jung TD, Chamberlain KR, Minoshima S, Koeppe RA, Fig LM: **Brain activation in PTSD in response to trauma-related stimuli.** *Biol Psychiatry* 1999, **45**:817-826.

5. Shin LM, Orr SP, Carson MA, Rauch SL, Macklin ML, Lasko NB, Peters PM, Metzger LJ, Dougherty DD, Cannistraro PA, Alpert NM, Fischman AJ, Pitman RK: **Regional cerebral blood flow in the amygdala and medial prefrontal cortex during traumatic imagery in male and female Vietnam veterans with PTSD.** *Arch Gen Psychiatry* 2004, **61**:168-176.

6. Stein MB, Goldin PR, Sareen J, Zorrilla LT, Brown GG: **Increased amygdala activation to angry and contemptuous faces in generalized social phobia.** *Arch Gen Psychiatry* 2002, **59**:1027-1034.

7. Straube T, Kolassa I T, Glauer M, Mentzel HJ, Miltner WH: **Effect of task conditions on brain responses to threatening faces in social phobics: an event-related functional magnetic resonance imaging study.** *Biol Psychiatry* 2004, **56**:921-930.

8. Straube T, Mentzel HJ, Miltner WH: **Neural mechanisms of automatic and direct processing of phobogenic stimuli in specific phobia.** *Biol Psychiatry* 2006, **59**:162-170.

9. Anderson AK, Christoff K, Panitz D, De Rosa E, Gabrieli JD: **Neural correlates of the automatic processing of threat facial signals.** *J Neurosci* 2003, **23**:5627-5633.

10. Breiter HC, Etcoff NL, Whalen PJ, Kennedy WA, Rauch SL, Buckner RL, Strauss MM, Hyman SE, Rosen BR: **Response and habituation of the human amygdala during visual processing of facial expression.** *Neuron* 1996, **17**:875-887.

11. Büchel C, Morris J, Dolan RJ, Friston KJ: **Brain systems mediating aversive conditioning: an event-related fMRI study.** *Neuron* 1998, **20**:947-957.

12. Straube T, Mentzel HJ, Miltner WH: **Waiting for spiders: brain activation during anticipatory anxiety in spider phobics.** *Neuroimage* 2007, **37**:1427-1436.

13. Straube T, Pohlack S, Mentzel HJ, Miltner WH: **Differential amygdala activation to negative and positive emotional pictures during an indirect task.** *Behav Brain Res* 2008, **191**:285-288.

14. Vuilleumier P, Armony JL, Driver J, Dolan RJ: **Effects of attention and emotion on face processing in the human brain: an event-related fMRI study.** *Neuron* 2001, **30**:829-841.

15. Bishop SJ, Jenkins R, Lawrence AD: **Neural processing of fearful faces: effects of anxiety are gated by perceptual capacity limitations.** *Cereb Cortex* 2007, **17**:1595-1603.

16. Lim SL, Padmala S, Pessoa L: **Affective learning modulates spatial competition during low-load attentional conditions.** *Neuropsychologia* 2008, **46**:1267-1278.

17. Pessoa L, McKenna M, Gutierrez E, Ungerleider LG: **Neural processing of emotional faces requires attention.** *Proc Natl Acad Sci USA* 2002, **99**:11458-11463.

18. Straube T, Weiss T, Mentzel HJ, Miltner WH: **Time course of amygdala activation during aversive conditioning depends on attention.** *Neuroimage* 2007, **34**:462-469.

19. Lavie N: **Perceptual Load as a Necessary Condition for Selective Attention.** *J Exp Psychol: Hum Percept Perform* 1995, **21**:451-468.

20. Lavie N: **Distracted and confused?: selective attention under load.** *Trends Cogn Sci* 2005, **9**:75-82.

21. Eysenck MW, Derakshan N, Santos R, Calvo MG: **Anxiety and cognitive performance: attentional control theory.** *Emotion* 2007, **7**:336-353.

22. Posner MI, Petersen SE: **The attention system of the human brain.** *Annu Rev Neurosci* 1990, **13**:25-42.

23. Pessoa L, Padmala S, Morland T: **Fate of unattended fearful faces in the amygdala is determined by both attentional resources and cognitive modulation.** *Neuroimage* 2005, **28**:249-255.

24. Lavie N, Ro T, Russell C: **The role of perceptual load in processing distractor faces.** *Psych Sci* 2003, **14**:510-515.

25. Mathews A, Mackintosh B: **A cognitive model of selective processing in anxiety.** *Cogn Ther Res* 1998, **22**:539-560.

26. Pull CB: **Recent trends in the study of specific phobias.** *Curr Opin Psychiatr* 2008, **21**:43-50.

27. Larson CL, Schaefer HS, Siegle GJ, Jackson CA, Anderle MJ, Davidson RJ: **Fear is fast in phobic individuals: amygdala activation in response to fear-relevant stimuli.** *Biol Psychiatry* 2006, **60**:410-417.

28. Wendt J, Lotze M, Weike AI, Hosten N, Hamm AO: **Brain activation and defensive response mobilization during sustained exposure to phobia-related and other affective pictures in spider phobia.** *Psychophysiology* 2008, **45**:205-215.

29. LeDoux JE: **Emotion circuits in the brain.** *Annu Rev Neurosci* 2000, **23**:155-184.

30. Sabatinelli D, Bradley MM, Fitzsimmons JR, Lang PJ: **Parallel amygdala and inferotemporal activation reflect emotional intensity and fear relevance.** *Neuroimage* 2005, **24**:1265-1270.

31. Schienle A, Schäfer A, Walter B, Stark R, Vaitl D: **Brain activation of spider phobics towards disorder-relevant, generally disgust- and fear-inducing pictures.** *Neurosci Lett* 2005, **388**:1-6.

32. Straube T, Glauer M, Dilger S, Mentzel HJ, Miltner WH: **Effects of cognitive-behavioral therapy on brain activation in specific phobia.** *Neuroimage* 2006, **29**:125-135.

33. Alpers GW, Gerdes AB, Lagarie B, Tabbert K, Vaitl D, Stark R: **Attention and amygdala activity: an fMRI study with spider pictures in spider phobia.** *J Neural Transm* 2009, **116**:747-757.

34. American Psychiatric Association: *Diagnostic and Statistical Manual of Mental Disorders.* 4 edition. Washington, DC, USA: American Psychiatric Association; 1995.

35. Wittchen HU, Zaudig M, Fydrich T, SKID: *Strukturiertes Klinisches Interview für DSM-IV* Göttingen, Germany: Hogrefe; 1997.

36. Klorman R, Weerts TC, Hastings JE, Melamed BG, Lang PJ: **Psychometric description of some specific-fear questionnaires.** *Behav Ther* 1974, **5**:401-409.

37. Laux L, Glanzmann P, Schaffner P, Spielberger CD: *State-Trait-Angstinventar (STAI)* Weinheim, Germany: Beltz; 1981.

38. Öhman A, Soares JJ: **On the automatic nature of phobic fear: conditioned electrodermal responses to masked fear-relevant stimuli.** *J Abnorm Psychol* 1993, **102**:121-132.

39. Soares JJ, Öhman A: **Preattentive processing, preparedness and phobias: effects of instruction on conditioned electrodermal responses to masked and non-masked fear-relevant stimuli.** *Behav Res Ther* 1993, **31**:87-95.

40. Lancaster JL, Rainey LH, Summerlin JL, Freitas CS, Fox PT, Evans AC, Toga AW, Mazziotta JC: **Automated labeling of the human brain: a preliminary report on the development and evaluation of a forward-transform method.** *Hum Brain Mapp* 1997, **5**:238-242.

41. Lancaster JL, Woldorff MG, Parsons LM, Liotti M, Freitas CS, Rainey L, Kochunov PV, Nickerson D, Mikiten SA, Fox PT: **Automated Talairach atlas labels for functional brain mapping.** *Hum Brain Mapp* 2000, **10**:120-131.

42. Straube T, Mentzel HJ, Miltner WH: **Common and distinct brain activation to threat and safety signals in social phobia.** *Neuropsychobiology* 2005, **52**:163-168.

43. Adolphs R, Gosselin F, Buchanan TW, Tranel D, Schyns P, Damasio AR: **A mechanism for impaired fear recognition after amygdala damage.** *Nature* 2005, **433**:68-72.

44. Straube T, Dietrich C, Mothes-Lasch M, Mentzel HJ, Miltner WH: **The volatility of the amygdala response to masked fearful eyes.** *Hum Brain Mapp* 2010, **31**:1601-1608.

45. Davis M, Whalen PJ: **The amygdala: vigilance and emotion.** *Mol Psychiatry* 2001, **6**:13-34.

46. Amaral DG, Insausti R: **Retrograde transport of D-[H-3]-aspartate injected into the monkey amygdaloid complex.** *Exp Brain Res* 1992, **88**:375-388.

47. Anderson AK, Phelps EA: **Lesions of the human amygdala impair enhanced perception of emotionally salient events.** *Nature* 2001, **411**:305-309.

48. Lipka J, Miltner WH, Straube T: **Vigilance for threat interacts with amygdala responses to subliminal threat cues in specific phobia.** *Biological Psychiatry* 2011 **70**:472-478.

49. Vuilleumier P, Armony JL, Driver J, Dolan RJ: **Effects of attention and emotion on face processing in the human brain: an event-related fMRI study.** *Neuron* 2001, **30**:829-841, 200.

50. Gamer M, Bartosz Z, Büchel C: **Different amygdala subregions mediate valence-related and attentional effects of oxytocin in humans.** *Proc Natl Acad Sci USA* 2010, **107**:9400-9405.

51. Holland PC, Gallagher M: **Amygdala circuitry in attentional and representational processes.** *Trends Cog Sci* 1999, **3**:65-73.

52. Kapp BS, Whalen PJ, Supple WF, Pascoe JP: **Amygdaloid contributions to conditioned arousal and sensory information processing.** In *The Amygdala: Neurobiological Aspects of Emotion, Memory, and Mental Dysfunction.* Edited by: Aggleton JP. New York, USA: Wiley-Liss; 1992:229-254.
53. Watts FN, Sharrock R: **Questionnaire dimensions of spider phobia.** *Behav Res Ther* 1984, **22**:575-580.
54. Quadflieg S, Mohr A, Mentzel HJ, Miltner WH, Straube T: **Modulation of the neural network involved in the processing of anger prosody: the role of task-relevance and social phobia.** *Biol Psychol* 2008, **78**:129-137.
55. Schmidt S, Mohr A, Miltner WH, Straube T: **Task-dependent neural correlates of the processing of verbal threat-related stimuli in social phobia.** *Biol Psychol* 2010, **84**:304-312.

Brain white matter microstructure alterations in adolescent rhesus monkeys exposed to early life stress: associations with high cortisol during infancy

Brittany R Howell[1,2*], Kai M McCormack[2,3], Alison P Grand[2], Nikki T Sawyer[4], Xiaodong Zhang[2], Dario Maestripieri[5], Xiaoping Hu[6] and Mar M Sanchez[1,2]

Abstract

Background: Early adverse experiences, especially those involving disruption of the mother-infant relationship, are detrimental for proper socioemotional development in primates. Humans with histories of childhood maltreatment are at high risk for developing psychopathologies including depression, anxiety, substance abuse, and behavioral disorders. However, the underlying neurodevelopmental alterations are not well understood. Here we used a nonhuman primate animal model of infant maltreatment to study the long-term effects of this early life stress on brain white matter integrity during adolescence, its behavioral correlates, and the relationship with early levels of stress hormones.

Methods: Diffusion tensor imaging and tract based spatial statistics were used to investigate white matter integrity in 9 maltreated and 10 control animals during adolescence. Basal plasma cortisol levels collected at one month of age (when abuse rates were highest) were correlated with white matter integrity in regions with group differences. Total aggression was also measured and correlated with white matter integrity.

Results: We found significant reductions in white matter structural integrity (measured as fractional anisotropy) in the corpus callosum, occipital white matter, external medullary lamina, as well as in the brainstem of adolescent rhesus monkeys that experienced maternal infant maltreatment. In most regions showing fractional anisotropy reductions, opposite effects were detected in radial diffusivity, without changes in axial diffusivity, suggesting that the alterations in tract integrity likely involve reduced myelin. Moreover, in most regions showing reduced white matter integrity, this was associated with elevated plasma cortisol levels early in life, which was significantly higher in maltreated than in control infants. Reduced fractional anisotropy in occipital white matter was also associated with increased social aggression.

Conclusions: These findings highlight the long-term impact of infant maltreatment on brain white matter structural integrity, particularly in tracts involved in visual processing, emotional regulation, and somatosensory and motor integration. They also suggest a relationship between elevations in stress hormones detected in maltreated animals during infancy and long-term brain white matter structural effects.

Keywords: Early life stress, Adolescence, Rhesus monkeys, Diffusion tensor imaging

* Correspondence: bcopp@emory.edu
[1]Department of Psychiatry & Behavioral Sciences, Emory University, 101 Woodruff Circle, WMB Suite 4000, Atlanta, GA 30322, USA
[2]Yerkes National Primate Research Center, Emory University, 954 Gatewood Road NE, Atlanta, GA 30329, USA
Full list of author information is available at the end of the article

Background

Childhood maltreatment is a serious health problem due to both adverse physical and psychopathological outcomes. Adverse outcomes associated with maltreatment include anxiety and mood disorders, substance abuse, conduct disorder, poor impulse control, increased aggression, and other social deficits [1-5]. Infant abuse is not exclusive to humans, but also occurs in wild and captive populations of nonhuman primates, including macaques, chimpanzees, baboons and marmosets [6]. Studies in rhesus monkeys have shown that infant maltreatment also results in socioemotional and stress physiology deficits [7-12] that resemble those seen in maltreated children.

The alterations in behavior and stress physiology exhibited by victims of maltreatment (both human and nonhuman) are hypothesized to be caused by stress-induced differences in brain development, particularly of neural circuits regulating those functions. Studies in humans utilizing MRI have shown alterations in the volumes of specific brain regions including the hippocampus, amygdala, and prefrontal cortex (PFC) in adults with histories of maltreatment [13-18]. Studies investigating alterations in children and adolescents are more inconsistent, and have found more diffuse neural alterations including reductions in temporal, frontal, and parietal cortical volumes as well as decreased corpus callosum (CC) and general cortical white matter (WM) volumes [3,19-22]. This, and additional evidence, supports the view that maturation of brain WM is particularly sensitive to early life stress/adversity [23-27], possibly due to the dramatic developmental changes in myelinated WM, and fiber tracts in general, that occur from childhood through adulthood in both humans [28-35] and nonhuman primates [36-38].

Diffusion tensor imaging (DTI) is a noninvasive, quantitative variation of structural magnetic resonance imaging (MRI) used to measure diffusion of water in the brain. When diffusion is unrestricted, the motion of the water molecules is isotropic, or equal in all directions. However, diffusion is restricted along the axons of myelinated WM tracts, resulting in anisotropic (preferential in one direction) diffusion. The strength of this directional diffusion can be quantified using measures such as fractional anisotropy (FA). Higher FA indicates an increase in the microstructural integrity of the tract, which can be due to several factors, such as increases in myelin thickness, axonal density/diameter, axon neurofilaments/microtubule density, and spread or coherence of fiber orientation in a given voxel [39-42]. Other diffusion properties can be examined to complement investigations of FA because as they provide additional information regarding the mechanisms underlying microstructural differences [43-45]. In particular, radial diffusivity (RD), which

quantifies water diffusion perpendicular to the axon and decreases with increased myelination [45-48], and axial diffusivity (AD), which measures diffusivity parallel to the fibers and increases with axonal microorganization, density and caliber, but is not affected by myelin thickness [49,50], can provide valuable information when measured in parallel to FA.

Although the neurobiological mechanisms underlying differences in FA and its functional effects on axonal tract efficiency are not completely understood, there is strong evidence of overall increases in FA (that is tract integrity) in major brain fiber tracts during primate development, although the maturational rates are tract-specific [28,29,33-36]. The role of brain WM tract integrity in behavioral control, particularly during development, is being recognized as an important mechanism underlying behavioral alterations [51] due to its effects on timing and speed of intercellular communication; for example increased tract integrity via increased myelin can increase information transfer via faster conduction speed along the axon [52,53]. Thus, increases in regional FA have been associated with behavioral training and learning [47,48,54-58] and cognitive skills in typically developing children, so that, in general, increased FA has been related to improved behavioral performance [53]. Decreases in FA thought to underlie the poor outcomes related to early stress/adversity have been reported [23,24,26,27,59]. Decreases in FA have also been observed in several psychopathologies including anxiety disorders [60], major depression [61,62], and bipolar disorder [63]. However, increases in FA have also been associated with psychopathology [64-66] and region-specific increases in FA have also been reported in some models of early stress [67,68], suggesting that adverse early experiences affect WM integrity in complex ways, which may depend on factors such as age of exposure, severity of experience/symptoms, and so on.

Prospective studies assessing the impact of childhood maltreatment on brain WM development and the potential mechanisms involved are difficult to perform in children. The goal of the present study was to use DTI to address these questions using a well-established rhesus monkey model of infant maltreatment. In particular we investigated the long-term effects of this adverse early experience on brain WM and behavior during adolescence, and its potential association with stress-induced elevations in cortisol during infancy. Infant maltreatment in this model is comprised of (1) physical abuse, operationalized as violent behaviors exhibited by the mother towards the infant, which reacts with overt signs of distress, and (2) high rates of infant rejection, which is a physically undamaging behavior consisting of pushing the infant away when it solicits contact from the mother, but that also causes infant distress [7,69].

Using this model we have previously reported increased emotional reactivity in maltreated infants and juveniles [7,9,70] and social alterations including delayed independence from the mother and less play during infancy [6,71], as well as increased social aggression during adolescence [72]. Alterations in the hypothalamic-pituitary-adrenal (HPA) stress neuroaxis have also been reported in this maltreatment model, including elevated basal plasma cortisol levels at one month of age, when abuse rates were highest [8,9], which in some cases remain elevated for the first year of life, in parallel with increased stress reactivity [11], and pituitary changes (that is blunted adrenocorticotropic hormone (ACTH) responses to corticotropin-releasing hormone (CRH) administration) that confirmed HPA axis overactivity during infancy [12].

Given all this evidence, in this study we used DTI and tract-based spatial statistics (TBSS) to investigate the long-term effects of infant maltreatment on brain WM tract integrity during adolescence and whether they were related to the increased cortisol levels detected in maltreated animals during their first month of life. WM tract integrity was measured by FA, in parallel with RD and AD measures to aid with the interpretation of the local microstructural mechanisms involved [36,43,45,47,48,54,55,73-75]. In order to assess potential functional correlates of maltreatment-related brain differences, we also examined the associations between brain WM tract integrity and measures of social behavior, in particular aggression, based on reports that it is increased in adolescent maltreated animals as compared to controls [72]. Given the associations reported between early adverse experiences and reduced brain WM tract integrity in children and adolescents, particularly in cortico-limbic tracts and association cortices, including prefrontal-temporal connections [23-25,68,76], we hypothesized that maltreated monkeys would have lower FA in these tracts than control animals. Based on the role of these cortico-limbic tracts in social and emotional regulation, we also hypothesized that lower WM tract integrity would be associated with increased aggression.

Methods

Subjects and housing

Nineteen adolescent rhesus monkeys (*Macaca mulatta*) living in four large social groups were used in these studies. Each group consisted of 2 to 3 adult males and 18 to 49 adult females with their sub-adult and juvenile offspring. The groups were housed in outdoor enclosures with access to climate-controlled indoor housing areas located at the Yerkes National Primate Research Center (YNPRC) Field Station, in Lawrenceville, GA, USA. Subjects were given commercially available primate chow

(Purina Mills Int., Lab Diets, St. Louis, MO, USA) supplemented with fresh fruit twice daily, and water was available *ad libitum*. All procedures were approved by the Emory University Institutional Animal Care and Use Committee in accordance with the Animal Welfare Act and the US Department of Health and Human Services 'Guide for Care and Use of Laboratory Animals'.

Of the nineteen subjects in this study, nine experienced maternal maltreatment in the form of physical abuse early in infancy (five females and four males; see operational definition below and in previous publications) [7,12] and the other ten subjects were non-maltreated controls (six females and four males). Following behavioral definitions, observation protocols, and inclusion/exclusion criteria described in detail in previous publications using this same group of nineteen animals [7,9], infant abuse was operationalized as at least three occurrences of the following violent behaviors by the mother towards the infant during the first three months of life: dragging the infant by the tail or leg while running or walking, crushing the infant against the ground with both hands, throwing the infant with one hand while standing or walking, stepping on the infant with one or both feet, sitting on the infant, roughly grooming by forcing the infant to the ground and pulling out the infant's hair causing distress calls, or carrying the infant with one arm away from the mother's body thus not allowing the infant to cling [7,12,69]. As mentioned in the Introduction section, all of these abusive behaviors caused distress in the infants, who experienced an average of one and a half events of abuse per hour during their first month of life [7]. Maltreated infants also experienced intense maternal rejection, which involved pushing away the infant when it solicited contact from its mother [7], hence the use of the term maltreatment rather than simply abuse. Subjects in the control and maltreated groups were matched for age, sex, and maternal dominance rank whenever possible so that the two groups did not significantly differ in any of these variables.

HPA axis basal activity: cortisol in infancy

Basal blood samples were collected at sunrise from all subjects when they were one month old, coincident with the highest rates of abuse [7], following published protocols [9,12,77]. Plasma concentrations of cortisol were measured in duplicate 10 μL aliquots by radio-immunoassay using commercially available kits (Diagnostic Systems Laboratories, DSL, Webster, TX, USA). Although we have already reported elsewhere that maltreated animals have greater plasma cortisol levels at one month of age than controls [8,9], these cortisol concentrations were used in the current study to examine their correlations with brain structural measures during adolescence (see details below).

Behavioral data collection during adolescence

Social behavior was collected around four years of age (close to 48 months) from observation towers located in the corners above each subjects' social home compound. Data was collected between 7 and 11 am, when animals are most active, using an established rhesus ethogram [78] with modifications [70]. This behavioral data was collected by three trained observers using binoculars and handheld computers (Palm IIIxe, Palm Inc., Sunnyvale, CA, USA) programmed to collect durations, frequencies, and sequences of behavior [79]. Inter-observer reliability was calculated prior to real time collection of behavior, by having each observer watch and record behavior from videos until percent agreement reached at least 90% and Cohen's Kappa was greater than 0.8.

Frequency of aggressive behaviors was measured using five hours of focal observations in each animal (five separate sessions, one hour each). Behaviors categorized as aggression included biting, grabbing, pinning, threatening and chasing of others in the group. A composite score of the frequencies of all of these behaviors was used to calculate the frequency of total aggression used in the analysis as rates per hour. Although increased social aggression has been reported in these maltreated animals as a separate and more extensive study of affiliative and agonistic behavior in these animals [72], total aggression rates per hour (average of contact and non-contact aggression) data were used in the current study to examine its associations with brain structural measures collected at similar ages (see details below).

In vivo neuroimaging

T1-Weighted MRI acquisition and template construction Imaging data was acquired during adolescence, beginning at four years of age (range: 48 to 55 months; mean ± SEM scan ages were: maltreated animals = 51.99 ± 0.6 months, controls = 51.98 ± 0.57 months). The scanning age was not different between control and maltreated animals, as described in the Results section. Structural (T1-weighted MRI) images were acquired during the same scanning session as the DTI scans on a 3 T Siemens Trio scanner (Siemens Medical Solutions USA, Inc., Malvern, PA, USA) at the YNPRC Imaging Center using a transmit and receive volume coil (Siemens CP Extremity Coil, Siemens Medical Solutions USA, Inc., Malvern, PA, USA) and a magnetization prepared rapid gradient echo (MPRAGE) sequence with the following parameters: TI/TR/TE = 950/3000/3.3 ms; flip angle = 8 degree; total scan time = 38 min; FOV = 116 mm × 116 mm × 96 mm, with a 192 × 192 × 160 matrix and 4 averages; voxel size: 0.6 × 0.6 × 0.6 mm^3. A T1 template was constructed from these scans using the methods described for rhesus monkeys by McLaren and colleagues [80]. Briefly, first a single subject

was affinely registered to the rhesus monkey atlas developed at the University of Wisconsin [80] resulting in a single subject in Wisconsin 112RM-SL rhesus atlas space (the target image), which is in the brain coordinate space of the Saleem-Logothetis rhesus stereotaxic atlas [81]. Each of the other subjects was then affinely registered to the target image and all of these images (now in atlas space) were averaged. This first-run template was then used as the target for a second round of affine registrations and averages resulting in a 0.5 × 0.5 × 0.5 mm^3, study-specific average T1 image that was used as a template for the analyses described below (Figure 1).

DTI data acquisition, preprocessing, and analysis

Whole brain DTI data was acquired using a dual spin-echo, segmented (multi-shot) diffusion-weighted echo-planar imaging (EPI) sequence with the acquisition parameters: TR/TE = 6,000/90 ms, 4 shots, b: 0, 1,000 s/mm^2, FOV = 96 mm × 96 mm, slice thickness = 1.5 mm with zero gap, voxel size = 1.5 × 1.5 × 1.5 mm^3, 30 slices, 64 × 64 matrix, 30 directions, and 4 averages.

The DTI data was corrected for B0 inhomogeneity-induced distortion [82] and eddy current effects [83] using the FSL software (FMRIB Center, University of Oxford, Oxford, UK) [84]. FA, RD, and AD were calculated using the diffusion analysis tools in FSL [84] (Figure 2). The TBSS tool in FSL [85] was used as a voxel-wise approach to identify the centers of all major WM tracts present in all subjects, therefore reducing the number of multiple comparisons. TBSS first nonlinearly registers each subject's FA image to the template image (the study specific T1 template produced as described above, resulting in a final image resolution of 0.5 × 0.5 × 0.5 mm^3). These images were then averaged to create a mean FA image from which a mean FA skeleton was created (see Figure 2B) using a user-defined FA threshold. The threshold applied in the current study was 0.2 to avoid inclusion of small peripheral white matter, and is a common threshold used for this type of analysis [85], and has been previously used by our group in studies in rhesus monkeys [68]. To reduce the effects of misregistration on the FA values contained within each subjects' skeletonized data, the TBSS software searches the voxels surrounding the mean FA skeleton in each subjects' registered FA image to assign the highest local FA value for each subject to the skeleton (for complete description see [85]). This ensures that despite the fact that the mean FA skeleton does not exactly cover the same anatomical regions in all subjects, the FA values contained in each subject's skeletonized data do represent the centers of the major WM tracts of each individual subject. These FSL diffusion analysis tools have been previously applied with success to rhesus brain DTI data by our group [68,86] and others [87-90].

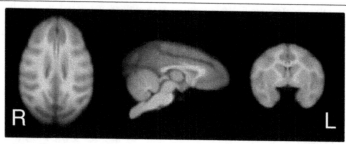

Figure 1 Study specific template of four and a half-year-old rhesus monkeys produced using iterative affine registrations and averaging as previously described [78].

Statistical analyses

Statistical analysis of FA, RD, and AD data

A voxel-wise two-group t-test was performed on the skeletonized FA data using the Randomise tool in FSL [84] to determine regions with significant differences between the maltreated and control groups. Results were considered significant at P-value less than 0.005 (uncorrected, but using a minimum cluster volume of 10 μL, approximately 4.5 significant contiguous voxels in native diffusion space) due to the relatively low spatial resolution. Results (significant clusters of > 4.5 contiguous significant voxels in native diffusion space) were displayed in the T1 study-specific template described above, registered to the Wisconsin 112RM-SL rhesus atlas [80,91], which is in the coordinate space of the Saleem-Logothetis rhesus brain stereotaxic atlas [81].

Binary masks were created for the clusters showing group FA differences. The mean RD and AD values were calculated within these regions, following previously published approaches [54,68,84]. A two-group t-test was performed on these values to determine the effects of infant maltreatment on RD and AD in those clusters with significant FA differences to aid in identifying the underlying microstructural mechanisms of the differences in tract integrity (significance level was set at $P < 0.05$). The mean FA calculated for each cluster was also used to examine its correlations with infant cortisol and adolescence aggression data using Pearson correlation (see details below).

Correlations between FA and biobehavioral measures (cortisol and aggression)

Because we were interested in examining the associations between infant cortisol levels and long-term alterations in tract integrity (that is, FA) detected as a consequence of this early adverse experience, as well as functional correlates of FA group differences during adolescence, we performed Pearson product moment correlation analyses restricted to those regions (clusters) where group differences in FA were detected above. Control and maltreated groups were included together in the correlation analyses between FA and basal plasma cortisol levels at one month of age and aggression during adolescence. Statistical significance level was set at $P < 0.05$.

Results

Group differences in FA

No differences in scanning age were detected between maltreated and control animals ($P = 0.99$; Student t-test). Significantly lower FA ($P < 0.005$, uncorrected, cluster volume ≥10 μL) was observed in maltreated animals, in comparison to controls, in six clusters: (1) one in WM located in the lateral portion of the medial midbody of the CC [92] (Figure 3A); (2) one in right occipital WM (Figure 4A); (3) two clusters in left occipital WM (Figures 5A and 6A), which, along with the cluster located in right occipital WM could include the inferior longitudinal fasciculus (ILF) or possibly short intra-

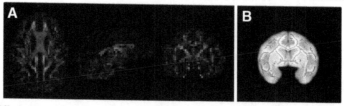

Figure 2 Representative diffusion tensor imaging (DTI) in four and a half-year-old rhesus monkeys. (A) Fractional anisotropy (FA) color map. Red represents left-right oriented fibers, blue represents dorsal-ventral oriented fibers, and green represents anterior-posterior oriented fibers. (B) Mean FA skeleton displayed on study specific template.

occipital fiber systems; (4) one in the WM dorsal to the left hippocampus and lateral to the pulvinar nucleus, which could correspond to the external medullary lamina (EML) (Figure 7A); and (5) one in the brainstem, in a location that matches the position of central tegmental tract (CTT) (Figure 8). No regions were found in which the maltreated animals had significantly higher FA than controls.

Group differences in RD and AD in regions with significant FA effects

The mean RD and AD values were calculated for each of the clusters with significant group differences in FA. In all clusters, except for the brainstem cluster, decreased FA was accompanied by an increase in RD, suggesting that the difference in FA was due to decreased myelin [42,45-48,93,94]. No differences in AD were observed in any of the clusters with FA effects.

Correlations of biobehavioral measures with FA

As mentioned above, our group has previously reported elevated plasma cortisol levels during infancy (at one month of age) [9], as well as increased aggression towards group mates during adolescence (at approximately four years of age) in the maltreated animals, which are the focus of this study, in comparison to controls [8,9,72]. Therefore, only results of the correlations between FA and these biobehavioral measures are presented here. The mean FA value of each cluster in which significant group differences in this measure were found was correlated with infant basal cortisol and frequency of aggressive behaviors during adolescence. Neither RD nor AD values were included in the correlation analyses because they are components of, and thus correlated with, FA.

Negative correlations between FA and infant cortisol were found in all clusters except for the one in the brainstem (see Table 1) (Figures 3B, 4B, 5B, 6B, and 7B). A negative correlation (Table 1) between aggression and FA was also found in one of the clusters in left occipital WM (Figure 6C), but in none of the other clusters examined.

Discussion

The main goal of this study was to examine the long-term consequences of infant maltreatment on brain WM tracts of adolescent rhesus monkeys and to determine whether they were related to the elevated cortisol levels reported in these maltreated animals during infancy [8,9]. We also examined whether alterations in brain WM microstructure were related to the increased aggressive behavior previously reported in the maltreated animals during adolescence [72]. To do this we used measures of microstructural integrity, specifically FA, RD, and AD, calculated from DTI scans. We chose this technique because of its sensitivity to changes in WM microstructure, such as myelin thickness and axon/microtubule density [39-41]. These are neuronal characteristics that can affect the timing and speed of intercellular communication [52,53], and can therefore affect behavior [51]. FA increases significantly in brain WM tracts throughout primate development, and is accompanied by decreases in RD and few changes in AD [28,29,34-36]. These developmental changes in measures of axon microstructure suggest a global increase in tract integrity mainly due to increases in myelin from childhood to adulthood. Brain region-specific increases in FA are also observed after training on visuo-motor tasks [58] and with acquirement of new cognitive skills, such as reading and math, in parallel to decreases in RD, but

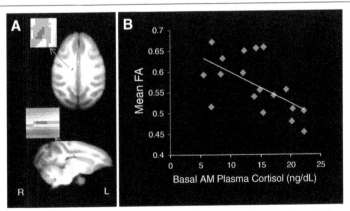

Figure 3 Maltreated animals have reduced fractional anisotropy (FA) in the corpus callosum. (A) Cluster of voxels (red) in right corpus callosum represents the region where maltreated animals had significantly lower FA than controls ($p < 0.005$, uncorrected, $\geq 10 \mu L$ volume). In insets, green represents the mean FA skeleton. **(B)** FA in the corpus callosum is negatively correlated with basal cortisol at one month of age ($r = -0.512$, $P = 0.025$).

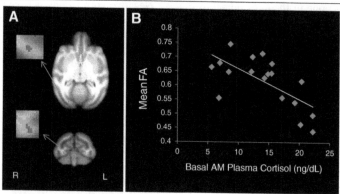

Figure 4 Maltreated animals have reduced fractional anisotropy (FA) in right occipital white matter (WM). **(A)** Cluster of voxels (red) in right occipital WM where maltreated animals had significantly lower FA than controls ($P < 0.005$, uncorrected, $\geq 10 \,\mu$L volume). In insets, green represents the mean FA skeleton. **(B)** FA in right occipital WM is negatively correlated with basal cortisol at one month of age ($r = -0.561$, $P = 0.012$).

no changes in AD [47,48,53,56]. This suggests that these experience-related and region-specific increases in FA are due to increases in myelin and underlie behavioral and cognitive improvements. In contrast, reduced FA, associated in most regions with elevated cortisol during infancy and with increased concurrent aggression in one of the clusters, was detected here in adolescent rhesus monkeys that experienced infant maltreatment. Our findings are consistent with previous reports in human individuals that experienced childhood maltreatment [25,27] or other forms of early life stress [23,24] and in other nonhuman primate models of adversity [26], as well as in several mood and anxiety disorders [66,95], with significant overlap with the regions affected in the current study.

To our knowledge, this is the first DTI study to examine the long-term effects of infant maltreatment on brain WM tract integrity in a nonhuman primate model. It is also the first to examine the associations of brain structural alterations with infant cortisol elevations and concurrent social behavior. Our findings show alterations in brain WM tract integrity measured using DTI in adolescent rhesus monkeys with histories of infant maltreatment. Decreased WM integrity (that is, FA) was found in maltreated subjects in the CC, occipital WM, EML, and brainstem, in comparison to controls. These regional FA decreases were paralleled by increases in RD, but no changes in AD, suggesting that the alterations in tract microstructural integrity in these brain regions were likely due to reduced myelin [42,45-48,93,94]. An

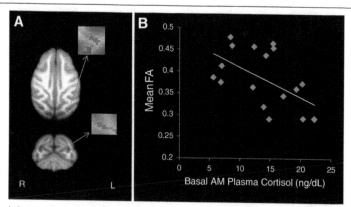

Figure 5 Maltreated animals have reduced fractional anisotropy (FA) in left occipital white matter (WM) (left occipital cluster 1). **(A)** Cluster of voxels (red) in left occipital WM where maltreated animals had significantly lower FA than controls ($P < 0.005$, uncorrected, $\geq 10 \,\mu$L volume). In insets, green represents the mean FA skeleton. **(B)** FA in left occipital WM is negatively correlated with basal cortisol at one month of age ($r = -0.483$, $P = 0.036$).

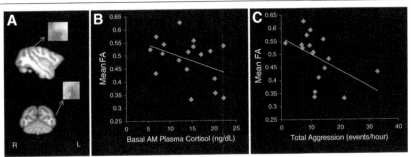

Figure 6 Maltreated animals have reduced fractional anisotropy (FA) in **left occipital white matter (WM) (left occipital cluster 2). (A)** Cluster of voxels (red) in left occipital WM where maltreated animals had significantly lower FA than controls (*P* < 0.005, uncorrected, ≥ 10 μL volume). In insets, green represents the mean FA skeleton. **(B)** FA in left occipital WM is negatively correlated with basal cortisol at one month of age (r = −0.479, *P* = 0.038). **(C)** FA in left occipital WM is negatively correlated with total aggression in adolescence (r = −0.465, *P* = 0.045).

exception was the brainstem cluster, where no RD differences were found between groups. Basal plasma cortisol levels measured when the individuals were one month old, when abuse rates were highest [7], were negatively correlated with FA in all regions except for the brainstem cluster. This suggests that maltreatment at that early age caused stress-induced elevations in cortisol that could have potentially contributed to the long-term brain WM alterations reported. However, future studies are needed to examine causality in this relationship.

One of the clusters with lower FA in maltreated animals than controls was located in the lateral aspect of the medial midbody of the CC [92]. The CC is the largest WM tract in the brain conveying interhemispheric fibers important for integration of information between cortical regions in both hemispheres [96]. Because these fibers are some of the last to myelinate [31,32,36,37], finding alterations in the CC is consistent with the view that areas undergoing active myelination or other

protracted developmental processes are especially vulnerable to environmental experience [97,98]. Alterations in the CC have also been reported in several studies of maltreated children, with reduced CC volume reported in maltreated children [99,100], a difference that appears to be related to a failure to show the typical age-related increase in volume [101]. Reduced CC size has also been reported in adults with histories of childhood maltreatment [102], suggesting that these CC alterations are persistent. Decreased FA in the CC of maltreated children [103] and adults who have experienced various forms of early life stress [104] has also been reported. The findings of the current study are also consistent with findings of reduced CC size in other nonhuman primate models of adverse early experience [92]. Our findings of reduced WM integrity in the CC medial midbody region, which carries some prefrontal but mostly frontal motor and somatosensory fibers [105], could result in group differences in integration of motor and somatosensory

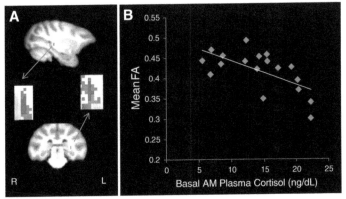

Figure 7 Maltreated animals have reduced fractional anisotropy (FA) in **white matter (WM) dorsal to the hippocampus and lateral to the pulvinar nucleus. (A)** Cluster of voxels (red) where maltreated subjects had significantly lower FA than controls (*P* < 0.005, uncorrected, ≥ 10 μL) seems to correspond to the external medullary lamina (EML). In insets, green represents the mean FA skeleton. **(B)** FA in the EML is negatively correlated with basal cortisol at one month of age (r = −0.637, *P* = 0.003).

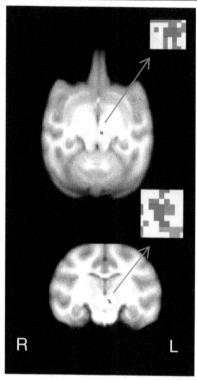

Figure 8 Maltreated animals have reduced fractional anisotropy (FA) in brainstem white matter (WM). The cluster of voxels (red) in left brainstem WM where maltreated animals had significantly lower FA than controls (P < 0.005, uncorrected, ≥ 10 μL) could correspond to the central tegmental tract (CTT). In insets, green represents the mean FA skeleton.

information. The reduced interhemispheric integration reported here and in human studies of childhood maltreatment could contribute to behavioral alterations and psychopathology, an idea supported by similar CC alterations reported in anxiety and mood disorders [106].

The location of the three clusters identified in occipital WM suggest that the tracts affected could include short intra-occipital fiber systems (possibly part of the forceps

Table 1 Correlations of fractional anisotropy (FA), one month cortisol, and total aggression in adolescence

Cluster location	Month 1 cortisol		Total aggression	
	r	P	r	P
Corpus callosum	−0.512	0.025[a]	−0.31	0.181
Right occipital	−0.561	0.012[a]	−0.113	0.645
Left occipital 1	−0.483	0.036[a]	−0.281	0.244
Left occipital 2	−0.479	0.038[a]	−0.465	0.045[a]
EML	−0.637	0.003[a]	−0.254	0.293
Brainstem	−0.315	0.189	−0.317	0.118

Pearson correlation analysis was used. [a]P < 0.05 was considered significant.

major, an interhemispheric tract that connects occipital cortices in both hemispheres), and/or the caudal portion of the ILF, a long cortico-cortical association tract that courses through occipital, parietal, and temporal cortices [96]. However, this can't be corroborated without running additional tractography analyses. Interestingly, reduced FA has been reported in the forceps major of adolescents with histories of child maltreatment [27] and in the caudal portion of the ILF in adolescents that witnessed domestic violence as children [107]. The ILF is part of the ventral visual pathway which is important for object identification [108], face processing [109], and emotional memory [110,111]. Along these lines, alterations in WM microstructure of the ILF have been observed in several mood and anxiety disorders. For example, decreased FA in the ILF at the level of the occipital lobe has also been found in patients with depression [112,113] and bipolar disorder [114,115]. Thus, it is possible that decreases in microstructural integrity of occipital WM, likely involving the ILF, could affect visual and face processing, as well as emotion/mood processes.

The negative correlation of FA with aggressive behavior detected in occipital WM is difficult to explain. Most neuroimaging studies involving neural substrates of aggression implicate structural and/or functional abnormalities in frontal brain circuits [116,117],although many of these studies have been done in patients with schizophrenia. Decreased FA in the anterior commissure (AC) has also been reported in violent youth with bipolar disorder, and FA in the AC was negatively correlated with aggression [118]. However, this study was done in a clinical population making it difficult to integrate with the findings reported here. Increased occipital WM volume has been reported in adult violent offenders [119], but to our knowledge no other occipital alterations have been associated with aggression. Interestingly, a recent study comparing neural systems supporting social cognition in chimpanzees and bonobos reported that chimpanzees (known to be more aggressive than bonobos) had higher FA in occipital WM and bigger occipital GM volumes than bonobos [120], suggesting a potential association between aggression and FA in occipital WM in these species. The discrepancy of the directionality of the correlation with our findings could be explained by factors such as species-specific differences in neural substrates of aggression, or age at measurement. Given the paucity of research on the neural substrates of aggression, particularly in children, the interpretation of our findings is difficult. The visual cortices located near the cluster in which FA and aggression were correlated are part of attentional networks [121], and thus alterations in these circuits could reflect more general alterations in attention that might be better reflected by other behaviors not measured in the current study. It also has to be noted that our small sample size is a limitation for these studies, which might have been underpowered to detect other significant associations.

The WM cluster located lateral to the pulvinar thalamic nucleus and dorsal to the hippocampus seems to be the EML based on rhesus brain atlases [81]. The EML contains both thalamo-cortical and cortico-thalamic fibers connecting the thalamus with parietal, temporal, occipital, cingulate, motor and PFC [96]. Although without performing tractography it is difficult to precisely identify the specific thalamic nuclei and cortical regions connected by the affected tracts, based on the rostro-caudal location of this cluster the fibers affected likely connect the thalamus with occipital or temporal cortices [96]. Interestingly, thalamo-cortical systems modulate amygdala activity, and are involved in the perception of fear [122]. Cortico-thalamic circuits are implicated in the pathogenesis of mood disorders [123]. Thus, our findings of reduced structural integrity in EML suggest potential alterations in cortico-thalamic and thalamo-cortical circuits that could contribute to deficits in emotional regulation reported above in maltreated animals.

The brainstem cluster where FA was lower in maltreated animals than controls was difficult to identify anatomically due to the low MRI contrast in this region. However, as described above, its location matches the position of the CTT [124]. The CTT is a pathway containing descending fibers from midbrain nuclei that project to the olivary complex, as well as ascending fibers originating in the pontine and medullary reticular formation that project to the thalamus [125]. These are brainstem pathways that carry and coordinate somatosensory and somatomotor information. MRI studies report lesions in the CTT in neurodegenerative and neurodevelopmental disorders, linked with motor and cognitive deficits [126]. This was the only region where group differences in FA (lower in maltreated subjects than in controls) were not related to the increased levels of cortisol during infancy in the maltreated animals, suggesting that the effects of maltreatment on this WM could be associated with other aspects of the early experience.

There are limitations to the DTI method as applied here. Most are due to the low spatial resolution of the diffusion data acquired in the relatively small rhesus brain. At this resolution partial voluming effects can make interpreting or finding results difficult. The TBSS analysis applied here addresses this limitation by using only voxels from the centers of large WM tracts in individual subjects. Partial voluming can also make registration difficult, which is another reason why we used the nonlinear registration built into the TBSS processing pipeline to perform our voxelwise analyses. The low angular resolution (that is, the small number of directions acquired for the DTI data), especially when combined with the low spatial resolution of our data, also makes accurate probabilistic tractography difficult, which is why it was not performed in these studies. Tractography would be helpful in future studies to determine the exact tracts affected in the clusters with group differences, although it would not help in determining the directionality of the affected fibers.

The correlations between infant cortisol and WM integrity found in the current study suggest that early life stress has long-term effects on brain WM in regions previously reported as vulnerable to childhood maltreatment in humans, and that are also altered in anxiety and mood disorders. One possible mechanism could be through the effects of elevated levels of glucocorticoids (GCs), in this case cortisol, on the development of WM [127]. Oligodendrocytes that form the myelin sheath express both intracellular glucocorticoid and mineralocorticoid receptors [128], and recent evidence suggests that GCs suppress proliferation of oligodendrocyte precursor cells in GM and WM [129]. Developmental studies also provide evidence that GCs modulate oligodendrocyte differentiation and myelogenesis via regulation of key oligodendroglial proteins such as myelin basic protein (MBP) [130], and that the effects of synthetic GCs differ as function of gestational age, with decreases in MBP immunoreactivity and numbers of oligodendrocytes associated with younger ages of GC exposure [131]. Taken together, these studies suggest that myelination is sensitive to GCs during development, making it possible for early life stress, via elevated cortisol levels, to affect brain WM development. The associations detected in our studies between decreased FA and basal cortisol levels at one month are consistent with this possibility, although the causality of this relationship needs to be tested in future studies. Due to the strong role of brain WM in behavioral control, for example, [132], GC-induced alterations in brain WM development could potentially lead to the alterations reported in maltreated monkeys, including increased aggression. Our findings also open new questions and hypotheses that need to be empirically tested. Does maltreatment lead to altered function of the affected circuits? When do these differences emerge and how they unfold? Prospective, longitudinal studies beginning at birth are necessary to address these important developmental questions in the context of maltreatment to determine the most beneficial timing and type of potential treatments, as well as intervention and prevention strategies.

Conclusions

The results of the current study suggest that early life stress in the form of infant maltreatment has long-term effects on brain WM in regions that are vulnerable to childhood maltreatment in humans, and that are also altered in anxiety and mood disorders. These findings highlight the long-term impact of infant maltreatment on brain white matter structural integrity, particularly in tracts involved in visual processing, emotional regulation, and somatosensory and motor integration. They also suggest a relationship between long-term brain white matter structural effects and elevations in stress hormones detected in maltreated animals during infancy, as well as aggression during adolescence.

Abbreviations
AC: Anterior commissure; ACTH: Adrenocorticotropic hormone; AD: Axial diffusivity; CC: Corpus callosum; CCT: Entral tegmental tract; CRH: Corticotropin releasing hormone; DTI: Diffusion tensor imaging; EML: External medullary lamina; EPI: Echo planar imaging; FA: Fractional anisotropy; FMRIB: Oxford Centre for Functional MRI of the Brain; FSL: FMRIB Software Library; GC: Glucocorticoid; GM: Gray matter; HPA: Hypothalamic-pituitary-adrenal axis; ILF: Inferior longitudinal fasciculus; MPRAGE: Magnetization prepared rapid gradient echo; MRI: Magnetic resonance imaging; PFC: Prefrontal cortex; RD: Radial diffusivity; TBSS: Tract based spatial statistics; WM: White matter; YNPRC: Yerkes National Primate Research Center.

Competing interests
The authors declare that they have no competing interests.

Authors' contributions
BRH carried out the processing and analyses of the DTI data, and drafted the manuscript. KM, APG, and NTS developed the experimental design of the aggression studies and collected and analyzed the data. MMS developed the experimental design of the overall studies, and some of the grant proposals that funded them. She also participated in the collection and analysis of the cortisol and DTI data and in the writing of the manuscript. DM participated in the experimental design of some of the studies and developed one of the grant proposals that funded them. XH and XZ developed the DTI scanning sequences used here for the rhesus monkey brain. All authors read and approved the final manuscript.

Acknowledgements
We would like to thank Anne Glenn, Richelle Scales, and the Animal/Veterinary Care staff at the Yerkes National Primate Research Center Field Station for their invaluable help in collecting the data presented. We would also like to thank Dr. Gwenaëlle Douaud (FMRIB) and Matt Glasser for their help in applying the TBSS methodology to monkeys. The project described was supported by Grant Numbers MH65046 (MMS), MH62577 (DM), P50 MH078105, MH091645, and F31 MH086203 (BRH) from the National Institute of Mental Health (NIMH) and NICHD055255 from the National Institute of Child Health and Human Development. The content is solely the responsibility of the authors and does not necessarily represent the official views of the NIMH, NICHD or the National Institutes of Health. The project was also funded by the National Center for Research Resources P51RR165 (YNPRC Base grant) and is currently supported by the Office of Research Infrastructure Programs/OD P51OD11132. The YNPRC is fully accredited by the American for the Assessment and Accreditation of Laboratory Care, International.

Author details
[1]Department of Psychiatry & Behavioral Sciences, Emory University, 101 Woodruff Circle, WMB Suite 4000, Atlanta, GA 30322, USA. [2]Yerkes National Primate Research Center, Emory University, 954 Gatewood Road NE, Atlanta, GA 30329, USA. [3]Department of Psychology, Spelman College, 350 Spelman Lane, Box 209, Atlanta, GA 30314, USA. [4]Department of Natural Sciences, Clayton State University, 2000 Clayton State Boulevard, Morrow, GA 30260, USA. [5]Department of Comparative Human Development, University of Chicago, 5730 South Woodlawn Avenue, Chicago, IL 60637, USA. [6]Biomedical Imaging Technology Center, Emory University, 1760 Haygood Drive, Room W232, Atlanta, GA 30322, USA.

References
1. Glaser D: Child abuse and neglect and the brain - a review. J Child Psychol Psychiatry 2000, 41:97–116.
2. Teicher MH, Andersen SL, Polcari A, Anderson CM, Navalta CP: Developmental neurobiology of childhood stress and trauma. Psychiatr Clin North Am 2002, 25:397–426. vii-viii.
3. Teicher MH, Andersen SL, Polcari A, Anderson CM, Navalta CP, Kim DM: The neurobiological consequences of early stress and childhood maltreatment. Neurosci Biobehav Rev 2003, 27:33–44.
4. Gunnar M, Quevedo K: The neurobiology of stress and development. Annu Rev Psychol 2007, 58:145–173.
5. Weber K, Rockstroh B, Borgelt J, Awiszus B, Popov T, Hoffmann K, Schonauer K, Watzl H, Propster K: Stress load during childhood affects psychopathology in psychiatric patients. BMC Psychiatry 2008, 8:63.
6. Maestripieri D, Carroll KA: Risk factors for infant abuse and neglect in group-living rhesus monkeys. Psychol Sci 1998, 9:143–145.
7. McCormack K, Sanchez MM, Bardi M, Maestripieri D: Maternal care patterns and behavioral development of rhesus macaque abused infants in the first six months of life. Dev Psychobiol 2006, 48:537–550.
8. Sanchez MM: The impact of early adverse care on HPA axis development: nonhuman primate models. Horm Behav 2006, 50:623–631.
9. McCormack K, Newman T, Higley J, Maestripieri D, Sanchez M: Serotonin transporter gene variation, infant abuse, and responsiveness to stress in rhesus macaque mothers and infants. Horm Behav 2009, 55:538–547.
10. Sanchez M, Pollak S: Socio-emotional development following early abuse and neglect: challenges and insights from translational research. In Handbook of Developmental Social Neuroscience. Edited by de Haan M, Gunnar MR. New York, NY: Guilford Press; 2009:497–520.
11. Koch H, McCormack K, Sanchez MM, Maestripieri D: The development of the hypothalamic-pituitary-adrenal axis in rhesus monkeys: effects of age, sex, and early experience. Dev Psychobiol 2013: in press.
12. Sanchez MM, McCormack K, Grand AP, Fulks R, Graff A, Maestripieri D: Effects of sex and early maternal abuse on adrenocorticotropin hormone and cortisol responses to the corticotropin-releasing hormone challenge during the first three years of life in group-living rhesus monkeys. Dev Psychopathol 2010, 22:45–53.
13. Bremner JD: Long-term effects of childhood abuse on brain and neurobiology. Child Adolesc Psychiatr Clin N Am 2003, 12:271–292.
14. Bremner JD: Neuroimaging of childhood trauma. Semin Clin Neuropsychiatry 2002, 7:104–112.
15. Bremner JD: Traumatic stress: effects on the brain. Dialogues Clin Neurosci 2006, 8:445–461.
16. van Harmelen A-L, van Tol M-J, van der Wee NJ, Veltman DJ, Aleman A, Spinhoven P, van Buchem MA, Zitman FG, Penninx BW, Elzinga BM: Reduced medial prefrontal cortex volume in adults reporting childhood emotional maltreatment. Biol Psychiatry 2010, 68:832–838.
17. Dannlowski U, Stuhrmann A, Beutelmann V, Zwanzger P, Lenzen T, Grotegerd D, Domschke K, Hohoff C, Ohrmann P, Bauer J: Limbic scars: long-term consequences of childhood maltreatment revealed by functional and structural magnetic resonance imaging. Biol Psychiatry 2012, 71:286–293.
18. Teicher MH, Anderson CM, Polcari A: Childhood maltreatment is associated with reduced volume in the hippocampal subfields CA3, dentate gyrus, and subiculum. Proc Natl Acad Sci U S A 2012, 109:E563–E572.
19. Hanson JL, Chung MK, Avants BB, Shirtcliff EA, Gee JC, Davidson RJ, Pollak SD: Early stress is associated with alterations in the orbitofrontal cortex: a tensor-based morphometry investigation of brain structure and behavioral risk. J Neurosci 2010, 30:7466–7472.
20. Hanson JL, Chung MK, Avants BB, Rudolph KD, Shirtcliff EA, Gee JC, Davidson RJ, Pollak SD: Structural variations in prefrontal cortex mediate the relationship between early childhood stress and spatial working memory. J Neurosci 2012, 32:7917–7925.
21. De Brito SA, Viding E, Sebastian CL, Kelly PA, Mechelli A, Maris H, McCrory EJ: Reduced orbitofrontal and temporal grey matter in a community sample of maltreated children. J Child Psychol Psychiatry 2013, 54:105–112.

22. Edmiston EE, Wang F, Mazure CM, Guiney J, Sinha R, Mayes LC, Blumberg HP: Corticostriatal-limbic gray matter morphology in adolescents with self-reported exposure to childhood maltreatment. Arch Pediatr Adolesc Med 2011, 165:1069–1077.

23. Govindan RM, Behen ME, Helder E, Makki MI, Chugani HT: Altered water diffusivity in cortical association tracts in children with early deprivation identified with tract-based spatial statistics (TBSS). Cereb Cortex 2010, 20:561–569.

24. Eluvathingal TJ, Chugani HT, Behen ME, Juhasz C, Muzik O, Maqbool M, Chugani DC, Makki M: Abnormal brain connectivity in children after early severe socioemotional deprivation: a diffusion tensor imaging study. Pediatrics 2006, 117:2093–2100.

25. Choi J, Jeong B, Rohan ML, Polcari AM, Teicher MH: Preliminary evidence for white matter tract abnormalities in young adults exposed to parental verbal abuse. Biol Psychiatry 2009, 65:227–234.

26. Coplan JD, Abdallah CG, Tang CY, Mathew SJ, Martinez J, Hof PR, Smith EL, Dwork AJ, Perera TD, Pantol G, et al: The role of early life stress in development of the anterior limb of the internal capsule in nonhuman primates. Neurosci Lett 2010, 480:93–96.

27. Huang H, Gundapuneedi T, Rao U: White matter disruptions in adolescents exposed to childhood maltreatment and vulnerability to psychopathology. Neuropsychopharmacology 2012, 37:2693–2701.

28. Asato MR, Terwilliger R, Woo J, Luna B: White matter development in adolescence: a DTI study. Cereb Cortex 2010, 20:2122–2131.

29. Lebel C, Walker L, Leemans A, Phillips L, Beaulieu C: Microstructural maturation of the human brain from childhood to adulthood. Neuroimage 2008, 40:1044–1055.

30. Giedd JN, Stockman M, Weddle C, Liverpool M, Alexander-Bloch A, Wallace GL, Lee NR, Lalonde F, Lenroot RK: Anatomic magnetic resonance imaging of the developing child and adolescent brain and effects of genetic variation. Neuropsychol Rev 2010, 20:349–361.

31. Deoni SC, Mercure E, Blasi A, Gasston D, Thomson A, Johnson M, Williams SC, Murphy DG: Mapping infant brain myelination with magnetic resonance imaging. J Neurosci 2011, 31:784–791.

32. Gao W, Lin W, Chen Y, Gerig G, Smith J, Jewells V, Gilmore J: Temporal and spatial development of axonal maturation and myelination of white matter in the developing brain. AJNR Am J Neuroradiol 2009, 30:290–296.

33. Westlye LT, Walhovd KB, Dale AM, Bjørnerud A, Due-Tønnessen P, Engvig A, Grydeland H, Tamnes CK, Østby Y, Fjell AM: Life-span changes of the human brain white matter: diffusion tensor imaging (DTI) and volumetry. Cereb Cortex 2010, 20:2055–2068.

34. Barnea-Goraly N, Menon V, Eckert M, Tamm L, Bammer R, Karchemskiy A, Dant CC, Reiss AL: White matter development during childhood and adolescence: a cross-sectional diffusion tensor imaging study. Cereb Cortex 2005, 15:1848–1854.

35. Schneider JF, Il'yasov KA, Hennig J, Martin E: Fast quantitative diffusion-tensor imaging of cerebral white matter from the neonatal period to adolescence. Neuroradiology 2004, 46:258–266.

36. Shi Y, Short SJ, Knickmeyer RC, Wang J, Coe CL, Niethammer M, Gilmore JH, Zhu H, Styner MA: Diffusion tensor imaging-based characterization of brain neurodevelopment in primates. Cereb Cortex 2012, 23:36–48.

37. Malkova L, Heuer E, Saunders RC: Longitudinal magnetic resonance imaging study of rhesus monkey brain development. Eur J Neurosci 2006, 24:3204–3212.

38. Gibson KR: Myelination and behavioral development: a comparative perspective on questions of neotony, altriciality, and intelligence. In Brain Maturation And Cognitive Development: Comparative And Cross-Cultural Perspectives. Edited by Gibson KR, Petersen AC. Hawthorne, NY: Aldine de Gruyter; 1991:29–63.

39. Beaulieu C: The basis of anisotropic water diffusion in the nervous system - a technical review. NMR Biomed 2002, 15:435–455.

40. Mamata H, Jolesz FA, Maier SE: Characterization of central nervous system structures by magnetic resonance diffusion anisotropy. Neurochem Int 2004, 45:553–560.

41. Concha L, Livy DJ, Beaulieu C, Wheatley BM, Gross DW: In vivo diffusion tensor imaging and histopathology of the fimbria-fornix in temporal lobe epilepsy. J Neurosci 2010, 30:996–1002.

42. Choe AS, Stepniewska I, Colvin DC, Ding Z, Anderson AW: Validation of diffusion tensor MRI in the central nervous system using light

microscopy: quantitative comparison of fiber properties. NMR Biomed 2012, 25:900–908.

43. Burzynska AZ, Preuschhof C, Backman L, Nyberg L, Li SC, Lindenberger U, Heekeren HR: Age-related differences in white matter microstructure: region-specific patterns of diffusivity. Neuroimage 2010, 49:2104–2112.

44. Bosch B, Arenaza-Urquijo EM, Rami L, Sala-Llonch R, Junque C, Sole-Padulles C, Pena-Gomez C, Bargallo N, Molinuevo JL, Bartres-Faz D: Multiple DTI index analysis in normal aging, amnestic MCI and AD. Relationship with neuropsychological performance. Neurobiol Aging 2012, 33:61–74.

45. Bennett IJ, Madden DJ, Vaidya CJ, Howard DV, Howard JH Jr: Age-related differences in multiple measures of white matter integrity: a diffusion tensor imaging study of healthy aging. Hum Brain Mapp 2010, 31:378–390.

46. Zhang J, Jones M, DeBoy CA, Reich DS, Farrell JA, Hoffman PN, Griffin JW, Sheikh KA, Miller MI, Mori S, Calabresi PA: Diffusion tensor magnetic resonance imaging of Wallerian degeneration in rat spinal cord after dorsal root axotomy. J Neurosci 2009, 29:3160–3171.

47. Hu Y, Geng F, Tao L, Hu N, Du F, Fu K, Chen F: Enhanced white matter tracts integrity in children with abacus training. Hum Brain Mapp 2011, 32:10–21.

48. Keller TA, Just MA: Altering cortical connectivity: remediation-induced changes in the white matter of poor readers. Neuron 2009, 64:624–631.

49. Kumar R, Nguyen HD, Macey PM, Woo MA, Harper RM: Regional brain axial and radial diffusivity changes during development. J Neurosci Res 2012, 90:346–355.

50. Kumar R, Macey PM, Woo MA, Harper RM: Rostral brain axonal injury in congenital central hypoventilation syndrome. J Neurosci Res 2010, 88:2146–2154.

51. Fields RD: White matter in learning, cognition and psychiatric disorders. Trends Neurosci 2008, 31:361–370.

52. Lang EJ, Rosenbluth J: Role of myelination in the development of a uniform olivocerebellar conduction time. J Neurophysiol 2003, 89:2259–2270.

53. Paus T: Growth of white matter in the adolescent brain: myelin or axon? Brain Cogn 2010, 72:26–35.

54. Tang YY, Lu Q, Fan M, Yang Y, Posner MI: Mechanisms of white matter changes induced by meditation. Proc Natl Acad Sci U S A 2012, 109:10570–10574.

55. Taubert M, Villringer A, Ragert P: Learning-related gray and white matter changes in humans: an update. Neuroscientist 2012, 18:320–325.

56. Engvig A, Fjell AM, Westlye LT, Moberget T, Sundseth O, Larsen VA, Walhovd KB: Memory training impacts short-term changes in aging white matter: a longitudinal diffusion tensor imaging study. Hum Brain Mapp 2011, 33:2390–2406.

57. Tang YY, Lu Q, Geng X, Stein EA, Yang Y, Posner MI: Short-term meditation induces white matter changes in the anterior cingulate. Proc Natl Acad Sci U S A 2010, 107:15649–15652.

58. Scholz J, Klein MC, Behrens TE, Johansen-Berg H: Training induces changes in white-matter architecture. Nat Neurosci 2009, 12:1370–1371.

59. Frodl T, Carballedo A, Fagan AJ, Lisiecka D, Ferguson Y, Meaney JF: Effects of early-life adversity on white matter diffusivity changes in patients at risk for major depression. J Psychiatry Neurosci 2012, 37:37–45.

60. Phan KL, Orlichenko A, Boyd E, Angstadt M, Coccaro EF, Liberzon I, Arfanakis K: Preliminary evidence of white matter abnormality in the uncinate fasciculus in generalized social anxiety disorder. Biol Psychiatry 2009, 66:691–694.

61. Cullen KR, Klimes-Dougan B, Muetzel R, Mueller BA, Camchong J, Houri A, Kurma S, Lim KO: Altered white matter microstructure in adolescents with major depression: a preliminary study. J Am Acad Child Adolesc Psychiatry 2010, 49:173–183.

62. Kieseppä T, Eerola M, Mäntylä R, Neuvonen T, Poutanen V-P, Luoma K, Tuulio-Henriksson A, Jylhä P, Mantere O, Melartin T: Major depressive disorder and white matter abnormalities: a diffusion tensor imaging study with tract-based spatial statistics. J Affect Disord 2010, 120:240–244.

63. Kafantaris V, Kingsley P, Ardekani B, Saito E, Lencz T, Lim K, Szeszko P: Lower orbital frontal white matter integrity in adolescents with bipolar I disorder. J Am Acad Child Adolesc Psychiatry 2009, 48:79–86.

64. Taylor WD, Hsu E, Krishnan K, MacFall JR: Diffusion tensor imaging: background, potential, and utility in psychiatric research. Biol Psychiatry 2004, 55:201–207.

65. Thomason ME, Thompson PM: Diffusion imaging, white matter, and psychopathology. Annu Rev Clin Psychol 2011, 7:63–85.

66. Ayling E, Aghajani M, Fouche JP, van der Wee N: Diffusion tensor imaging in anxiety disorders. Curr Psychiatry Rep 2012, 14:197–202.

67. Katz M, Liu C, Schaer M, Parker KJ, Ottet MC, Epps A, Buckmaster CL, Bammer R, Moseley ME, Schatzberg AF, et al: **Prefrontal plasticity and stress inoculation-induced resilience.** Dev Neurosci 2009, **31**:293–299.

68. Howell BR, Godfrey J, Gutman DA, Michopoulos V, Zhang X, Nair G, Hu X, Wilson ME, Sanchez MM: **Social subordination stress and serotonin transporter polymorphisms affect the development of brain white matter tracts and behavior in juvenile female macaques.** Cereb Cortex 2013: in press.

69. Maestripieri D: **Parenting styles of abusive mothers in group-living rhesus macaques.** Anim Behav 1998, **55**:1–11.

70. Maestripieri D, Higley JD, Lindell SG, Newman TK, McCormack KM, Sanchez MM: **Early maternal rejection affects the development of monoaminergic systems and adult abusive parenting in rhesus macaques (Macaca mulatta).** Behav Neurosci 2006, **120**:1017–1024.

71. Maestripieri D, Jovanovic T, Gouzoules H: **Crying and infant abuse in rhesus monkeys.** Child Dev 2000, **71**:301–309.

72. Grand AP, Sawyer NT, Maestripieri D, Sanchez MM, McCormack KM: *The long-term impact of maternal maltreatment on affiliative, aggressive, and defensive behavior in rhesus macaques [abstract].* West Palm Beach, FL: 31th Meeting of the American Society of Primatologists; 2008.

73. Metwalli NS, Benatar M, Nair G, Usher S, Hu X, Carew JD: **Utility of axial and radial diffusivity from diffusion tensor MRI as markers of neurodegeneration in amyotrophic lateral sclerosis.** Brain Res 2010, **1348**:156–164.

74. Shamy JL, Carpenter DM, Fong SG, Murray EA, Tang CY, Hof PR, Rapp PR: **Alterations of white matter tracts following neurotoxic hippocampal lesions in macaque monkeys: a diffusion tensor imaging study.** Hippocampus 2010, **20**:906–910.

75. Wheeler-Kingshott CA, Cercignani M: **About "axial" and "radial" diffusivities.** Magn Reson Med 2009, **61**:1255–1260.

76. Hanson JL, Adluru N, Chung MK, Alexander AL, Davidson RJ, Pollak SD: **Early neglect is associated with alterations in white matter integrity and cognitive functioning.** Child Dev 2013:. in press.

77. Sanchez MM, Noble PM, Lyon CK, Plotsky PM, Davis M, Nemeroff CB, Winslow JT: **Alterations in diurnal cortisol rhythm and acoustic startle response in nonhuman primates with adverse rearing.** Biol Psychiatry 2005, **57**:373–381.

78. Altmann SA: **A field study of the sociobiology of rhesus monkeys.** Ann N Y Acad Sci 1962, **102**:338–435.

79. Graves FC, Wallen K: **Androgen-induced yawning in rhesus monkey females is reversed with a nonsteroidal anti-androgen.** Horm Behav 2006, **49**:233–236.

80. McLaren DG, Kosmatka KJ, Oakes TR, Kroenke CD, Kohama SG, Matochik JA, Ingram DK, Johnson SC: **A population-average MRI-based atlas collection of the rhesus macaque.** Neuroimage 2009, **45**:52–59.

81. Saleem KS, Logothetis NK: *A combined MRI and Histology Atlas of the Rhesus Monkey Brain in Stereotaxic Coordinates.* London, UK: Elsevier Science; 2012.

82. Jezzard P, Balaban RS: **Correction for geometric distortion in echo planar images from B0 field variations.** Magn Reson Med 1995, **34**:65–73.

83. Mangin JF, Poupon C, Clark C, Le Bihan D, Bloch I: **Distortion correction and robust tensor estimation for MR diffusion imaging.** Med Image Anal 2002, **6**:191–198.

84. Smith SM, Jenkinson M, Woolrich MW, Beckmann CF, Behrens TE, Johansen-Berg H, Bannister PR, De Luca M, Drobnjak I, Flitney DE, et al: **Advances in functional and structural MR image analysis and implementation as FSL.** Neuroimage 2004, **23**(Suppl 1):S208–S219.

85. Smith SM, Jenkinson M, Johansen-Berg H, Rueckert D, Nichols TE, Mackay CE, Watkins KE, Ciccarelli O, Cader MZ, Matthews PM, Behrens TE: **Tract-based spatial statistics: voxelwise analysis of multi-subject diffusion data.** Neuroimage 2006, **31**:1487–1505.

86. Hecht EE, Gutman DA, Preuss TM, Sanchez MM, Parr LA: **Rilling JK: process versus product in social learning: comparative diffusion tensor imaging of neural systems for action execution-observation matching in macaques, chimpanzees, and humans.** Cereb Cortex 2012, **23**:1014–1024.

87. Bendlin BB, Canu E, Willette A, Kastman EK, McLaren DG, Kosmatka KJ, Xu G, Field AS, Colman RJ, Coe CL, et al: **Effects of aging and calorie restriction on white matter in rhesus macaques.** Neurobiol Aging 2011, **2319**:e2311–2311.

88. Makris N, Papadimitriou GM, van der Kouwe A, Kennedy DN, Hodge SM, Dale AM, Benner T, Wald LL, Wu O, Tuch DS, et al: **Frontal connections and**

89. Willette AA, Bendlin BB, McLaren DG, Canu E, Kastman EK, Kosmatka KJ, Xu G, Field AS, Alexander AL, Colman RJ, et al: **Age-related changes in neural volume and microstructure associated with interleukin-6 are ameliorated by a calorie-restricted diet in old rhesus monkeys.** Neuroimage 2010, **51**:987–994.

90. Willette AA, Coe CL, Colman RJ, Bendlin BB, Kastman EK, Field AS, Alexander AL, Allison DB, Weindruch RH, Johnson SC: **Calorie restriction reduces psychological stress reactivity and its association with brain volume and microstructure in aged rhesus monkeys.** Psychoneuroendocrinology 2011, **37**:903–916.

91. McLaren DG, Kosmatka KJ, Kastman EK, Bendlin BB, Johnson SC: **Rhesus macaque brain morphometry: a methodological comparison of voxel-wise approaches.** Methods 2010, **50**:157–165.

92. Sanchez MM, Hearn EF, Do D, Rilling JK, Herndon JG: **Differential rearing affects corpus callosum size and cognitive function of rhesus monkeys.** Brain Res 1998, **812**:38–49.

93. Song SK, Sun SW, Ramsbottom MJ, Chang C, Russell J, Cross AH: **Dysmyelination revealed through MRI as increased radial (but unchanged axial) diffusion of water.** Neuroimage 2002, **17**:1429–1436.

94. Song SK, Sun SW, Ju WK, Lin SJ, Cross AH, Neufeld AH: **Diffusion tensor imaging detects and differentiates axon and myelin degeneration in mouse optic nerve after retinal ischemia.** Neuroimage 2003, **20**:1714–1722.

95. Drevets WC: **Neuroimaging studies of mood disorders.** Biol Psychiatry 2000, **48**:813–829.

96. Schmahmann JD, Pandya DN: *Fiber Pathways of the Brain.* Oxford New York: Oxford University Press; 2006.

97. Davison AN, Dobbing J: **Myelination as a vulnerable period in brain development.** Br Med Bull 1966, **22**:40–44.

98. Rice D, Barone S Jr: **Critical periods of vulnerability for the developing nervous system: evidence from humans and animal models.** Environ Health Perspec 2000, **108**:511.

99. De Bellis MD, Keshavan MS, Shifflett H, Iyengar S, Beers SR, Hall J, Moritz G: **Brain structures in pediatric maltreatment-related posttraumatic stress disorder: a sociodemographically matched study.** Biol Psychiatry 2002, **52**:1066–1078.

100. Teicher MH, Dumont NL, Ito Y, Vaituzis C, Giedd JN, Andersen SL: **Childhood neglect is associated with reduced corpus callosum area.** Biol Psychiatry 2004, **56**:80–85.

101. De Bellis MD, Keshavan MS: **Sex differences in brain maturation in maltreatment-related pediatric posttraumatic stress disorder.** Neurosci Biobehav Rev 2003, **27**:103–117.

102. Kitayama N, Brummer M, Hertz L, Quinn S, Kim Y, Bremner JD: **Morphologic alterations in the corpus callosum in abuse-related posttraumatic stress disorder: a preliminary study.** J Nerv Ment Dis 2007, **195**:1027–1029.

103. Jackowski AP, Douglas-Palumberi H, Jackowski M, Win L, Schultz RT, Staib LW, Krystal JH, Kaufman J: **Corpus callosum in maltreated children with posttraumatic stress disorder: a diffusion tensor imaging study.** Psychiatry Res 2008, **162**:256–261.

104. Paul R, Henry L, Grieve SM, Guilmette TJ, Niaura R, Bryant R, Bruce S, Williams LM, Richard CC, Cohen RA, Gordon E: **The relationship between early life stress and microstructural integrity of the corpus callosum in a non-clinical population.** Neuropsychiatr Dis Treat 2008, **4**:193–201.

105. Lamantia AS, Rakic P: **Cytological and quantitative characteristics of four cerebral commissures in the rhesus monkey.** J Comp Neurol 1990, **291**:520–537.

106. Drevets WC, Price JL, Furey ML: **Brain structural and functional abnormalities in mood disorders: implications for neurocircuitry models of depression.** Brain Struct Funct 2008, **213**:93–118.

107. Choi J, Jeong B, Polcari A, Rohan ML, Teicher MH: **Reduced fractional anisotropy in the visual limbic pathway of young adults witnessing domestic violence in childhood.** Neuroimage 2012, **59**:1071–1079.

108. Mishkin M, Ungerleider LG, Macko KA: **Object vision and spatial vision: two cortical pathways.** Trends Neurosci 1983, **6**:414–417.

109. Fox CJ, Iaria G, Barton JJS: **Disconnection in prosopagnosia and face processing.** Cortex 2008, **44**:996–1009.

110. Habib M: **Visual hypoemotionality and prosopagnosia associated with right temporal lobe isolation.** Neuropsychologia 1986, **24**:577–582.

Brain white matter microstructure alterations in adolescent rhesus monkeys exposed to early...

169

111. Ross ED: **Sensory-specific amnesia and hypoemotionality in humans and monkeys: Gateway for developing a hodology of memory.** *Cortex* 2008, **44**:1010–1022.

112. Versace A, Almeida JRC, Quevedo K, Thompson WK, Terwilliger RA, Hassel S, Kupfer DJ, Phillips ML: **Right orbitofrontal corticolimbic and left corticocortical white matter connectivity differentiate bipolar and unipolar depression.** *Biol Psychiatry* 2010, **68**:560–567.

113. Liao Y, Huang X, Wu Q, Yang C, Kuang W, Du M, Lui S, Yue Q, Chan RCK, Kemp GJ: **Is depression a disconnection syndrome? Meta-analysis of diffusion tensor imaging studies in patients with MDD.** *J Psychiatry Neurosci* 2012, **37**:110180.

114. Bruno S, Cercignani M, Ron MA: **White matter abnormalities in bipolar disorder: a voxel-based diffusion tensor imaging study.** *Bipolar Disord* 2008, **10**:460–468.

115. Zanetti MV, Jackowski MP, Versace A, Almeida JRC, Hassel S, Duran FLS, Busatto GF, Kupfer DJ, Phillips ML: **State-dependent microstructural white matter changes in bipolar I depression.** *Eur Arch Psychiatry Clin Neurosci* 2009, **259**:316–328.

116. Dolan MC: **What imaging tells us about violence in anti-social men.** *Crim Behav Ment Health* 2010, **20**:199–214.

117. Hoptman MJ, Antonius D: **Neuroimaging correlates of aggression in schizophrenia: an update.** *Curr Opin Psychiatry* 2011, **24**:100–106.

118. Saxena K, Tamm L, Walley A, Simmons A, Rollins N, Chia J, Soares JC, Emslie GJ, Fan X, Huang H: **A preliminary investigation of corpus callosum and anterior commissure aberrations in aggressive youth with bipolar disorders.** *J Child Adolesc Psychopharmacol* 2012, **22**:112–119.

119. Tiihonen J, Rossi R, Laakso MP, Hodgins S, Testa C, Perez J, Repo-Tiihonen E, Vaurio O, Soininen H, Aronen HJ: **Brain anatomy of persistent violent offenders: more rather than less.** *Psychiatry Res* 2008, **163**:201–212.

120. Rilling JK, Scholz J, Preuss TM, Glasser MF, Errangi BK, Behrens TE: **Differences between chimpanzees and bonobos in neural systems supporting social cognition.** *Soc Cogn Affect Neurosci* 2012, **7**:369–379.

121. Bisley JW: **The neural basis of visual attention.** *J Physiol* 2011, **589**:49–57.

122. Das P, Kemp AH, Liddell BJ, Brown KJ, Olivieri G, Peduto A, Gordon E, Williams LM: **Pathways for fear perception: modulation of amygdala activity by thalamo-cortical systems.** *Neuroimage* 2005, **26**:141–148.

123. Price JL, Drevets WC: **Neural circuits underlying the pathophysiology of mood disorders.** *Trends Cogn Sci* 2012, **16**:61–71.

124. Snider RS, Lee JC: *A Stereotaxic Atlas of the Monkey Brain: (Macaca Mulatta).* Chicago: University of Chicago Press; 1961.

125. Carpenter WB, Sutin J: *Human Neuroanatomy.* 8th edition. Baltimore, MD: Williams and Wilkins; 1983.

126. Shioda M, Hayashi M, Takanashi J-i, Osawa M: **Lesions in the central tegmental tract in autopsy cases of developmental brain disorders.** *Brain Dev* 2011, **33**:541–547.

127. Jauregui-Huerta F, Ruvalcaba-Delgadillo Y, Gonzalez-Castaneda R, Garcia-Estrada J, Gonzalez-Perez O, Luquin S: **Responses of glial cells to stress and glucocorticoids.** *Curr Immunol Rev* 2010, **6**:195.

128. Bohn MC, Howard E, Vielkind U, Krozowski Z: **Glial cells express both mineralocorticoid and glucocorticoid receptors.** *J Steroid Biochem Mol Biol* 1991, **40**:105–111.

129. Alonso G: **Prolonged corticosterone treatment of adult rats inhibits the proliferation of oligodendrocyte progenitors present throughout white and gray matter regions of the brain.** *Glia* 2000, **31**:219–231.

130. Kumar S, Cole R, Chiappelli F, de Vellis J: **Differential regulation of oligodendrocyte markers by glucocorticoids: post-transcriptional regulation of both proteolipid protein and myelin basic protein and transcriptional regulation of glycerol phosphate dehydrogenase.** *Proc Natl Acad Sci U S A* 1989, **86**:6807–6811.

131. Antonow-Schlorke I, Helgert A, Gey C, Coksaygan T, Schubert H, Nathanielsz PW, Witte OW, Schwab M: **Adverse effects of antenatal glucocorticoids on cerebral myelination in sheep.** *Obstet Gynecol* 2009, **113**:142–151.

132. Nagy Z, Westerberg H, Klingberg T: **Maturation of white matter is associated with the development of cognitive functions during childhood.** *J Cogn Neurosci* 2004, **16**:1227–1233.

Functional anomalies in healthy individuals with a first degree family history of major depressive disorder

Francesco Amico[1,2*], Angela Carballedo[1,2,3], Danuta Lisiecka[1,2], Andrew J Fagan[4], Gerard Boyle[4] and Thomas Frodl[1,2,3,4]

Abstract

Background: Individuals with major depressive disorder (MDD) process information with a bias towards negative stimuli. However, little is known on the link between vulnerability to MDD and brain functional anomalies associated with stimulus bias.

Methods: A cohort of 38 subjects, of which 14 were patients with acute MDD and 24 were healthy controls (HC), were recruited and compared. The HC group included 10 healthy participants with a first degree family history of depression (FHP) and 14 volunteers with no family history of any psychiatric disease (FHN). Blood oxygen level dependence signals were acquired from functional magnetic resonance imaging (fMRI) during performance in a dot-probe task using fearful and neutral stimuli. Reaction times and the number of errors were also obtained.

Results: Although MDD patients and HC showed no behavioral difference, the MDD group exhibited smaller activation in the left middle cingulum. The MDD group also showed smaller activation in the left insula when compared to the HC group or the FHN group. Finally, FHP participants exhibited higher activation in the right Heschl's gyrus compared to FHN participants.

Conclusions: The present study shows that family risk for MDD is associated with increased activation in the Heschl's gyrus. Our results also suggest that acute MDD is linked to reduced activation in the insula and anterior cingulate cortex during processing of subliminal, not recognizable, masked fearful stimuli. Further research should confirm these results in a larger cohort of participants.

Introduction

Most conceptions of the relationship between mood and emotions suggest that moods may potentiate matching emotional reactions (for example, irritable mood facilitates angry reactions [1]). Depressed individuals show more attention towards negative, anxiogenic stimuli [2] which has also been found to be a risk factor for developing major depressive disorder (MDD) [3]. Importantly, functional magnetic resonance imaging (fMRI) studies have demonstrated activation anomalies in both MDD patients and in patients at risk for depression during presentation of fearful images [4,5].

Interestingly, similar results have been found in healthy individuals with family history of depression (FHP) when compared to healthy individuals without any family history of the disease (FHN). FHP subjects exhibit impairment in emotion recognition [6] and have been shown to have higher amygdala and nucleus accumbens activation in response to the presentation of fearful faces when compared to age-matched FHN controls, in line with previous findings showing that FHP subjects have significantly elevated waking salivary cortisol when compared to FHN subjects [7]. However, when face viewing is accompanied by a constrained attention task (that is, having to rate nose width on the face and subjective fear while viewing the face), the differences between FHP and FHN subjects disappear whilst prefrontal activity increases [8]. This suggests that FHP subjects may be

* Correspondence: famico@tcd.ie
[1]Department of Psychiatry, Trinity College Dublin, College Green, Dublin 2, Ireland
Full list of author information is available at the end of the article

Functional anomalies in healthy individuals with a first degree family history of major...

171

able to normalize emotion-related neural functions by focusing their attention and that face-viewing with unconstrained attention may leave room for aberrant psychological processes associated with the risk for developing MDD [8]. However, both behavioral and event related potential (ERP) studies have identified subtle deficits in selective attention among FHP individuals that may affect their ability to adequately regulate emotion under stressful circumstances [9].

In order to investigate the interplay between cognitive and emotion processing in both FHP and FHN participants, a masked emotion task combined with a cognitive task known to elicit cognitive processing bias in MDD might be useful to reveal performance differences between these two groups. In this context, neuropsychological studies in a task called 'dot-probe' suggest that depression is associated with an attentional bias towards negative information [10] and that effortful cognitive control of negative emotions can reduce the bias towards fearful stimuli [11]. Neuroimaging dot-probe studies suggest that unmasked fearful faces facilitate visual processing [12,13] and that the amygdala modulates fear responses in the occipital cortex [14]. Further, previous fMRI studies on participants performing in the dot-probe task (for example, [12]) have shown that the amygdala directs spatial attention to backward masked fearful faces through a network of brain structures that include the left anterior cingulate cortex (CC), right superior temporal sulcus and right lingual gyrus [15-17]. Other research in the dot-probe task has shown that individuals with MDD cannot avoid attending negative information in their environment [18] and FHP individuals attend selectively to sad faces [19]. Importantly, there is evidence that effortful control modulates the relationship between negative affectivity and attentional bias in the dot-probe task, with low levels of effortful control and high levels of negative affectivity predicting a preference for threat stimuli [11]. With respect to the fact that, when viewing subliminal masked stimuli, participants do not focus their attention on the masked stimuli, the dot-probe task is highly interesting because it might elicit activity associated with vulnerability to MDD [8]. However, to the best of our knowledge, little or no research has investigated putative functional anomalies in the brain showing during performance in this task in either MDD or FHP individuals.

In the present study, we hypothesized that patients with MDD compared to HC subjects, but also FHP subjects compared to FHN subjects, exhibit differences in emotional processing of fearful versus neutral stimuli when attention is biased during performance in a dot-probe task. Based on previous fMRI findings (for example, [17]) in a similar behavioral task [8,20-24], we selected the CC, amygdala, insula and prefrontal cortex as primary regions

where we expected significant differences between groups to appear.

Methods
Participant recruitment

A cohort of 38 subjects aged between 18 and 65 was recruited. The healthy family history positive subjects (FHP, n = 10) were unaffected first-degree relatives of patients formally diagnosed with MDD according to the fourth edition of the Diagnostic and Statistical Manual of Mental Disorders (DSM-IV) and treated at the South-West Mental Health Services in Dublin, Ireland. However, the FHP subjects recruited were not the relatives of the MDD patients that participated in the study. Family history of MDD was assessed by a psychiatrist through a structured interview. Participants were asked whether any of their first degree relatives had been diagnosed with a psychiatric disease or had ever displayed symptoms of psychosis. Healthy volunteers without a history of psychiatric illness (FHN, n = 14) were recruited from the local community via announcements. The MDD group consisted of 14 patients with acute MDD attending our clinical outpatient services (Table 1). Of these, 4 were currently drug-free and came as new patients to our service, three received escitalopram, one fluoxetine, two venlafaxine, one venlafaxine plus mirtazapine, one sertraline plus mirtazapine, one sertraline, and one duloxetine plus mirtazapine.

For all subjects, a structured written observer interview and a structured interview carried out by two psychiatrists were used to assess demographic variables and medical history. Exclusion criteria were previous head injury with loss of consciousness, cortisol medication in their medical history, previous alcohol or substance abuse, co-morbidity with other mental illnesses, personality disorders, neurological or psychiatric disorder (Axis I or Axis II) or age over 65 years. No subject had ever received electroconvulsive therapy before investigation or took any psychotropic medications.

All participants included in the study filled out the following self- and observer-rated scales: the 21-item version of the Hamilton Depression Rating Scale for Depression [25], the Montgomery-Åsberg Depression Rating Scale [26], Beck's Depression Inventory [27] and the Structured Clinical Interviews for DSM-IV (SCID)-I [28] for psychiatric diseases and SCID-II [29] for personality assessment.

Handedness was determined by the Edinburgh Handedness Inventory [30]. Written informed consent was obtained from all subjects subsequent to a detailed description of the study. The study design, approved by the ethics committee of the Adelaide and Meath Hospital incorporating the National Children's Hospital and St. James' Hospitals, was prepared in accordance with the

Table 1 Demographic and clinical data of participants

	FHN (n = 14)		FHP (n = 10)		MDD (n = 14)				
							X^2	df	P
Gender (female/male)	4/10		6/4		9/5		4.1	2/36	0.12
Handedness (right/left/ambidextrous)	14/0/0		8/2/0		12/1/1		5	4/34	0.3
	Mean	SD	Mean	SD	Mean	SD	F	df	P
Age (years)	35	9.4	33	10	41.2	10.3	2.2	2/36	ns
Weight (kg)	74	18	63.3	5	73.6	13	1.9	2/36	ns
Illness duration (years)	-	-	-	-	16	10	-	-	-
HDRS score	0.7	0.9	4.8	5.3	24.8	5	125	2/36	< 0.001[a]
Age of onset	-	-	-	-	25	11	-	-	-
	Median	MR	Median	MR	Median	MR	4.7	df	P
Alcohol intake per week (g)	16	16	60	26	28	18	4.6	2/36	ns
Cigarettes per day	0	15	1	23.5	0	21	5.7	2/36	ns

[a]There was a difference between the MDD patients and either the FHN (P < 0.001) or the FHP (P < 0.001) subjects in the HDRS; [b]F-score from analysis of variance. df: degrees of freedom; MDD: patients with major depressive disorder; FHN: healthy participants without family history of MDD; FHP: healthy participants with family history of MDD; HDRS: Hamilton Depression Rating Scale for Depression; ns: not significant; SD: standard deviation, X^2: Chi-squared score, MR: Mean Rank

Statistical analysis of clinical and demographic characteristics

Clinical and demographic data were analyzed using SPSS-16. Differences in gender and handedness were analyzed using Chi-square tests (see Table 1). Differences in age, weight and height were computed using a one-way analysis of variance (ANOVA). As alcohol intake (g/day) and the number of cigarettes smoked per day were found to be non-normally distributed, medians were calculated and a Kruskal-Wallis test was used to evaluate statistical differences between groups.

Behavioral data

Behavioral measures analyzed included mean reaction time (RT) and the number of errors (that is, an error being made when the dot was indicated in the wrong

side of the screen). Two conditions were compared: 'fear same' (dot and fearful face presented on the same side of the screen) and 'fear opposite' (dot and fearful face presented on opposite sides of the screen). There were a total of 19 'fear opposite' trials and 31 'fear same' trials for each participant. These trials were randomly selected by the presentation software. Unfortunately, due to a recording failure during the scanning sessions, some behavioral data were lost. Only the data that could be fully retrieved were included in the analysis (see Table 2). Both RTs and the number of errors for each condition were submitted to an ANOVA. A Bonferroni test was used for post hoc comparisons.

fMRI data acquisition

Functional images were acquired on a 3-Tesla MRI scanner (Philips Achieva, The Netherlands). The MRI protocol consisted of the acquisition of a high resolution three-dimensional T1-weighted structural dataset

Table 2 Mean reaction times and total number of errors for conditions 'neutral' and 'fear'

	FHN (n = 10)		FHP (n = 7)		MDD (n = 5)				
	Mean	SD	Mean	SD	Mean	SD	F^c	df	P
Neutral same[a]	4932	1076	4936	745	5342	606	0.402	2/20	0.67
Neutral opposite[b]	4903	1406	4818	697	5455	466	0.6	2/20	0.56
Fear same[a]	4589	721	4767	690	5582	684	4.4	2/20	0.05
Fear opposite[b]	5122	586	4734	710	5121	643.5	1.25	2/20	0.31
Fear (right+left)	4756	956	4728	700	5672	600	0.81	2/20	0.46
Neutral (right+left)	9835	2454	9754	1436	10797	1040	0.51	2/20	0.60
Number of errors	7	6.6	3.9	8	16.4	35	0.70	2/20	0.51

[a]Dot and fearful face presented on the same side of the screen; [b]dot and fearful face presented in opposite sides of the screen; [c] F-score from analysis of variance. df: degrees of freedom; MDD: patients with major depressive disorder; FHN: healthy participants without family history of MDD; FHP healthy participants with family history of MDD; SD: standard deviation.

[spoiled gradient recalled sequence with repetition time (TR)/echo time (TE) = 8.5/3.9 ms and 1 mm spatial resolution], followed by an fMRI experiment [spin-echo echo-planar imaging (SE-EPI) sequence with TR/TE = 2000/35 ms, in-plane resolution = 3 × 3 mm, 4.8 mm slice thickness, 304 dynamic scans each with 2 s duration].

Twenty five slices [dynamic scan time: 304, field of view: reference line: 230 mm, aperture: 230 mm, Fourier with a Hanning window (FH): 120 mm] covered the whole brain. Slices were positioned on the connecting line between the anterior and posterior commissure.

Dot-probe task

Color mixed-race facial identities including 12 (6 male and 6 female) fearful and 12 (6 male and 6 female) neutral expressions [31] were randomly presented on a screen. A 7th neutral female face from the same database was used as a mask. Each trial started with a fixation cross lasting between 1,000 and 2,500 ms. Next, a stimulus (randomly selected from neutral and fearful stimuli) was presented for 33 ms on the left or right visual field (LVF and RVF, respectively) and immediately masked by two neutral faces simultaneously presented (100 ms) on each visual field. Projections of masks were followed by a LVF or RVF target dot (750 ms) presentation with a jittered (500 ms to 2,000 ms) inter-trial interval. Subjects were required to respond as soon as possible by pressing a 'right' or 'left' button on a computer keyboard, according to the position of the target dot on the visual field. All participants were administered a practice trial. The total duration of the task was 10 minutes.

fMRI data analysis

Standard preprocessing procedures were performed in SPM8 (Wellcome Trust Centre for Neuroimaging). The first six scans were not used to allow for T1 equilibration. The EPI images were then realigned to the first volume in order to correct for head movements. Realignment parameters were inspected visually to identify any potential subjects with head movement > 4.8 mm (slice thickness). Each participant's structural image was co-registered to the mean of the motion-corrected functional images using a 12-parameter affine transformation. Image slice time was corrected to TR/2. The structural images were segmented according to the standard procedure in SPM8 [32]. Spatial normalization to standard 3 mm × 3 mm × 3 mm Montreal Neurological Institute (MNI) space was then applied to functional images in order to allow for inter-subject analysis. Finally, these images were smoothed using an 8 mm full width at half maximum Gaussian kernel. Statistical parametric maps were calculated using a general linear model based on a voxel-by-voxel method [33].

First level single subject statistical parameter maps were created for each condition using the general linear model in SPM8. After parameter estimation, the following two contrasts were created: 'fear' > 'neutral' (F > N) and 'fear' < 'neutral' (F < N). Subsequently, these were entered into a full factorial second level analysis model using three groups (MDD, FHP and FHN) as factors. Age and gender were entered as cofactors. The statistical threshold was set to $P < 0.05$, with whole brain family-wise error (FWE) correction for multiple comparisons. Moreover, we reported differences with $P < 0.001$ in predefined regions of interest.

Results
Demographic data
The MDD group scored higher in the Hamilton Depression scale than either the FHN ($P < 0.001$) or FHP group ($P < 0.001$). No age, gender or handedness difference was found between groups (Table 1).

Behavioral data
There was no significant difference between groups for either the RTs or the number of errors (Table 2).

fMRI data (Table 3)
Contrast F > N
MDD patients exhibited smaller activation than healthy controls (HC) in the left middle cingulum (T = 3.82, $P = 0.041$, FWE corrected for multiple comparisons) and left insula (T = 4.19, $P < 0.001$, uncorrected), which also showed a trend for significance after correction for multiple comparisons ($P = 0.072$) (Figure 1). Smaller activation in the left insula was also found in the MDD group when compared to the FHN group (T = 4.43, $P = 0.033$, FWE corrected for multiple comparisons). Further, MDD patients had smaller activation in the left post-central gyrus when compared to FHN participants (T = 3.59, $P < 0.001$, uncorrected), although this difference did not survive FWE correction. Finally, the FHP group had greater activation in the right Heschl's gyrus when compared to the FHN group (T = 4.60, $P = 0.018$, FWE corrected for multiple comparisons) (Figure 2).

Contrast F < N
The FHP group had smaller activation in the right Heschl's gyrus (T = 5.22, $P = 0.002$, FWE corrected for multiple comparisons) when compared to the FHN group.

Discussion
While being presented with masked fearful stimuli, our participants showed significant differences in areas that are thought to play a key role in emotion processing, namely the CC and insula. Further, our results suggest a link between family history of MDD and functional anomalies in the Heschl's gyrus.

Table 3 Paired comparisons between healthy controls (HC, n = 24), family history negative healthy participants (FHN, n = 14), family history positive healthy participants (FHP, n = 10) and patients with major depressive disorder (MDD, n = 14)

Contrast	Comparison	Region	Region of interest P (FWE correction)	Ke	T	Puncorrected	x	y	z
F > N	MDD < HC	Left middle cingulum	0.041 (cluster corr.)	71	3.82	< 0.001	-15	-28	37
		Left insula	0.072	8	4.19	< 0.001	-27	29	7
	MDD < FHN	Left insula	< 0.033	11	4.43	< 0.001	-27	29	7
		Left post-central gyrus	ns	29	3.59	< 0.001	-27	-28	37
	MDD > FHN	-	ns	-	-	ns	-	-	-
	MDD < FHP	-	ns	-	-	ns	-	-	-
	MDD > FHP	-	ns	-	-	ns	-	-	-
	FHP > FHN	Right Heschl's gyrus	0.018	17	4.60	< 0.001	51	-28	13
	FHP < FHN	-	ns	-	-	ns	-	-	-
F < N	FHP < FHN	Right Heschl's gyrus	0.002	26	5.22	< 0.001	51	-28	13
	MDD < FHP	-	ns	-	-	ns	-	-	-
	MDD > FHP	-	ns	-	-	ns	-	-	-

F > N: "fear" > "neutral" contrast; F < N: "fear" < "neutral" contrast; FWE: family wise error correction; Ke: number of significant voxels; ns: not significant; T: t-value; x, y, z: coordinates in the Montreal Neurological Institute system.

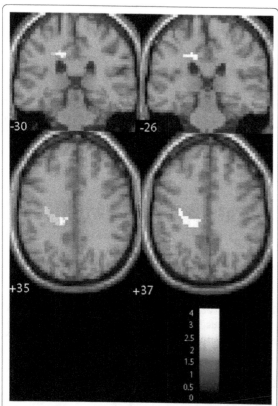

Figure 1 Coronal and axial sections displaying activation differences between major depressive disorder (MDD) patients and healthy controls (HC) in the left middle cingulum (T = 3.82, PFWE = 0.041) and left insula (T = 4.19, P < 0.001, uncorrected). FWE: whole brain family-wise error correction.

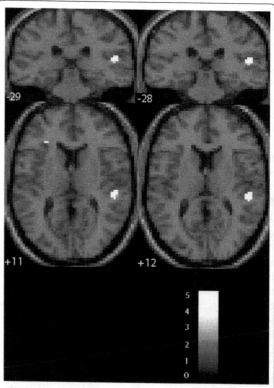

Figure 2 Coronal and axial sections displaying activation differences between family history positive (FHP) and family history negative (FHN) participants in the right Heschl's gyrus (T = 4.60, PFWE = 0.01). FWE: whole brain family-wise error correction.

MDD patients showed reduced activity in the left middle CC when compared to the HC group, adding to previous findings suggesting an important role of CC anomalies in the diagnosis of anxiety disorders and/or depression [34]. In particular, this effect was observed when fearful facial expressions elicited stronger activation, in line with earlier fMRI research suggesting a role for the CC in orienting spatial attention to crude threat signals [8,17]. In this study, we found no effect in the amygdalae for all participants, suggesting a more direct involvement of the CC in attention recruitment during performance in the dot-probe task. This result might also agree with previous findings showing an involvement of the CC in shaping emotional expectancy in both healthy individuals and patients with MDD [35]. Interestingly, we found no effect in the prefrontal cortex, which contrasts with previous research showing prefrontal anomalies in both MDD and healthy participants with family history of MDD [8,24,36]. Our findings might suggest that our version of the dot-probe task is not sensitive to prefrontal activation anomalies in either MDD or FHP subjects, in line with previous research on the dot-probe task showing the involvement of the anterior CC, amygdalae, temporal and occipital cortices [12,13]. Although these results might need replication, an important consideration is to be made when comparing our data to previous findings in similar experimental contexts: while in the study of Monk *et al.* [8] participants were required to consciously shift their attention towards a specific feature of the stimulus presented (that is, participants were asked to rate the size of the nose in a given face), in the dot-probe task, stimulus perception is subliminal (emotional stimuli are masked by neutral stimuli). This might have an effect on how attention is recruited and might explain why, in our study, we detected no prefrontal effect. Previous research [15,17,37] has shown that the CC plays a key role in directing attention when an individual is not conscious of an emotional facial stimulus being presented. Further, recent ERP findings suggest that backward masked fearful face-elicited spatial attention facilitates behavior and modulates the early stage of facial processing [38].

Interestingly, when compared to the FHN group, the FHP group exhibited activation differences in the right Heschl's gyrus. In this area, FHP participants had greater activation for contrast F > N and smaller activation for contrast F < N. The Heschl's gyrus is a subregion of the superior temporal gyrus that, apart from being functionally involved in auditory processing, plays an important role in emotional processing, theory of mind and empathy [39,40]. Volumetric reductions in this area have been found in MDD patients, even after recovery from the

disease [41]. Moreover, similar results have also been shown in bipolar disorder patients [42]. Our results implicate activation differences in superior temporoparietal areas between individuals with and without family history of MDD during exposure to fearful facial expressions. As only the right hemisphere was involved, our findings might also suggest a lateralization effect. This is perhaps in line with previous fMRI research suggesting a role of the right Heschl's gyrus during exposure to emotional (auditory) stimuli [43] and showing that the activation of auditory processing regions specialized for language, like the Heschl's gyrus, can be detected during performance in tasks requiring visual perception of the human face [44]. This might support the belief that this cortical area plays a role in acquired dynamic audiovisual integration mechanisms in the left superior temporal sulcus [44]. In this context, our results suggest a non-task specific role of the Heschl's gyrus in facial emotion processing, which is perhaps lost in MDD.

It is certainly interesting that MDD patients and FHP participants showed activation anomalies in different cortical areas, when compared to FHN participants. However, in the present study, these two groups consisted of unrelated individuals and whether MDD affects functional aberrances already detected before its onset in FHP subjects should be determined by future longitudinal studies.

The present study has a number of limitations. The subject sample was probably too small to reveal behavioral differences across groups. Additionally, the total number of HC participants was almost double than the number of MDD patients. This surely had an effect on our results. For example, our raw data suggested that MDD patients made considerably more errors than the HC group, although this could not be supported by statistical significance. Increasing the participant sample and having a comparable number of HC versus MDD participants would probably have yielded more definitive results. Further research in a larger sample of participants is also needed to confirm our RT analysis and comparisons (the RTs of some participants were lost due to a system failure).

Importantly, in the present study, we did not include images displaying faces conveying positive (happy) emotions. For this reason, we cannot rule out that our fMRI findings simply reflected brain activation associated with the presentation of emotional stimuli. In this regard, further fMRI research should aim at comparing brain activation relative to both happy and fearful faces. Participants were asked after scanning whether they could recognize subliminal images and confirmed that they did not detect them. Employing a detection task within the session would have been difficult, because participants already had to respond to the dots they saw after the shortly presented face images (100 ms). Further, future studies should also investigate correlations between behavioral and MRI data. Quite a substantial limitation of the present study is also represented by the inclusion of MDD patients with differences in medication which, as shown by previous fMRI research (for example, [23,45]), can affect brain activation. Finally, it also possible that the outcome of this research was affected by our recruitment method. We selected FHP participants as first-degree relatives of patients with well-known recurrent depression, but who did not necessarily take part in the study. As all the MDD patients recruited were assessed by the same psychiatrists, selecting relatives of MDD patients involved in the study might have contributed to ascertain family history of the disease in FHP participants. On the other hand, this would have introduced a genetic bias, whose selective effect on MRI data should be investigated in future research.

Conclusions

Our results suggest that, in the dot-probe task, FHP subjects exhibit altered activity in the right Heschl's gyrus associated with subliminal presentation of fearful stimuli, indicating that lateralized alteration in the functionality of this cortical area could be associated with a higher risk of becoming depressed, although this should be confirmed by longitudinal studies on a larger population sample. Moreover, in individuals with MDD, the CC might mediate a preference for negative emotions as delivered by subliminally presented human faces. Further research is surely needed to explore the correlation between cortical and/or subcortical anomalies and behavioral responses in a similar experimental setting and to investigate putative therapeutic effects of psycho- and pharmacotherapy on the activation anomalies we detected.

Abbreviations

ANOVA: analysis of variance; CC: cingulate cortex; DSM-IV: Diagnostic and Statistical Manual of Mental Disorders; SE-EPI: spin-echo echo-planar imaging; ERP: event related potential; FHN: family history negative; FHP: family history positive; fMRI: functional magnetic resonance imaging; FWE: family-wise error; HC: healthy control; LVF: left visual field; MDD: major depressive disorder; RVF: right visual field; RT: reaction time; TE: echo time; TR: repetition time.

Acknowledgements

We would like to thank Dr Mimi Liljholm, Dr Tobias Larsen and Daniel McNamee for their invaluable advice on behavioral data analysis. Also a special thanks to Prof. Hugh Garavan for kindly offering his behavioral testing facilities and Prof Fiona Newell for her constructive critique of our version of the dot-probe task.

Author details

[1]Department of Psychiatry, Trinity College Dublin, College Green, Dublin 2, Ireland. [2]Institute of Neuroscience, Trinity College Dublin, College Green, Dublin 2, Ireland. [3]Adelaide and Meath Hospital incorporating the National Children's Hospital, Tallaght, Dublin 24, Dublin, Ireland. [4]St James's Hospital, Centre of Advanced Medical Imaging (CAMI), James's Street, Dublin 8, Dublin, Ireland.

Authors' contributions

TF, AC and DL acquired MRI data. AF and GB supervised MRI data acquisition. FA and TF carried out data analysis and wrote the present manuscript. All authors read and approved the final manuscript.

Competing interests

The authors declare that they have no competing interests.

References

1. Rosenberg EL: Levels of analysis and the organization of affect. *Review of General Psychology* 1998, 2:247-270.
2. Hankin BL, Gibb BE, Abela JR, Flory K: Selective attention to affective stimuli and clinical depression among youths: role of anxiety and specificity of emotion. *J Abnorm Psychol* 2010, 119:491-501.
3. Williams LM, Gatt JM, Schofield PR, Olivieri G, Peduto A, Gordon E: 'Negativity bias' in risk for depression and anxiety: brain-body fear circuitry correlates, 5-HTT-LPR and early life stress. *Neuroimage* 2009, 47:804-814.
4. Chan SW, Norbury R, Goodwin GM, Harmer CJ: Risk for depression and neural responses to fearful facial expressions of emotion. *Br J Psychiatry* 2009, 194:139-145.
5. Harmer CJ, Mackay CE, Reid CB, Cowen PJ, Goodwin GM: Antidepressant drug treatment modifies the neural processing of nonconscious threat cues. *Biol Psychiatry* 2006, 59:816-820.
6. Joormann J, Gilbert K, Gotlib IH: Emotion identification in girls at high risk for depression. *J Child Psychol Psychiatry* 2010, 51:575-582.
7. Mannie ZN, Harmer CJ, Cowen PJ: Increased waking salivary cortisol levels in young people at familial risk of depression. *Am J Psychiatry* 2007, 164:617-621.
8. Monk CS, Klein RG, Telzer EH, Schroth EA, Mannuzza S, Moulton JL, Guardino M, Masten CL, McClure-Tone EB, Fromm S, Blair RJ, Pine DS, Ernst M: Amygdala and nucleus accumbens activation to emotional facial expressions in children and adolescents at risk for major depression. *Am J Psychiatry* 2008, 165:90-98.
9. Perez-Edgar K, Fox NA, Cohn JF, Kovacs M: Behavioral and electrophysiological markers of selective attention in children of parents with a history of depression. *Biol Psychiatry* 2006, 60:1131-1138.
10. Donaldson C, Lam D, Mathews A: Rumination and attention in major depression. *Behav Res Ther* 2007, 45:2664-2678.
11. Lonigan CJ, Vasey MW: Negative affectivity, effortful control, and attention to threat-relevant stimuli. *J Abnorm Child Psychol* 2009, 37:387-399.
12. Pourtois G, Schwartz S, Seghier ML, Lazeyras F, Vuilleumier P: Neural systems for orienting attention to the location of threat signals: an event-related fMRI study. *Neuroimage* 2006, 31:920-933.
13. Pourtois G, Grandjean D, Sander D, Vuilleumier P: Electrophysiological correlates of rapid spatial orienting towards fearful faces. *Cereb Cortex* 2004, 14:619-633.
14. Vuilleumier P, Richardson MP, Armony JL, Driver J, Dolan RJ: Distant influences of amygdala lesion on visual cortical activation during emotional face processing. *Nat Neurosci* 2004, 7:1271-1278.
15. Armony JL, Dolan RJ: Modulation of spatial attention by fear-conditioned stimuli: an event-related fMRI study. *Neuropsychologia* 2002, 40:817-826.
16. Bush G, Luu P, Posner MI: Cognitive and emotional influences in anterior cingulate cortex. *Trends Cogn Sci* 2000, 4:215-222.
17. Carlson JM, Reinke KS, Habib R: A left amygdala mediated network for rapid orienting to masked fearful faces. *Neuropsychologia* 2009, 47:1386-1389.
18. Mingtian Z, Xiongzhao Z, Jinyao Y, Shuqiao Y, Atchley RA: Do the early attentional components of ERPs reflect attentional bias in depression? It depends on the stimulus presentation time. *Clin Neurophysiol* 2011, 122:1371-1381.
19. Kujawa AJ, Torpey D, Kim J, Hajcak G, Rose S, Gotlib IH, Klein DN: Attentional biases for emotional faces in young children of mothers with chronic or recurrent depression. *J Abnorm Child Psychol* 2011, 39:125-135.
20. Townsend JD, Eberhart NK, Bookheimer SY, Eisenberger NI, Foland-Ross LC, Cook IA, Sugar CA, Altshuler LL: fMRI activation in the amygdala and the

Functional anomalies in healthy individuals with a first degree family history of major...

177

orbitofrontal cortex in unmedicated subjects with major depressive disorder. *Psychiatry Res* 2010, **183**:209-217.

21. Anderson IM, Juhasz G, Thomas E, Downey D, McKie S, Deakin JF, Elliott R: The effect of acute citalopram on face emotion processing in remitted depression: a pharmacoMRI study. *Eur Neuropsychopharmacol* 2011, **21**:140-148.

22. van Wingen GA, van Eijndhoven P, Tendolkar I, Buitelaar J, Verkes RJ, Fernandez G: Neural basis of emotion recognition deficits in first-episode major depression. *Psychol Med* 2011, **41**:1397-1405.

23. Fales CL, Barch DM, Rundle MM, Mintun MA, Mathews J, Snyder AZ, Sheline YI: Antidepressant treatment normalizes hypoactivity in dorsolateral prefrontal cortex during emotional interference processing in major depression. *J Affect Disord* 2009, **112**:206-211.

24. Fales CL, Barch DM, Rundle MM, Mintun MA, Snyder AZ, Cohen JD, Mathews J, Sheline YI: Altered emotional interference processing in affective and cognitive-control brain circuitry in major depression. *Biol Psychiatry* 2008, **63**:377-384.

25. Hamilton M: Standardised assessment and recording of depressive symptoms. *Psychiatr Neurol Neurochir* 1969, **72**:201-205.

26. Montgomery SA, Asberg M: A new depression scale designed to be sensitive to change. *Br J Psychiatry* 1979, **134**:382-389.

27. Beck AT, Ward CH, Mendelson M, Mock J, Erbaugh J: An inventory for measuring depression. *Arch Gen Psychiatry* 1961, **4**:561-571.

28. Spitzer RL, Williams JB, Gibbon M, First MB: The Structured Clinical Interview for DSM-III-R (SCID). I: History, rationale, and description. *Arch Gen Psychiatry* 1992, **49**:624-629.

29. Williams JB, Gibbon M, First MB, Spitzer RL, Davies M, Borus J, Howes MJ, Kane J, Pope HG Jr, Rounsaville B, Wittchen HU: The Structured Clinical Interview for DSM-III-R (SCID). II. Multisite test-retest reliability. *Arch Gen Psychiatry* 1992, **49**:630-636.

30. Oldfield RC: The assessment and analysis of handedness: the Edinburgh inventory. *Neuropsychologia* 1971, **9**:97-113.

31. Gur RC, Sara R, Hagendoorn M, Marom O, Hughett P, Macy L, Turner T, Bajcsy R, Posner A, Gur RE: A method for obtaining 3-dimensional facial expressions and its standardization for use in neurocognitive studies. *J Neurosci Methods* 2002, **115**:137-143.

32. Ashburner J, Friston KJ: Unified segmentation. *Neuroimage* 2005, **26**:839-851.

33. Friston KJ, Holmes AP, Worsley KJ, Polina J-P, Frith CD, Frackowiak RSJ: Statistical parametric maps in functional imaging: a general linear approach. *Hum Brain Mapp* 1994, **2**:189-210.

34. Clark DA, Beck AT: Cognitive theory and therapy of anxiety and depression: convergence with neurobiological findings. *Trends Cogn Sci* 2010, **14**:418-424.

35. Sharot T, Riccardi AM, Raio CM, Phelps EA: Neural mechanisms mediating optimism bias. *Nature* 2007, **450**:102-105.

36. Frokjaer VG, Vinberg M, Erritzoe D, Svarer C, Baare W, Budtz-Joergensen E, Madsen K, Madsen J, Kessing LV, Knudsen GM: High familial risk for mood disorder is associated with low dorsolateral prefrontal cortex serotonin transporter binding. *Neuroimage* 2009, **46**:360-366.

37. Bush G, Luu P, Posner MI: Cognitive and emotional influences in anterior cingulate cortex. *Trends Cogn Sci* 2000, **4**:215-222.

38. Carlson JM, Reinke KS: Spatial attention-related modulation of the N170 by backward masked fearful faces. *Brain Cogn* 2009, **73**:20-27.

39. Abu-Akel A, Shamay-Tsoory S: Neuroanatomical and neurochemical bases of theory of mind. *Neuropsychologia* 2011, **49**:2971-2984.

40. Dziobek I, Preissler S, Grozdanovic Z, Heuser I, Heekeren HR, Roepke S: Neuronal correlates of altered empathy and social cognition in borderline personality disorder. *Neuroimage* 2011, **57**:539-548.

41. Takahashi T, Yucel M, Lorenzetti V, Walterfang M, Kawasaki Y, Whittle S, Suzuki M, Pantelis C, Allen NB: An MRI study of the superior temporal subregions in patients with current and past major depression. *Prog Neuropsychopharmacol Biol Psychiatry* 2009, **34**:98-103.

42. Takahashi T, Malhi GS, Wood SJ, Yucel M, Walterfang M, Kawasaki Y, Suzuki M, Pantelis C: Gray matter reduction of the superior temporal gyrus in patients with established bipolar I disorder. *J Affect Disord* 2010, **123**:276-282.

43. Meyer M, Zysset S, von Cramon DY, Alter K: Distinct fMRI responses to laughter, speech, and sounds along the human peri-sylvian cortex. *Brain Res Cogn Brain Res* 2005, **24**:291-306.

44. Calvert GA, Campbell R: Reading speech from still and moving faces: the neural substrates of visible speech. *J Cogn Neurosci* 2003, **15**:57-70.

45. Bruhl AB, Kaffenberger T, Herwig U: Serotonergic and noradrenergic modulation of emotion processing by single dose antidepressants. *Neuropsychopharmacology* 2010, **35**:521-533.

Resting state amygdala-prefrontal connectivity predicts symptom change after cognitive behavioral therapy in generalized social anxiety disorder

Heide Klumpp[1,2,3*], Michael K Keutmann[2], Daniel A Fitzgerald[1,4], Stewart A Shankman[2,3] and K Luan Phan[1,2,3,4]

Abstract

Background: Aberrant amygdala-prefrontal interactions at rest and during emotion processing are implicated in the pathophysiology of generalized social anxiety disorder (gSAD), a common disorder characterized by fears of potential scrutiny. Cognitive behavioral therapy (CBT) is first-line psychotherapy for gSAD and other anxiety disorders. While CBT is generally effective, there is a great deal of heterogeneity in treatment response. To date, predictors of success in CBT for gSAD include reduced amygdala reactivity and increased activity in prefrontal regulatory regions (e.g., anterior cingulate cortex, ACC) during emotion processing. However, studies have not examined whether tonic (i.e., at rest) coupling of amygdala and these prefrontal regions also predict response to CBT.

Results: Twenty-one patients with gSAD participated in resting-state functional magnetic resonance imaging (fMRI) before 12 weeks of CBT. Overall, symptom severity was significantly reduced after completing CBT; however, the patients varied considerably in degree of symptom change. Whole-brain voxel-wise findings showed symptom improvement after CBT was predicted by greater right amygdala-pregenual ACC (pgACC) connectivity and greater left amygdala-pgACC coupling encompassing medial prefrontal cortex. In support of their predictive value, area under receiver operating characteristic curve was significant for the left and right amygdala-pgACC in relation to treatment responders.

Conclusions: Improvement after CBT was predicted by enhanced resting-state bilateral amygdala-prefrontal coupling in gSAD. Preliminary results suggest baseline individual differences in a fundamental circuitry that may underlie emotion regulation contributed to variation in symptom change after CBT. Findings offer a new approach towards using a biological measure to foretell who will most likely benefit from CBT. In particular, the departure from neural predictors based on illness-relevant stimuli (e.g., socio-emotional stimuli in gSAD) permits the development of biomarkers that reflect commonalities in the neurobiology of anxiety and mood disorders.

Keywords: Generalized social anxiety, fMRI, Treatment, Brain imaging, Rest

* Correspondence: hklumpp@psych.uic.edu
[1]Mood and Anxiety Disorders Research Program, Department of Psychiatry (HK, DAF, KLP), University of Illinois at Chicago, 1747 W. Roosevelt Rd, Chicago, IL 60608, USA
[2]Department of Psychology (HK, MKK, SAS, KLP), University of Illinois at Chicago, Chicago, IL, USA
Full list of author information is available at the end of the article

Background

Cognitive behavioral therapy (CBT) is empirically supported psychotherapy for generalized social anxiety disorder (gSAD), a common, debilitating illness marked by excessive fears of negative evaluation by others [1]. CBT primarily attempts to reduce symptoms via cognitive restructuring, an emotion regulation strategy aimed at decreasing thought-related negative affect, in conjunction with exposure exercises (e.g., facing anxiety-evoking situations). While generally effective, treatment response is varied with approximately 30% 40% of patients with gSAD not fully responding to CBT [2,3]. Findings from neuroimaging studies indicate heterogeneity in treatment outcome may relate in part to brain regions implicated in the pathophysiology of gSAD that are utilized by CBT.

Accumulating data indicate the amygdala, a key emotion processing region that mediates fear [4], plays a prominent role in gSAD. The amygdala has interconnections to prefrontal regions that down-regulate emotional reactivity (e.g., medial prefrontal cortex (mPFC); [5]). In gSAD, amygdala hyper-reactivity to salient signals has been demonstrated in addition to disturbances in regulatory regions (e.g., exaggerated or attenuated mPFC activation; [6]). Moreover, in the absence of stimuli presentation or task engagement (i.e., during rest), aberrant amygdala connectivity with prefrontal regulatory areas (e.g., anterior cingulate cortex (ACC), medial orbitofrontal cortex (mOFC)) has been observed [7-9]. Findings suggest phasic hyper-reactive amygdala responses to external information involve tonic disturbances in core amygdala-prefrontal circuitry [8] and that individual differences in such circuitry may factor into the likelihood of benefiting from CBT.

To date, studies of amygdala as a brain-based marker in predicting CBT response in gSAD appear to be limited to emotion perception tasks, and results have been mixed. For example, we recently showed less pre-CBT amygdala activity to emotional faces predicted CBT success [10]; however, other emotion processing studies of gSAD have not revealed amygdala effects [11,12]. Regarding prefrontal regions as predictors, we have observed a positive link between dorsal ACC and mOFC activity in gSAD during emotion processing and symptom improvement in CBT [10,12] even in the absence of amygdala findings [12]. However, it is not clear whether amygdala response contributed to symptom change as regions were examined in isolation as opposed to nodes in a network.

A means of increasing our understanding of amygdala-based circuitry as a biomarker in predicting who will likely respond to CBT is with resting-state functional MRI (rs-fMRI). An advantage of rs-fMRI is that it examines fundamental networks that are task independent but may underlie emotion and regulatory processes in the unprovoked state [13]. Therefore, the objective of this study was to use pre-CBT rs-fMRI to investigate the relationship between amygdala-prefrontal coupling and CBT success in gSAD. Based on the literature [10,12], we hypothesized greater rs-fMRI amygdala-ACC or amygdala-mOFC connectivity would correspond with CBT response.

Methods

Participants

All 21 participants (14 female, 7 male) with an average age of 28.3 9.4 years met criteria for gSAD based on the Structured Clinical Interview for DSM-IV (SCID) [14]. Symptom severity was assessed with the Liebowitz Social Anxiety Scale (LSAS) [15] administered by licensed clinicians, and depression level was measured with the Beck Depression Inventory [16]. Clinical Global Impression-Improvement (CGI-I; [17]), comprising a 7-point scale (1 = very much improved, 7 = worsening symptoms), was used to determine whether or not a patient responded to treatment.

All the participants were free of psychotropic medication, except for two who were on a stable dose of bupropion for at least 8 weeks prior to, and throughout, the study. Exclusion criteria included current or recent (within 6 months of study) comorbid major depressive disorder or recent substance abuse/dependence or any history of major psychiatric illness (e.g., bipolar, psychotic disorder).

The participants were between 18 and 55 years of age, right-handed, and free of current and past major medical or neurologic illness, as confirmed by a Board Certified physician. None of the participants tested positive for alcohol or illegal substances. The study protocol was approved by the Institutional Review Boards of the University of Michigan Medical School, and as per protocol, all the participants provided written informed consent.

The patients received 12 weeks of manualized individual CBT conducted by the same doctoral-level licensed clinical psychologist who has several years of training in CBT. A licensed clinical psychologist with both expertise in CBT and clinical trial investigations involving CBT provided supervision to ensure adherence to treatment. CBT encompassed psychoeducation, cognitive restructuring, *in vivo* exposures, and relapse prevention [18].

Resting-state fMRI

Padding with foam cushions was used to reduce head movement. The participants were instructed to fixate on a crosshair centrally displayed on the blank gray screen, relax, and let their mind wander without falling asleep for 8 min.

Functional imaging: acquisition and analysis

Magnetic resonance imaging (MRI) was performed on a 3 T GE Signa System (Milwaukee, WI) acquiring blood-oxygen-level-dependent (BOLD) images with a T2*-sensitive gradient-echo reverse spiral acquisition (3 mm

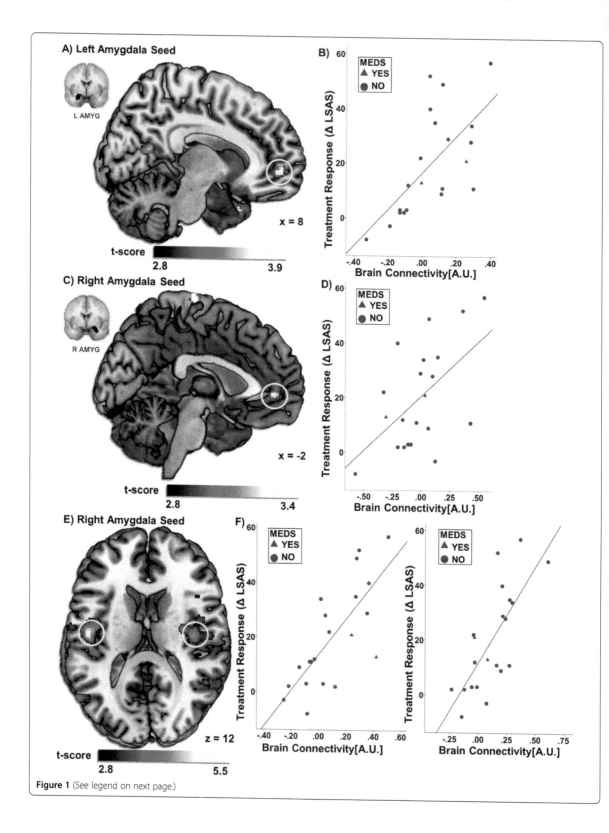

Figure 1 (See legend on next page.)

(See figure on previous page.)
Figure 1 Regressing LSAS change and scatterplot of regression analyses. (A) Regressing LSAS change ($\Delta_{PreTx-PostTx}$) while initial severity ($LSAS_{PreTx}$) is controlled for as a regressor of no interest; brain map depicts whole-brain analysis of covariance showing enhanced left amygdala-anterior cingulate cortex/medial prefrontal cortex coupling during rest in gSAD displayed on statistical t-map at $p < 0.005$. **(B)** Scatterplot of regression analyses depicting extracted measures of left amygdala-anterior cingulate cortex/medial prefrontal cortex connectivity and relation to change in social anxiety severity. **(C)** Regressing LSAS change ($\Delta_{PreTx-PostTx}$) while baseline severity ($LSAS_{PreTx}$) is controlled for as a regressor of no interest; brain map depicts whole-brain analysis of covariance showing enhanced right amygdala-anterior cingulate cortex connectivity during rest in gSAD displayed on statistical t-map at $p < 0.005$. **(D)** Scatterplot of regression analyses depicting extracted measures of right amygdala-anterior cingulate cortex coupling and relation to change in social anxiety severity. **(E)** Regressing LSAS change ($\Delta_{PreTx-PostTx}$) while initial severity ($LSAS_{PreTx}$) is controlled for as a regressor of no interest; brain map depicts whole-brain analysis of covariance showing enhanced right amygdala-bilateral insula connectivity during rest in gSAD displayed on statistical t-map at $p < 0.005$. **(F)** Scatterplot of regression analyses illustrating extracted measures of right amygdala-bilateral insula coupling and relation to change in social anxiety severity. LSAS, Liebowitz Social Anxiety Scale; CBT, cognitive behavioral therapy; gSAD, generalized social anxiety disorder.

43 axial slices; 2 s TR; 30 ms TE; 64 64 matrix; 220 mm FOV; 90 flip) optimized to minimize susceptibility artifacts in the medial temporal pole. High-resolution, T1-weighted anatomical scans (3D-SPGR; 9 ms TR; 1.8 ms TE; 15 flip; 256 256 matrix; 256 mm FOV, 1.2 mm 124 axial slices) were also acquired for precise anatomical localization and normalization.

Analyses were performed using the Functional Connectivity (CONN) toolbox [19], which employs routines from the Statistical Parametric Mapping software (SPM8; Wellcome Trust Centre for Neuroimaging, London, UK). Eight initial volumes from each resting-state run were discarded to allow for T1 equilibration effects. Images were realigned to correct for motion, corrected for errors in slice timing, spatially transformed to standard MNI space using the functional template provided with SPM8, resampled to 2-mm voxels, and smoothed with an 8-mm FWHM Gaussian kernel prior to statistical analysis. The participants had no movement greater than 2-mm translation or 2 rotation across the run. Effects of nuisance variables (global, white matter and CSF signals and movement parameters) were reduced following the CompCor strategy [20]; data were band-pass filtered to 0.01 0.09 Hz.

Temporal correlations of the resting-state BOLD signal time series were examined between the left and right amygdala seed regions (anatomically derived regions of interest from the Automated Anatomical Labeling (AAL) toolbox [21]) and the rest of the brain. During second-level processing, LSAS change ($\Delta_{PreTx-PostTx}$) was regressed with initial severity ($LSAS_{PreTx}$) controlled for as a regressor of no interest. The ACC and medial OFC regions of interest were examined at the whole-brain level with significance defined as $p < 0.005$ uncorrected with more than 20 contiguous voxels per cluster (>160 volume mm^3) to strike a balance between type I and II errors [22]. The AAL atlas [21,23] was used to identify regions of interest (ROIs) and other significant whole-brain findings across subjects.

To clarify the directionality and magnitude of baseline amygdala-prefrontal connectivity related to change in symptom severity, 10-mm-diameter spherical ROIs were generated around the peak activation of a whole-brain cluster. Subsequently, parameter estimates (β weights and arbitrary units (au)) were extracted from the ROIs for each participant and submitted to Pearsons correlations and scatterplots in the Statistical Package for the Social Sciences (SPSS version 20; Chicago, IL). Additionally, the parameter estimates were used to calculate the area under a receiver operating characteristic (ROC) curve in SPSS to assess the predictive value of *a priori* connectivity results in terms of CBT responders based on CGI-I. Apart from fMRI, we performed a regression analysis in SPSS to examine whether demographic factors (i.e., age, gender, education level) independently effected LSAS change ($\Delta_{PreTx-PostTx}$).

Results
Treatment effects on social anxiety
Symptom severity assessed by LSAS significantly decreased from an average of 71.6 11.9 to 51.5 19.5 ($t = 4.87$, $p < 0.001$). The clinical cutoff is ≥ 60 for gSAD [24]; therefore, results point to a significant overall improvement with variation in degree of symptom change. Additionally, depression level which was in the minimal range [16] at the start of CBT (11.7 8.3) significantly decreased (5.0 6.0) ($t = 4.60$, $p < 0.001$). Based on the CGI-I, about 70% of the patients with gSAD (15 of 21) were responders as they were rated to be very much improved or much improved (CGI-I score of 1 or 2) whereas 6 patients had a CGI-I score of >2 post-treatment and were thus considered non-responders. Regression analysis findings were not significant for age, gender, or education level (all $ps > 0.05$).

fMRI
For the right amygdala, LSAS change ($\Delta_{PreTx-PostTx}$) was predicted by more baseline connectivity with the left pregenual ACC (pgACC) (i.e., anterior cingulum) [(−4, 48, 0), $z = 2.90$, volume = 392 mm^3; $r = 0.55$, $p < 0.010$] (Figure 1). Area under an ROC curve regarding the right amygdala-pgACC was 0.80 in the context of CBT

responders which was significant ($p < 0.04$). Similar pgACC results were observed for the left amygdala [(10, 52, −2), $z = 3.30$, volume = 928 mm^3; $r = 0.66$, $p < 0.001$] though here the cluster extended to the medial prefrontal cortex (i.e., frontal medial orbital gyrus) volume = 712 mm^3 (Figure 1). Again, area under the curve (i.e., 0.83) was significant ($p < 0.02$). As to regions beyond *a priori* prefrontal areas, we observed symptom improvement robustly corresponded with bilateral insula (i.e., rolandic operculum) coupling [left: (−36, −30, 26), $z = 4.00$, volume = 2,648 mm^3; $r = 0.75$, $p < 0.001$; right: (30, −10, 18), $z = 4.14$, volume = 2,192 mm^3; $r = 0.74$, $p < 0.001$] related to the right amygdala. Area under the curves concerning the right amygdala-left insula and right amygdala-right insula were significant (i.e., 0.84, $p < 0.02$; 0.80, $p < 0.04$, respectively) (Figure 1). For completeness, we report all results outside regions of interest in Table 1.

Discussion

As hypothesized, clinical improvement following CBT in the patients with gSAD was predicted by greater pretreatment amygdala connectivity with prefrontal regions implicated in controlling emotion. Specifically, greater symptom reduction was foretold by increased pre-CBT right amygdala-pgACC and left amygdala-pgACC/mPFC coupling, a circuit involved in emotion processing and regulation [25,26]. In support of its predictive capacity, ROC results pertaining to CBT responder based on a CGI-I cutoff were also significant. Pointing to the potential relevance of the circuit as a brain predictor and/ or target for treatment is a resting-state study showing lower amygdala-ACC/mPFC connectivity in gSAD correlated with social anxiety severity and that deficient coupling was enhanced by an acute challenge of the neuropeptide oxytocin [9]. Together, findings indicate intrinsic amygdala-medial prefrontal interactions may play a role in predicting the likelihood of responding to an intervention in gSAD. Findings expand on emotion activation paradigms that have demonstrated associations between increases in ACC or mOFC activity before treatment and improvement after CBT in gSAD [10,12]. Further study is needed to examine whether phasic (e.g., task/emotion-based) in combination with tonic (i.e., at rest) biomarkers can be used to predict response to CBT.

Beyond prefrontal regions of interest, symptom change was foretold by more and less connectivity in an extensive network indicative of the regions interconnected with the amygdala (e.g., insula, occipital lobe, middle temporal gyrus, superior frontal gyrus, parahippocampal gyrus; [27]) in addition to wide-scale coupling within and between networks exhibited at rest [13]. We did not have *a priori* hypotheses for these regions and, therefore,

hesitate to interpret these preliminary, exploratory findings. Nevertheless, it is interesting to note symptom improvement also positively corresponded with the right amygdala-insula (i.e., rolandic operculum) coupling and, based on ROC findings, served as a good estimate of treatment response. The insula is proposed to play a role in anxiety disorders [28,29], which is supported by observations of exaggerated insula reactivity to emotional stimuli in gSAD relative to healthy controls [6]. In the context of treatment for gSAD, we observed insula hyper-reactivity to threat relevant stimuli decreased after CBT [12]; however, task-based pre-CBT insula activity to threat has not yet been shown to predict symptom change in gSAD [10-12]. Our findings suggest that in the absence of external stimuli, baseline emotion processing circuitry appears to function as a predictor. More study is needed to understand how the intrinsic amygdala-insula and other resting-state networks beyond *a priori* regions might be utilized by CBT.

Conclusions

First, our study is not without important limitations. These include a relatively small sample size which increases risk for type II errors. Second, 2 of the 21 participants with gSAD were taking bupropion. Even though the medication was stable before the study and remained unchanged during the study, and these participants did not serve as outliers in *a priori* findings as indicated by scatterplots, any influence it may have had on other outcomes cannot be ruled out. Third, the lack of a waitlist group to serve as a control for changes in symptoms unrelated to treatment reduces our ability to draw firm conclusions about neural predictors of CBT response. Fourth, replication in an independent sample is necessary before conclusions can be made as to the clinical relevance of our findings. Fifth, connectivity results were limited to the bilateral amygdala. Future studies may want to seed prefrontal regions implicated in emotion regulation (e.g., dorsolateral, dorsomedial prefrontal cortex; orbitofrontal cortex; anterior cingulate cortex; [5]) to examine their relationship with the amygdala and ability to predict CBT success. Sixth, the lack of independent evaluators of treatment fidelity and symptom change warrants replication and further investigation. Despite limitations, findings suggest individual differences in intrinsic amygdala-prefrontal connectivity can help explain the heterogeneity in response to CBT in gSAD. Findings also indicate resting-state fMRI may be a useful approach in identifying brain-based biomarkers in treatment response. Among the advantages of resting-state biomarkers is the ease of application across other internalizing psychopathologies that may have common pathophysiology and for which CBT is an empirically validated treatment option (e.g., post-traumatic stress disorder, major depressive disorder).

Table 1 Whole-brain voxel-wise regression: relation between pre-treatment to post-treatment change in social anxiety severity, controlling for pre-treatment severity

Region	MNI coordinates			Volume (mm³)	Z
	x	y	z		
Right amygdala					
Positive correlation	R rolandic operculum				
R rolandic operculum	30	−10	18	2,192	4.14
L rolandic operculum	−36	−30	26	2,648	4.00
L middle temporal gyrus	−58	−66	12	800	3.67
L angular gyrus	−36	−70	48	552	3.38
R frontal inferior triangularis	48	26	10	760	3.26
L middle temporal gyrus	−66	−34	2	608	3.18
L paracentral lobule	−8	−20	78	344	3.15
R middle frontal gyrus	26	34	34	408	2.96
L anterior cingulum	−4	48	0	392	2.90
Negative correlation — L parahippocampal gyrus	−14	2	−18	528	4.01
L temporal pole superior gyrus	−26	14	−26	440	4.00
R hippocampus	24	−10	−20	328	3.98
R frontal superior orbital gyrus	16	16	−18	264	3.73
R gyrus rectus	6	32	−18	760	3.69
R frontal superior gyrus	16	66	26	360	3.64
R frontal middle orbital gyrus	38	42	−10	512	3.64
R frontal superior medial gyrus	10	40	56	352	3.48
L cerebellum	−4	−40	−18	336	3.33
L frontal middle orbital gyrus	−22	58	−10	296	3.04
L fusiform gyrus	−32	−18	−18	360	2.18
Left amygdala					
Positive correlation — L calcarine gyrus	−12	−60	16	1,136	4.44
R temporal pole middle gyrus	32	18	−36	344	3.58
R anterior cingulum	10	52	−2	928	3.30
R frontal medial orbital gyrus				712	3.30
L middle occipital gyrus	−38	−78	20	344	3.27
R calcarine gyrus	8	−58	14	464	3.06
Negative correlation — L caudate	−18	−14	18	224	4.67
R frontal middle orbital gyrus	36	64	−4	1,104	4.05
L frontal middle gyrus	−44	20	48	1,104	3.97
R inferior occipital gyrus	36	−64	−8	472	3.87
L cerebellum	−42	−80	−22	784	3.77
R frontal superior medial gyrus	6	42	52	1,744	3.74
R frontal superior gyrus	14	68	24	576	3.68
R cerebellum	4	−48	−44	432	3.60
R frontal superior orbital gyrus	18	38	−16	376	3.53
R frontal inferior orbital gyrus	36	38	−12	480	3.47
L frontal middle orbital gyrus	−22	52	−10	360	3.36
R superior parietal lobule	20	−62	60	440	3.21
L cerebellum	−18	−90	−30	200	3.15
R inferior temporal gyrus	56	−66	−8	296	3.00
R frontal middle gyrus	42	16	54	168	2.84

All listed clusters are significant at $p < 0.005$ (uncorrected) with a threshold of greater than 160 volume (mm³).
Areas showing *a priori* hypothesized treatment-related predictors are bolded.
MNI Montreal Neurological Institute, *Z* Z-score.

Abbreviations

CBT: cognitive behavioral therapy; gSAD: generalized social anxiety disorder; ACC: anterior cingulate cortex; mOFC: medial orbitofrontal cortex; rs-fMRI: resting-state functional magnetic resonance imaging; DSM-IV: diagnostic and statistical manual of mental disorders fourth edition; SCID: Structured Clinical Interview for DSM Disorders; LSAS: Liebowitz Social Anxiety Scale; BDI: Beck Depression Inventory; CGI-I: Clinical Global Impression-Improvement; BOLD: blood-oxygen-level-dependent; 3T: 3.0 Tesla; GE: general electric; T2: spin-spin relaxation time; TR: repetition time; TE: echo time; ms: millisecond; mm: millimeter; FOV: field of view; 3D-SPGR: three-dimensional spoiled gradient-recalled acquisition in steady state; FWHM: full width at half maximum; CSF: cerebrospinal fluid; CompCor: component-based noise correction method; Hz: Hertz; β: beta; pgACC: pregenual anterior cingulate cortex; mPFC: medial prefrontal cortex; PreTx: pre-treatment; PostTx: post-treatment; AAL: automated anatomical labeling; ROI: region of interest; SPSS: Statistical Package for the Social Sciences; ROC: receiver operating characteristic; au: arbitrary units.

Competing interests

The authors declare that they have no competing interests.

Authors contributions

HK conceived and designed the study, conducted the statistical analysis, data interpretation, and wrote the manuscript. MKK and DAF conducted the neuroimaging analyses and participated in the data interpretation and drafting of the manuscript. SAS participated in the data interpretation and drafting of the manuscript. KLP conceived and designed the study, conducted the data interpretation, and participated in the drafting of the manuscript. All authors read and approved the final manuscript.

Acknowledgements

This work was supported by grants from the National Institutes of Health and National Institute of Mental Health (MH076198 to KLP and MH093679 to HK).

Author details

[1]Mood and Anxiety Disorders Research Program, Department of Psychiatry (HK, DAF, KLP), University of Illinois at Chicago, 1747 W. Roosevelt Rd, Chicago, IL 60608, USA. [2]Department of Psychology (HK, MKK, SAS, KLP), University of Illinois at Chicago, Chicago, IL, USA. [3]Department of Psychiatry (HK, SAS, KLP), University of Illinois at Chicago, Chicago, IL, USA. [4]Mental Health Service (DAF, KLP), Jesse Brown VA Medical Center, Chicago, IL, USA.

References

1. American Psychiatric Association: *Diagnostic and Statistical Manual of Mental Disorders, Fourth Edition: DSM-IV-TR*. Washington, D.C.: American Psychiatric Association; 2000.
2. Heimberg RG, Liebowitz MR, Hope DA, Schneier FR, Holt CS, Welkowitz LA, Juster HR, Campeas R, Bruch MA, Cloitre M, Fallon B, Klein DF: **Cognitive behavioral group therapy vs phenelzine therapy for social phobia: 12-week outcome.** *Arch Gen Psychiatry* 1998, **55:**1133 1141.
3. Davidson JRT, Foa EB, Huppert JD, Keefe FJ, Franklin ME, Compton JS, Zhao N, Connor KM, Lynch TR, Gadde KM: **Fluoxetine, comprehensive cognitive behavioral therapy, and placebo in generalized social phobia.** *Arch Gen Psychiatry* 2004, **61:**1005 1013.
4. LeDoux JE: **Emotion circuits in the brain.** *Annu Rev Neurosci* 2000, **23:**155 184.
5. Banks SJ, Eddy KT, Angstadt M, Nathan PJ, Phan KL: **Amygdala-frontal connectivity during emotion regulation.** *Soc Cogn Affect Neurosci* 2007, **2:**303 312.
6. Brhl AB, Delsignore A, Komossa K, Weidt S: **Neuroimaging in social anxiety disorder a meta-analytic review resulting in a new neurofunctional model.** *Neurosci Biobehav Rev* 2014, **47C:**260 280.
7. Hahn A, Stein P, Windischberger C, Weissenbacher A, Spindelegger C, Moser E, Kasper S, Lanzenberger R: **Reduced resting-state functional connectivity between amygdala and orbitofrontal cortex in social anxiety disorder.** *Neuroimage* 2011, **56:**881 889.
8. Prater KE, Hosanagar A, Klumpp H, Angstadt M, Phan KL: **Aberrant amygdala-frontal cortex connectivity during perception of fearful faces and at rest in generalized social anxiety disorder.** *Depress Anxiety* 2013, **30:**234 241.
9. Dodhia S, Hosanagar A, Fitzgerald DA, Labuschagne I, Wood AG, Nathan PJ, Phan KL: **Modulation of resting-state amygdala-frontal functional connectivity by oxytocin in generalized social anxiety disorder.** *Neuropsychopharmacol Off Publ Am Coll Neuropsychopharmacol* 2014, **39:**2061 2069.
10. Klumpp H, Fitzgerald DA, Angstadt M, Post D, Phan KL: **Neural response during attentional control and emotion processing predicts improvement after cognitive behavioral therapy in generalized social anxiety disorder.** *Psychol Med* 2014, **44:**3109 3121.
11. Doehrmann O, Ghosh SS, Polli FE, Reynolds GO, Horn F, Keshavan A, Triantafyllou C, Saygin ZM, Whitfield-Gabrieli S, Hofmann SG, Pollack M, Gabrieli JD: **Predicting treatment response in social anxiety disorder from functional magnetic resonance imaging.** *JAMA Psychiatr* 2013, **70:**87 97.
12. Klumpp H, Fitzgerald DA, Phan KL: **Neural predictors and mechanisms of cognitive behavioral therapy on threat processing in social anxiety disorder.** *Prog Neuropsychopharmacol Biol Psychiatry* 2013, **45:**83 91.
13. Fox MD, Snyder AZ, Vincent JL, Corbetta M, Van Essen DC, Raichle ME: **The human brain is intrinsically organized into dynamic, anticorrelated functional networks.** *Proc Natl Acad Sci U S A* 2005, **102:**9673 9678.
14. First MB, Spitzer RL, Gibbon M, Williams JBW: *Structured Clinical Interview for DSM-IV Axis I Disorders, Clinician Version (SCID-CV)*. Washington, D.C: American Psychiatric Association; 1996.
15. Liebowitz MR: **Social phobia.** *Mod Probl Pharmacopsychiatry* 1987, **22:**141 173.
16. Beck AT, Steer RA, Ball R, Ranieri WF: **Comparison of beck depression inventories-IA and -II in psychiatric outpatients.** *J Pers Assess* 1996, **67:**588 597.
17. Busner J, Targum SD: **The clinical global impressions scale.** *Psychiatry* 2007, **4:**28 37.
18. Hope DA, Heimberg RG, Turk CL: *Managing Social Anxiety: A Cognitive-Behavioral Therapy Approach*. 1st edition. New York, USA: Oxford University Press; 2006.
19. Whitfield-Gabrieli S, Nieto-Castanon A: **Conn: a functional connectivity toolbox for correlated and anticorrelated brain networks.** *Brain Connect* 2012, **2:**125 141.
20. Behzadi Y, Restom K, Liau J, Liu TT: **A component based noise correction method (CompCor) for BOLD and perfusion based fMRI.** *Neuroimage* 2007, **37:**90 101.
21. Tzourio-Mazoyer N, Landeau B, Papathanassiou D, Crivello F, Etard O, Delcroix N, Mazoyer B, Joliot M: **Automated anatomical labeling of activations in SPM using a macroscopic anatomical parcellation of the MNI MRI single-subject brain.** *Neuroimage* 2002, **15:**273 289.
22. Lieberman MD, Cunningham WA: **Type I and type II error concerns in fMRI research: re-balancing the scale.** *Soc Cogn Affect Neurosci* 2009, **4:**423 428.
23. Lancaster JL, Woldorff MG, Parsons LM, Liotti M, Freitas CS, Rainey L, Kochunov PV, Nickerson D, Mikiten SA, Fox PT: **Automated Talairach atlas labels for functional brain mapping.** *Hum Brain Mapp* 2000, **10:**120 131.
24. Mennin DS, Fresco DM, Heimberg RG, Schneier FR, Davies SO, Liebowitz MR: **Screening for social anxiety disorder in the clinical setting: using the Liebowitz Social Anxiety Scale.** *J Anxiety Disord* 2002, **16:**661 673.
25. Etkin A, Egner T, Kalisch R: **Emotional processing in anterior cingulate and medial prefrontal cortex.** *Trends Cogn Sci* 2011, **15:**85 93.
26. Ongr D, Ferry AT, Price JL: **Architectonic subdivision of the human orbital and medial prefrontal cortex.** *J Comp Neurol* 2003, **460:**425 449.
27. Roy AK, Shehzad Z, Margulies DS, Kelly AMC, Uddin LQ, Gotimer K, Biswal BB, Castellanos FX, Milham MP: **Functional connectivity of the human amygdala using resting state fMRI.** *Neuroimage* 2009, **45:**614 626.
28. Paulus MP, Stein MB: **An insular view of anxiety.** *Biol Psychiatry* 2006, **60:**383 387.
29. Paulus MP, Stein MB: **Interoception in anxiety and depression.** *Brain Struct Funct* 2010, **214:**451 463.

Intolerance of uncertainty predicts fear extinction in amygdala-ventromedial prefrontal cortical circuitry

Jayne Morriss, Anastasia Christakou and Carien M. van Reekum[*]

Abstract

Background: Coordination of activity between the amygdala and ventromedial prefrontal cortex (vmPFC) is important for fear-extinction learning. Aberrant recruitment of this circuitry is associated with anxiety disorders. Here, we sought to determine if individual differences in future threat uncertainty sensitivity, a potential risk factor for anxiety disorders, underly compromised recruitment of fear extinction circuitry.

Twenty-two healthy subjects completed a cued fear conditioning task with acquisition and extinction phases. During the task, pupil dilation, skin conductance response, and functional magnetic resonance imaging were acquired. We assessed the temporality of fear extinction learning by splitting the extinction phase into early and late extinction. Threat uncertainty sensitivity was measured using self-reported intolerance of uncertainty (IU).

Results: During early extinction learning, we found low IU scores to be associated with larger skin conductance responses and right amygdala activity to learned threat vs. safety cues, whereas high IU scores were associated with no skin conductance discrimination and greater activity within the right amygdala to previously learned safety cues. In late extinction learning, low IU scores were associated with successful inhibition of previously learned threat, reflected in comparable skin conductance response and right amgydala activity to learned threat vs. safety cues, whilst high IU scores were associated with continued fear expression to learned threat, indexed by larger skin conductance and amygdala activity to threat vs. safety cues. In addition, high IU scores were associated with greater vmPFC activity to threat vs. safety cues in late extinction. Similar patterns of IU and extinction learning were found for pupil dilation. The results were specific for IU and did not generalize to self-reported trait anxiety.

Conclusions: Overall, the neural and psychophysiological patterns observed here suggest high IU individuals to disproportionately generalize threat during times of uncertainty, which subsequently compromises fear extinction learning. More broadly, these findings highlight the potential of intolerance of uncertainty-based mechanisms to help understand pathological fear in anxiety disorders and inform potential treatment targets.

Keywords: Intolerance of uncertainty, Fear extinction, Amygdala, Prefrontal, fMRI

Background

The modulation of affective responses to cues based on their current contextual relevance is crucial for preserving health and protecting against psychopathology [1–3]. Past animal and human research using classical fear conditioning paradigms has demonstrated an important role of the amygdala in fear acquisition and expression, and of the ventromedial prefrontal cortex (vmPFC) in fear extinction [4–6].

During fear acquisition, heightened amygdala activity and increased skin conductance have been observed in response to previously neutral cues that, through conditioning, come to be associated with aversive outcomes (conditioned stimulus, CS+, e.g. shock or tone) [4, 7, 8]. Subsequent extinction training, which involves repeated presentations of the CS+ without the aversive outcome, results in reduced amygdala and skin conductance responsivity over time [5, 9, 7]. The vmPFC is critical for the fear extinction process and the observed reduction in

* Correspondence: c.vanreekum@reading.ac.uk
Centre for Integrative Neuroscience and Neurodynamics, School of Psychology and Clinical Language Sciences, University of Reading, Earley Gate, Whiteknights Campus, RG6 6AH Reading, UK

amygdala and skin conductance responses to the CS+ over time [3]. For example, stimulation of the infralimbic cortex in rats, an area homologous to the human vmPFC, reduces responsiveness of amygdala neurons and defensive freezing behavior to conditioned tones [10]. In both humans and animals, increased vmPFC activity to the CS+ has been observed in late extinction phases [6, 11], and during subsequent extinction sessions, conducted a few days after initial fear acquisition [12, 13].

Current exposure therapies for anxiety disorders are based on fear extinction models. A large body of clinical and neurobiological research using fear extinction paradigms has shown that individuals with anxiety/trauma disorders are prone to delayed fear extinction learning or even resistance to fear extinction (for reviews see, [3, 14, 15]). For example, compared to healthy controls, anxiety patients show elevated autonomic nervous system and amygdala responding and reduced recruitment of the vmPFC to both threat and safety cues at the start of extinction and to threat cues across fear extinction learning [16, 11, 17, 18].

In addition to clinical samples, it is important to test fear extinction learning in non-clinically anxious individuals to appropriately separate those processes that are risk factors for anxiety disorder development from those that are consequential to an anxiety disorder. A series of recent studies have shown that individuals with high trait anxiety and genetic predisposition for anxiety exhibit the following: (1) exaggerated autonomic nervous system responding to both threat and safety cues in the early phase of extinction learning [9] and (2) sustained autonomic nervous system responding, sustained amygdala activation and atypical activation in the medial prefrontal cortex to threat cues from the early to late phase of fear extinction learning [19–21, 9]. Genetic evidence also points to similar temporal patterns of delayed fear extinction learning and increased risk for anxiety in both homozygote and heterozygote Met allele carriers of the brain-derived neurotrophic factor (BDNF) Val66Met genotype in mice [21–23] and humans [24, 21, 25]. Furthermore, both the phenotypic and genetic results in mice and humans appear to be specific to fear extinction learning rather than fear acquisition [19, 26, 20, 27, 21–24, 28], but see [27, 9], suggesting that individuals prone to developing an anxiety disorder have difficulty inhibiting learned threat cues and have a tendency to generalize threat to safety cues, rather than being more readily or strongly conditioned [26, 29].

Simple changes to the contingency at the start of fear extinction learning are inherently uncertain and ambiguous. Despite this, the majority of fear extinction studies have focused predominantly on self-reported trait anxiety [20, 19, 9] rather than self-reported intolerance of uncertainty (IU) [30], a key transdiagnostic factor in maintaining and mediating anxiety and depression [31–34]. IU is defined as a difficulty in accepting the possibility of future negative events, rendering ambiguous or even neutral cues as threatening. In the context of fear extinction learning, changes to contingency may exacerbate future threat uncertainty, resulting in threat responses to both learned threat and safety cues at the start of extinction, and continued threat responses to learned threat cues in late extinction for those individuals who find uncertainty anxiety-provoking. Given the extant literature, it seems pertinent to examine whether IU carries the association between trait anxiety and delayed fear extinction learning. Understanding associations between IU and fear extinction learning could help characterize IU-based maintenance of anxiety, with implications for targeted treatment [35, 34, 30].

Here, we used cued fear conditioning with acquisition and extinction phases to assess the relationship between individual differences in self-reported IU and in psychophysiological and neural correlates of fear extinction learning over time. We measured event-related fMRI, skin conductance response (SCR), pupil dilation and behavioral ratings whilst participants performed the conditioning task. We used an aversive sound as an unconditioned stimulus and visual shapes as conditioned stimuli, as in previous conditioning research [36, 13, 37, 19, 38, 4]. We hypothesized that, during extinction learning, threat uncertainty sensitivity would predict generalized fear expression to both learned threat and safety cues, and/or sustained fear expression to learned threat cues. Given that fear extinction paradigms are temporally sensitive [5, 13, 3, 21, 9, 20], we expected this effect to be indexed by the following: (1) larger responses in high IU individuals to both learned threat and safety cues in *early* fear extinction, across our physiological and behavioral measurements, including relatively higher amygdala activation; (2) sustained larger responses across measures in high IU individuals to learned threat cues vs. safety cues during *late* fear extinction. We further predicted (3) an association between vmPFC activation and the management of responses to threat vs. safety cues during extinction in low IU individuals. We tested the specificity of the involvement of IU by comparing it with broader measures of anxiety, such as Spielberger State-Trait Anxiety Inventory, Trait Version (STAIX-2) [39] and Penn State Worry Questionnaire (PSWQ) [40].

Methods

Participants

Twenty-two right-handed volunteers were recruited from the University of Reading and local area through advertizements (M age = 23.59, SD age = 2.75; 12 females and 10 males). All participants had normal or corrected to normal vision and were medication-free. Participants provided written informed consent and received a picture of their brain and £20 for their participation. The University of Reading's Research Ethics Committee approved the study protocol.

Conditioning task

Visual stimuli were presented through MRI-compatible VisualSystem head-coil mounted eye goggles (Nordic-NeuroLab, Bergen, Norway), which displayed stimuli at 60 Hz on an 800 × 600 pixel screen. Sound stimuli were presented through MRI-compatible AudioSystem headphones (NordicNeuroLab, Bergen, Norway). Participants used an MRI-compatible response box with their dominant right hand to respond.

Visual stimuli were blue and yellow squares with 183 × 183 pixel dimensions, resulting in a visual angle of 5.78° × 9.73°. The aversive sound stimulus consisted of a fear inducing female scream (sound number 277) from the International Affective Digitized Sound battery (IADS-2) and which has been normatively rated as unpleasant (M = 1.63, SD = 1.13) and arousing (M = 7.79, SD = 1.13) [41]. We used Audacity 2.0.3 software (http://audacity.sourceforge.net/) to shorten the female scream to 1000 ms in length and to amplify the sound by 15 dB, resulting in a 90-dB (±5 dB) sound.

The three learning phases were presented in three separate blocks. During the acquisition phase, one of two squares (i.e. blue or yellow, counterbalanced) was always paired with the aversive sound (CS+), whilst the other square was presented alone (CS–). In a subsequent extinction phase, both stimuli were presented unpaired (CS+, CS–). A third phase comprised partial reacquisition, where the CS+ square was paired with the sound 25 % of the time and the CS– remained unpaired (not reported here).

Participants were instructed to attend and listen to the stimulus presentations and provide a rating of the stimulus following each trial. The rating scale asked how 'uneasy' the participant felt after each stimulus presentation, where the scale ranged from 1 ('not at all') to 10 ('extremely').

The acquisition phase consisted of 24 trials (12 CS+, 12 CS–), the extinction phase 32 trials (16 CS+, 16 CS–) and the reacquisition phase 60 trials (8 CS+, 24 CS+_{unpaired}, 28 CS–; data not presented here) (see Fig. 1). Experimental trials were pseudo randomized into an order, which resulted in no more than three presentations of the same stimulus in a row. Colour-sound contingencies were counterbalanced across the sample.

Procedure

Participants arrived at the laboratory and were informed of the experimental procedures. First, participants completed a consent form as an agreement to take part in the study. Second, a hearing test was performed with an audiometer to check for normative hearing (e.g. 500–8000 Hz, below 30 dB). Third, participants completed a battery of cognitive tasks (results not reported here) and questionnaires on a computer outside of the scanner. Next, participants were taken to the MRI unit. We used a conditioning task inside the scanner, whilst concurrently recording ratings, electrodermal activity and pupil dilation. Participants were simply instructed to: (1) maintain attention to the task by looking and listening to the colored squares and sounds presented, (2) respond to the uneasiness scale using the button box and (3) to keep as still as possible. After scanning, participants rated the sound stimulus outside of the scanner.

Questionnaires

To assess emotional disposition, we presented the following six questionnaires on a computer: two versions of the Positive and Negative Affect Scales (PANAS-NOW; PANAS-GEN) [42], Spielberger State-Trait Anxiety Inventory, Trait Version (STAIX-2) [39], PSWQ [40], IU [43] and the Barratt Impulsiveness Scale (BIS-11) [44]. We focused on IU because of the intrinsic uncertainty within conditioning paradigms. Similar distributions and internal reliability of scores were found for the anxiety measures, IU (M = 53.04; SD = 15.68; range 27–85; α = .90), STAIX-2 (M = 40.33; SD = 7.92; range = 27–53; α = .85) and PSWQ

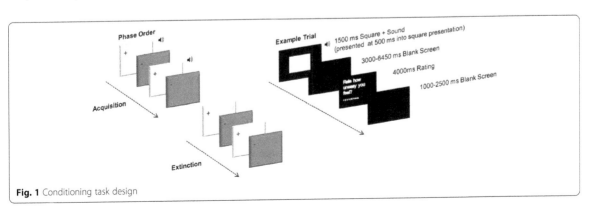

Fig. 1 Conditioning task design

(M = 41.47; SD = 11.10; range = 20–65; α = .90). We collected the other questionnaires to check for correlational consistency and specificity across anxiety measures as well as to check for outlying values on IU due to mood or impulsivity.

Sound stimulus rating
Participants rated the valence and arousal of the sound stimulus using 9-point Likert scales ranging from 1 (valence: negative; arousal: calm) to 9 (valence: positive; arousal: excited).

Behavioral data scoring and reduction
Rating data from the conditioning task were reduced for each participant by calculating their average responses for each experimental condition. Missing data points were excluded.

Physiological acquisition and reduction
Electrodermal recordings were obtained using ADInstruments (ADInstruments Ltd., Chalgrove, Oxfordshire) hardware and software. An ML138 Bio Amp connected to an ML870 PowerLab Unit Model 8/30 amplified the EDA signal, which were digitized through a 16-bit A/D converter at 1000 Hz. EDA was measured during the scanning session with MRI-safe MLT117F Ag/AgCl bipolar finger electrodes filled with NaCl electrolyte paste (Mansfield R & D, St Albans, Vermont, USA) that were attached to the distal phalanges of the index and middle fingers of the left hand. A constant voltage of 22 mV/ms at 75 Hz was passed through the electrodes, which were connected to a ML116 GSR Amp. SCR were scored when there was an increase of skin conductance level exceeding 0.03 microSiemens. The amplitude of each response was scored as the difference between the onset and the maximum deflection prior to the signal flattening out or decreasing. SCR onsets had to be within 7 s following each trial to be included. Trials with no discernible SCRs were scored zero. The first trial of each experimental phase was excluded, to reduce contamination of averages from the orienting response. SCR amplitudes were square root transformed to reduce skew. Trials with motion artefacts were discarded from the analysis. SCR magnitudes were calculated from remaining trials by averaging SCR square-root-transformed values for each condition.

Pupil dilation was recorded at a sample rate of 60 Hz through a built-in infrared camera on the head-coil mounted eye goggles (NordicNeuroLab, Bergen, Norway). PD data was averaged for each 1000 ms window following stimulus onset, resulting in five windows of 1000 ms each. These data were baseline corrected by subtracting 1000 ms preceding each stimulus onset from a blank screen. Trials were averaged per condition and time window for each participant.

Learning assessment
To assess whether participants learned the association between the neutral cue and aversive sound, we calculated conditioned response scores for behavioral ratings, pupil dilation and SCR magnitude in extinction. The conditioned response score was the first 2 CS+ trials and the first 2 CS− trials. A positive score indicated a larger response for CS+ vs. CS−, indexing successful conditioning. This type of learning assessment procedure is commonly reported in the fear extinction literature [30, 11, 6, 13]. To reduce subject attrition, we labelled subjects as learners if they had a positive conditioned response score for any measure. Based on the learning assessment criterion, we identified four potential non-learners out of the 22 participants. Since removing the data of these four subjects did not change the results reported here,[1] we retained the data of all participants.

Ratings and psychophysiology analysis
IU differences across extinction were assessed by conducting a condition (CS+, CS−) × time (early, late) × IU repeated measures ANCOVA for behavioral ratings, SCR magnitude and pupil dilation. IU was entered as a continuous mean centered predictor variable. The early part of extinction was defined as the first eight CS+ and eight CS− trials, and the last part of extinction was defined as the last eight CS+ and eight CS− trials. For pupil dilation, which was based on second-by-second averaging, we also included the factor window with five levels representing seconds post-stimulus onset. To check for specificity of findings with IU in extinction, we conducted a condition (CS+, CS−) × window × IU repeated measures ANCOVA on behavioral ratings, SCR magnitude and pupil dilation obtained in the acquisition phase.

We performed hierarchical regression analyses on the resulting significant SCR magnitude and pupil dilation difference scores (CS+ − CS− early; CS+ − CS− late; CS+ early − CS+ late; CS− early − CS− late) for extinction and the anxiety measures to test for IU-specific effects. We entered STAIX-2 and PSWQ in the first step and then IU in the second step.

MRI
Participants were scanned with a 3T Siemens Trio set up with a 12-channel head coil (Siemens Inc., Erlangen, Germany). Three T2*-weighted echo planar imaging (EPI) functional scans were acquired for each phase of the conditioning task consisting of 161, 208, and 380 volumes, respectively (TR = 2000 ms, TE = 30 ms, flip angle = 90°, FOV = 192 × 192 mm, 3 × 3 mm voxels, slice thickness 3 mm with an interslice gap of 1 mm, 30 axial slices, interleaved acquisition).

Following completion of the functional scans, fieldmap and structural scans were acquired, which comprised of a high-resolution T1-weighted anatomical scan (MP-RAGE, TR = 2020 ms, TE = 2.52 ms, flip angle = 90°, FOV = 256 × 256 mm, 1 × 1 × 1 mm voxels, slice thickness 1 mm, sagittal slices), two fieldmaps (TR = 488 ms, TE 1 = 4.98 ms, TE 2 = 7.38 ms, flip angle = 60°, FOV = 256 × 256 mm, slice thickness 4 mm with an interslice gap of 4 mm, 30 axial slices) and diffusion weighted images, which will not be further discussed here (TR = 6800 ms, TE = 93 ms, flip angle = 60°, FOV = 192 × 192 mm, slice thickness 2 mm with an interslice gap of 2 mm, b-value = 1000, 64 axial slices, 30 diffusion gradients).

fMRI analysis

FMRI analyses were carried out in Feat version 5.98 as part of FSL (FMRIB's Software Library, www.fmrib.ox. ac.uk/fsl). Brains were extracted from their respective T1 images by using the FSL brain extraction tool (BET) [45]. Distortion, slice timing and motion correction were applied to all extracted EPI volumes using FUGUE and MCFLIRT tools. Gaussian smoothing (FWHM 5 mm) and a 50 s high pass temporal filter were applied.

A first-level GLM analysis was carried out for each functional scan run from acquisition and extinction. Separate regressors were specified for the experimental conditions of primary interest in each learning phase (acquisition: CS+>CS−, extinction: CS+>CS−) by convolving a binary boxcar function with an ideal haemodynamic response (HR), which corresponded to the length of each trial (1500 ms). Regressors for the uneasiness rating period and six motion parameters were included to model out brain activity that was unrelated to the conditions of interest.

We defined two main effect contrasts to reveal fear extinction-related activity. To examine temporal effects across extinction, we contrasted (CS+ vs. CS−)$_{early}$ > (CS+ vs. CS−)$_{late}$. We defined early extinction as the first eight trials for CS+ and CS− and the last eight trials for CS+ and CS−. Particular focus is given to the temporal effects across extinction, given our predictions. We also examined the overall effect of CS+ vs. CS− during extinction for comparison against the extant literature. All contrasts were normalized and registered to MNI standard space using FLIRT [46]. Second-level GLM analysis consisted of regressors for the group mean and demeaned IU scores using FSL's FLAME stage 1 + 2 procedure. Whole-brain analysis was carried out using cluster thresholding with a z = 2.3 and a corrected p < 0.05.

We were specifically interested in the extent to which IU scores would be associated with the BOLD response in the amygdala and vmPFC for early and late extinction phases. Therefore, we performed small volume corrections on the left amygdala, right amygdala and vmPFC using cluster thresholding with a z = 2.3 and a corrected

p < 0.05 on the IU × (CS+ vs. CS−)$_{early}$ > (CS+ vs. CS−)$_{late}$ extinction contrast map. We used anatomically defined masks from the Harvard-Oxford cortical and subcortical structural atlases in FSL [47]. We selected the left amygdala, right amygdala and frontal medial cortex regions with a 50 % probability threshold. For control purposes, we also applied small volume corrections within the left amygdala, right amygdala and vmPFC on the IU × acquisition CS+ vs. CS− and the IU × extinction CS+ vs. CS− contrast maps.

To assess fear expression correspondence between the amygdala and psychophysiology measures, we correlated percent BOLD signal response from significant amygdala regions and SCR magnitude/pupil dilation.

We performed hierarchical regression analyses on the resulting statistical a priori regions of interest difference scores from extinction (CS+ − CS− early; CS+ − CS− late; CS+ early − CS+ late; CS− early − CS− late) and the anxiety measures to test for IU-specific effects, STAIX-2 and PSWQ in the first and then IU in the second step.

Results

One participant's data were removed from all analyses due to having an extreme IU score that was +3 SD from the group mean.

Questionnaires

As expected, the anxiety measures were positively correlated with each other, suggesting shared variance, IU with PSWQ, r(19) = .590, p = .005, IU with STAIX-2, r(19) = .619, p = .003, and PSWQ with STAIX-2, r(19) = .657, p = .001.

Ratings

Participants rated the sound stimulus serving as the US as negative (M = 3.52, SD = 1.63) and moderately arousing (M = 5.23, SD = 2.14). With respect to the uneasiness ratings (on a scale from 1 to 10), a main effect of condition was found for acquisition across all individuals, F(1,19) = 13.394, p = .002. During acquisition, participants significantly reported feeling more uneasy for the CS+ relative to the CS− trials, p = .002 (for descriptive statistics, see Table 1). We found no effect of condition or condition × time for the uneasiness ratings during extinction, p's > .1, F's < 1 (see Table 1). Results revealed no IU differences for uneasiness ratings for any of the experimental phases, p's > .3, F's > .1, max F = 1.015.

SCR magnitude

Seven subjects were removed from the SCR magnitude analysis due to six subjects not responding, which is not uncommon when recorded in an MRI setting (see 'Methods' section), and one subject with a recording error.

Table 1 Summary of means (SD) for each dependent measure as a function of condition and phase

Measure	Acquisition		Extinction		Early extinction		Late extinction	
	CS+	CS−	CS+	CS−	CS+	CS−	CS+	CS−
Physiological								
Square root transformed SCR magnitude (μS)	.27 (.17)**	.13 (.11)**	.16 (.13)*	.13 (.12)*	.20 (.17)	.14 (.11)	.13 (.14)	.11 (.14)
Pupil dilation (Δmm)	−.023 (.010)	−.024 (.010)	−.025 (.008)	−.024 (.013)	−.027 (.015)	−.026 (.018)	−.023 (.008)	−.023 (.022)
Behavioral								
Uneasiness rating (1–9)	3.61 (1.93)**	2.09 (1.50)**	1.67 (1.23)	1.75 (1.32)	1.84 (1.27)	1.88 (1.42)	1.49 (1.38)	1.41 (1.31)

Note: SCR magnitude (μS), skin conductance magnitude is measured in microSiemens. Pupil dilation (Δmm) is measured in delta millimetres. Significant comparisons are specified with *$p < .05$ and **$p < .01$

As expected, larger SCR magnitudes were found for CS+ vs. CS− during acquisition, $F(1,12) = 14.376$, $p = .003$ (see Table 1), but there was no interaction between condition × IU, $F(1,12) = .564$, $p = .467$.

During extinction, we found greater SCR magnitude for the CS+ vs. CS−, $F(1,12) = 5.369$, $p = .039$ (see Table 1), but no significant interaction effect between condition and time, $F(1,12) = 1.711$, $p = .215$. However, as predicted, we found a significant condition × time × IU interaction, $F(1,12) = 8.782$, $p = .012$. Further inspection of follow-up pairwise comparisons for early vs. late extinction at IU ±1 SD from the mean revealed that at the low IU end (1 SD below the IU mean) is associated with the commonly reported extinction pattern, including discrimination between CS+ and CS− in early extinction, $p = .026$, but no significant differences between CS+ and CS− in late extinction, $p = .139$ (see Fig. 2a). Furthermore, low IU is associated with a reduction in SCR magnitude to the CS+ from early to late extinction, $p = .006$, but not to the CS− from early to late extinction, $p = .425$. High IU (captured at 1 SD above the mean) is associated with the opposite pattern, with no significant differences between CS+ and CS− in early extinction, $p = .586$, but discrimination between CS+ and CS− in late extinction, $p = .014$ (see Fig. 2a). In addition, high IU is not associated with differences in SCR magnitude between CS+ from early to late extinction, $p = .525$, and CS− from early to late extinction, $p = .582$. No other significant main effects or interactions were found with IU, max $F = 3.552$, p's > .08.

We conducted hierarchical regression analyses on the effects that were significant in the ANCOVA above, creating difference scores by subtracting response to CS− from CS+. Hierarchical regression analyses of early and late SCR magnitude difference scores in extinction revealed mixed specificity with IU over the STAIX-2 and PSWQ measures: (1) CS+ − CS− early extinction, first step: $R^2 = .409$, $F(2,11) = 1.108$, $p = .364$, second step: $\Delta R^2 = .419$, $F(1,10) = .101$, $p = .757$, second step: (2) CS+ − CS− late extinction, first step: $R^2 = .390$, $F(2,11) = .986$, $p = .404$, second step: $\Delta R^2 = .755$, $F(1,10) = 9.737$ $p = .011$, and (3) CS+ early − CS+ late extinction, first step: $R^2 = .620$, $F(2,11) = 3.426$, $p = .70$, second step: $\Delta R^2 = .664$, $F(1,10) = 1.023$, $p = .336$.

Pupil dilation

One subject was removed from the pupil dilation analysis due to a recording error, leaving 20 participants. No effect of acquisition or extinction was found for the whole sample, p's > .1, Fs < .2, max $F = 1.615$ (see Table 1). We found a significant condition × time × IU interaction for pupil dilation during extinction, $F(1,18) = 7.921$, $p = .011$. Follow-up pairwise comparisons for early vs. late at IU ±1 SD from the mean showed this effect to be driven by high IU scores, which were associated with greater relative pupil constriction for CS− relative to CS+ at trend during early extinction, $p = .052$, but did not display significant differences between CS+ and CS− in late extinction, $p = .134$ (see Fig. 2b). Furthermore, high IU was characterized by an increase in pupil constriction to the CS+ from early to late extinction at trend, $p = .057$, but not to the CS− from early to late extinction, $p = .167$. Low IU scores (1 SD below the mean) were not associated with significant differences between condition and time, p's > .065 (see Fig. 2b). No other significant interactions were found with IU, p's > .1, max $F = 1.817$.

Following up on the significant effects from the ANCOVA above, hierarchical regression analyses of early and late pupil dilation difference scores in extinction revealed specificity for IU over the STAIX-2 and PSWQ measures: (1) CS+ − CS− early extinction, first step: $R^2 = .246$, $F(2,17) = .547$, $p = .589$, second step: $\Delta R^2 = .646$, $F(1,16) = 9.772$, $p = .007$, (2) CS+ early − CS+ late extinction, first step: $R^2 = .075$, $F(2,17) = .048$, $p = .953$, second step: $\Delta R^2 = .476$, $F(1,16) = 4.565$, $p = .048$.

fMRI

Likely because we had a large individual variation in response patterns during extinction, our whole-brain analyses did not yield significant BOLD differences in our a priori brain regions of interest often reported in the extinction literature [4, 5, 13, 6].[2] We did, however, find greater lateral occipital cortex and parietal lobule activation

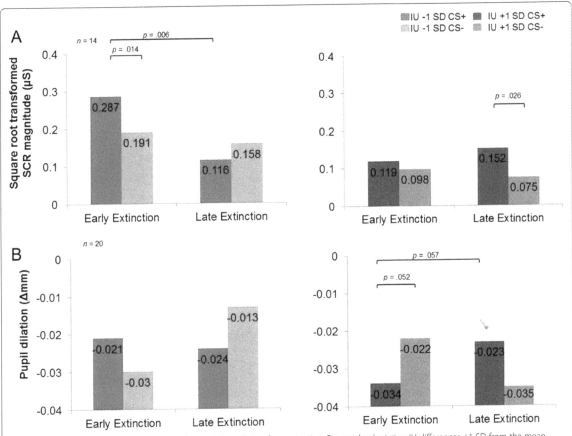

Fig. 2 Intolerance of uncertainty predicts psychophysiology during fear extinction. Bar graphs depicting IU differences ±1 SD from the mean during early and late extinction learning. **a** SCR magnitude and **b** pupil dilation. Low IU were associated with significantly greater SCR magnitude responses to CS+ vs. CS− in early extinction and no differences between stimuli in late extinction. High IU scorers showed no differences in SCR magnitude to CS+ and CS− stimuli in early extinction, and delayed discrimination in SCR magnitude to CS+ vs. CS− in late extinction. The pupil dilation results followed a similar pattern to the SCR magnitude results, albeit at trend. SCR magnitude (μS), skin conductance magnitude measured in microSiemens; Pupil dilation (Δmm) measured in delta millimetres

across extinction for the CS+ > CS− (see Table 2) as well as greater occipital pole activation in early extinction for the CS+ > CS−, relative to late extinction for the CS+ > CS−, suggesting increased attention for the conditioned stimulus.

As expected, areas within the right amygdala and the vmPFC significantly correlated with IU scores during extinction (see Table 2, Figs. 3 and 4). We performed follow-up correlations to identify the source of the interaction effect from the significant IU × (CS+ vs. CS−)$_{early}$ > (CS+ vs. CS−)$_{late}$ contrast. During early extinction, higher IU predicted increased activation to the CS−, relative to CS+ for the right amygdala cluster, $r(19) = −.58$, $p = .005$ (see Fig. 3). There were no significant effects of IU in the vmPFC cluster during early extinction however, $r(19) = −0.106$, $p = .646$. During late extinction, IU was positively associated with activation to the CS+ relative to the CS− for the right amygdala cluster, $r(19) = .47$,

$p = .030$ (see Fig. 3), and, unexpectedly, for the vmPFC cluster, $r(19) = .62$, $p = .002$ (see Fig. 4). In addition, higher IU predicted relative higher right amygdala activity from CS− early to CS− late, $r(19) = .631$, $p = .002$, suggesting generalization of threat to the CS− at the start of extinction. All other condition and time difference scores were not significant for the right amygdala and vmPFC, p's > .125. Furthermore, the BOLD response in areas associated with vigilance, such as the opercular cortex, cingulate gyrus, lateral occipital cortex and precentral gyrus, significantly differed over time as a function of IU scores during extinction (see Table 2).

A hierarchical regression analysis confirmed the significant extinction difference scores from the right amygdala and vmPFC were specific to IU vs. STAIX-2 and PSWQ; adding IU in the second step significantly improved the model: (1) right amygdala for CS+ − CS− early extinction, first step: $R^2 = .191$, $F(2,18) = .2.123$, $p = .149$, second step:

Table 2 Significant activation patterns in a priori regions of interest and other brain regions during extinction

Extinction	Brain region	BA	Voxels (mm³)	Max Z	Location of max Z		
					x	y	z
A priori regions							
(CS+ > CS−)$_{early}$ > (CS+ > CS−)$_{late}$ × IU	R amygdala		33	2.96	26	−8	−12
(CS− > CS+)$_{early}$ > (CS− > CS+)$_{late}$ × IU	R L vmPFC	10	40	2.92	−8	42	−16
Outside a priori regions							
CS+ > CS−	L lateral occipital cortex, inferior parietal lobule	7/39	439	3.31	−38	−60	44
(CS+ > CS−)$_{early}$ > (CS+ > CS−)$_{late}$	R occipital pole	18	643	3.88	34	−94	2
(CS− > CS+)$_{early}$ > (CS− > CS+)$_{late}$	R precentral gyrus, postcentral gyrus	3–4/6	504	3.49	38	−24	38
(CS− > CS+)$_{early}$ > (CS− > CS+)$_{late}$ × IU	Cingulate gyrus, juxtapositional lobule, precentral gyrus, postcentral gyrus, parietal lobule	3–7/40	4267	3.99	−2	−8	60
(CS− > CS+)$_{early}$ > (CS− > CS+)$_{late}$ × IU	R central opercular cortex	6	361	3.16	56	−2	6
(CS− > CS+)$_{early}$ > (CS− > CS+)$_{late}$ × IU	L parietal operculum cortex	40	304	3.16	−52	−28	14
(CS− > CS+)$_{early}$ > (CS− > CS+)$_{late}$ × IU	R parietal operculum cortex	40	292	3.33	56	−26	18
(CS− > CS+)$_{early}$ > (CS− > CS+)$_{late}$ × IU	L cerebellum		274	3.29	12	−70	−18
(CS− > CS+)$_{early}$ > (CS− > CS+)$_{late}$ × IU	R lateral occipital cortex	37	259	3.23	46	−60	−8

Note: clusters for small volume corrected a priori regions and whole-brain corrected regions outside a priori regions corrected for multiple comparisons at $p <$ 0.05. Location of cluster's maximum Z are in MNI space. BA Brodmann areas, R right, L left

$\Delta R^2 = .404$, $F(1,17) = 6.090$, $p = .025$, (2) right amygdala for CS+ − CS− late extinction, first step: $R^2 = .099$, $F(2,18) = .987$, $p = .392$, second step: $\Delta R^2 = .237$, $F(1,17) = 3.067$, $p = .098$, (3) right amygdala CS− early vs. CS− late extinction, first step: $R^2 = .334$, $F(2,18) = 1.127$, $p = .346$, second step: $\Delta R^2 = .642$, $F(1,17) = 8.692$, $p = .009$, and (4) vmPFC for CS+ vs. CS− late extinction, first step: $R^2 = .122$, $F(2,18) = 1.255$, $p = .309$, second step: $\Delta R^2 = .396$, $F(1,17) = 7.694$, $p = .013$.

We found no significant effects of IU during acquisition on a whole-brain basis or within the a priori ROIs. Furthermore, we found no significant effects of IU across the entire extinction phase (early and late collapsed) on a whole-brain basis, nor within the a priori ROIs.

Relationships between right amygdala and psychophysiology

Percent BOLD signal difference (CS+ vs. CS−) in the right amygdala correlated positively with SCR magnitude during early, $r(12) = .540$, $p = .046$, and late extinction, $r(12) = .652$, $p = .012$.(see Fig. 5). Percent BOLD signal in the right amygdala was not correlated with pupil dilation during early extinction, $r(18) = .540$, $p = .246$, but did correlate positively during late extinction, $r(18) = .540$, $p = .052$ (see Fig. 5).

Relationships between a priori ROIs and ratings

Uneasiness rating difference scores for early and late fear extinction did not significantly correlate with percent BOLD signal difference scores for early and late extinction in the a priori ROIs, p's > .35.

Discussion

We show that self-reported IU, a personality trait implicated in the maintenance of anxiety and depressive disorders [32, 33, 31], predicts psychophysiological and neural recruitment during fear extinction learning. Our data suggest that individuals who are sensitive to threat uncertainty (high IU) are prone to generalize threat, and have difficulty inhibiting learned threat cues, as indexed by heightened psychophysiology and by amygdala and vmPFC function during fear extinction learning. Importantly, our results highlight threat uncertainty sensitivity as a potential factor in the maintenance of extinction-resistant fear, seen in anxiety disorders. Furthermore, these fMRI results were specific to an association between extinction and IU, and did not generalize to other anxiety measures (STAIX-2, PSWQ) or associative learning phases (acquisition).

In early extinction, low IU was characterized by a discrimination of threat and safety cues, consistent with previous fear extinction studies [13, 6, 11] where SCR magnitude and right amygdala response was larger to threat cues, relative to safety cues. Expanding previous research on individual differences in trait anxiety [21, 19, 20, 9, 28, 27] and IU [30], high IU was associated with fear expression to both learned threat and safety cues in early extinction, indexed by indiscriminate SCR magnitude. Furthermore, high IU was associated with larger pupil dilation (at trend) and right amygdala activity to safety vs. threat cues in early extinction. These results suggest potential spill over of learned threat to safety cues in those who are sensitive to future threat uncertainty.

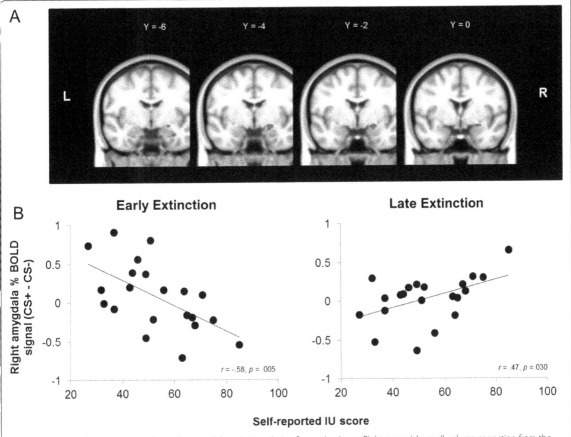

Fig. 3 Intolerance of uncertainty predicts right amygdala activation during fear extinction. **a** Right amygdala small volume correction from the $(CS- > CS+)_{early} > (CS- > CS+)_{late} \times IU$ contrast in extinction. **b** Significant correlations between percent signal change in the right amygdala for $CS+ - CS-$ and IU scores during early and late extinction. High IU was associated with threat-like responses in the amygdala to CS− in early extinction and to CS+ in late extinction. These findings suggest high IU scorers generalize threat when faced with uncertainty, resulting in compromised safety learning. MNI coordinates: *R* right, *L* left

During late extinction, low IU predicted reduced SCR magnitude and right amygdala activity to threat vs. safety cues, suggesting successful fear extinction, in line with previous extinction research [13, 11, 6]. However, high IU predicted larger SCR magnitude, pupil dilation (at trend) and right amygdala to threat vs. safety cues during late extinction, suggesting sustained fear expression to learned threat cues. Although we predicted low IU to be associated with increased vmPFC recruitment to threat vs. safety cues during early extinction, we instead found that high IU was associated with increased vmPFC activation in response to threat vs. safety cues in late extinction. Whilst this pattern was not predicted, it is similar to previous studies that report hyperactivity of the prefrontal cortex during fear extinction for trait anxious individuals [19] and during emotion regulation tasks for depressed patients [48]. Overall, these findings suggest that high IU is associated with slower discrimination of threat from safety cues, which subsequently compromises fear extinction learning.

Notably, we found the fear extinction learning results to be specific to IU, over other broader measures of trait anxiety and worry (STAIX-X2 and PSWQ). The specificity of IU was strongly supported by neural indices and partially supported in SCR magnitude and pupil dilation. Crucially, these results suggest uncertainty to be an important factor in maintaining learned fearful associations and hindering the formation of new safety associations. Furthermore, these data provide initial evidence that uncertainty may be the driver behind previous trait anxiety and fear extinction learning findings [19–21, 9]. These results call for further study of the neural basis underlying uncertainty-based maintenance of anxiety disorders, which may prove useful for clinicians in improving and developing therapies.

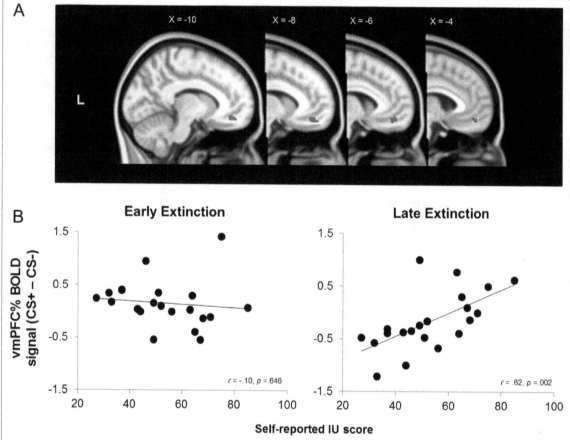

Fig. 4 Intolerance of uncertainty predicts vmPFC activation during fear extinction. **a** vmPFC small volume correction from the (CS– > CS+)$_{early}$ > (CS– > CS+)$_{late}$ × IU contrast in extinction. **b** Significant correlations between percent signal change in the vmPFC for CS+ – CS– and IU scores during early and late extinction. During late extinction, high IU scores were associated with increased recruitment of the vmPFC to the CS+, relative to the CS–, suggesting attempts to down regulate fearful associations. MNI coordinates: R right, L left

We found no evidence of IU predicting differential recruitment of brain regions involved in fear acquisition for the threat and safety cues. However, we used a 100 % reinforcement schedule in the acquisition phase, where the CS+ and US are confounded. Furthermore, the 100 % reinforcement schedule is very certain and unambiguous. Therefore, high IU individuals are not generally more aroused to the US and do not generalize fear to CS– cues during acquisition, at least during 100 % reinforcement. Further work needs to specifically test whether high IU individuals also show discriminatory deficits during the acquisition of conditioned fear [30].

Individual differences in IU were reflected in physiological and brain indices during extinction. However, self-reported arousal ratings did not reflect individual differences in IU in our sample. Divergence between self-reported and neural measures are often reported, perhaps due to lack of direct mapping between behavior and brain activity or to a lack of sensitivity of self-report metrics to

capture such individual differences. Interestingly, neural indices during fear extinction were better predicted by IU, over self-reported uneasiness ratings. Such findings suggest IU to be a more suitable predictor of neutral activity during fear extinction than moment-to-moment subjective ratings of uneasiness. However, the lack of relationship between neural activity and subjective ratings may be simply due to the time between phasic cue events and rating periods.

Conclusions

We found individual differences in IU to specifically predict fear extinction capacity and associated responsivity in psychophysiology and amygdala-vmPFC circuitry. Individuals with high IU scores exhibited exaggerated amygdala and psychophysiology responses to both threat and safety cues during fear extinction. These findings suggest reduced flexibility in amygdala-vmPFC circuitry for high IU individuals. Importantly, these results were specific to

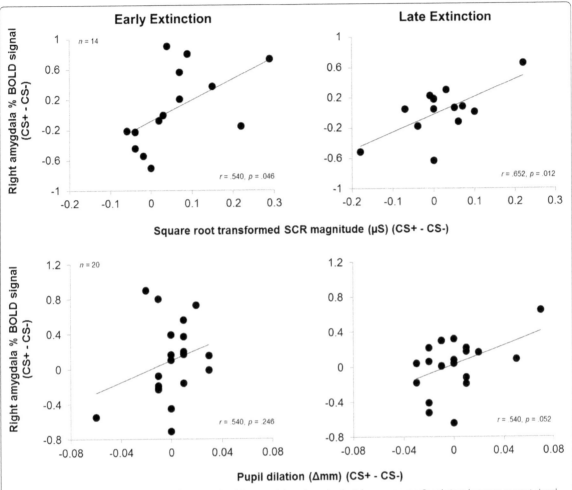

Fig. 5 Correlations between percent signal change in the right amygdala and psychophysiology measures. Correlations between percent signal change in the right amygdala and psychophysiology measures. The response in the right amygdala is significantly correlated with SCR magnitude and at trend with pupil dilation, suggesting correspondence between measures of fear expression. SCR magnitude (μS), skin conductance magnitude measured in microSiemens; pupil dilation (Δmm) measured in delta millimetres

IU, highlighting an opportunity for further examination of IU in relation to: (1) current exposure-based therapies, and (2) focused forms of anxiety disorder treatment that target uncertainty-based maintenance of anxiety/fear, such as intolerance of uncertainty therapy [34, 35].

Endnotes

[1] Results do not change when non-learners are removed: the main effect of condition for SCR magnitude during fear extinction learning, without non-learners $F(1,10) = 7.624$, $p = .020$. Condition × time × IU interaction for SCR magnitude during fear extinction learning without non-learners, $F(1,10) = 8.380$, $p = .016$. Extinction CS+ – CS– difference scores for early and late extinction in the right amygdala correlated with IU: early extinction

without non-learners, $r(15) = -.66$, $p = .003$. Late extinction without non-learners, $r(15) = .71$, $p = .001$.

[2] The CS+ > CS– contrast map revealed vmPFC (approx. 20 voxels) and left amygdala (approx. 4 voxels) clusters at sub-threshold, $z = 2.0$, $p = .045$.

Abbreviations

Ag/AgCl: silver/silver chloride; ANCOVA: analysis of covariance; BOLD: blood oxygenation level dependent; CS+/CS: conditioned stimulus; EPI: echo planar imaging; FLAME: FMRIB's local analysis of mixed effects; FLIRT: FMRIB's linear image registration tool; FMRI: functional magnetic resonance imaging; FMRIB: Oxford Centre for Functional Magnetic Resonance Imaging of the Brain; FOV: field of view; FSL: FMRIB software library; FUGUE: FMRIB's utility for geometrically unwarping EPIs; GLM: general linear model; IADS-2: international affective digitized sound battery 2; IU: intolerance of uncertainty; M: mean; MCFLIRT: motion correction using FMRIB's linear image registration tool; MNI: Montreal neurological institute; PSWQ: Penn State Worry Questionnaire; SCR: skin conductance response; SD: standard deviation; STAIX-2: Spielberger State-Trait Anxiety Inventory; TR: repetition time; vmPFC: ventromedial prefrontal cortex.

Competing interests

The authors declare that they have no competing interests.

Authors' contributions

JM carried out the study, performed the statistical analyses and drafted the manuscript. JM, AC and CvR designed the study. AC and CvR revised the manuscript. All authors read and approved the final manuscript.

Acknowledgements

This research was supported by the Centre for Integrative Neuroscience and Neurodynamics (CINN) at the University of Reading and by a Medical Research Council (MRC) doctoral studentship (MR/J003980/1) awarded to Jayne Morriss. The authors thank the participants who took part in this study and members of the CINN, Dave Johnson, BJ Casey, and the reviewers of the manuscript for their advice. For inquires about access to the data, please contact Jayne Morriss and Carien van Reekum.

References

1. Davidson RJ. Affective style and affective disorders: perspectives from affective neuroscience. Cognition & Emotion. 1998;12(3):307–30.
2. Frijda NH. The emotions. Cambridge: Cambridge University Press; 1986.
3. Milad MR, Quirk GJ. Fear extinction as a model for translational neuroscience: ten years of progress. Annu Rev Psych. 2012;63:129–51.
4. Büchel C, Morris J, Dolan RJ, Friston KJ. Brain systems mediating aversive conditioning: an event-related fMRI study. Neuron. 1998;20(5):947–57.
5. LaBar KS, Gatenby JC, Gore JC, LeDoux JE, Phelps EA. Human amygdala activation during conditioned fear acquisition and extinction: a mixed-trial fMRI study. Neuron. 1998;20:937–45.
6. Milad MR, Wright CI, Orr SP, Pitman RK, Quirk GJ, Rauch SL. Recall of fear extinction in humans activates the ventromedial prefrontal cortex and hippocampus in concert. Bio Psych. 2007;62(5):446–54.
7. Knight DC, Smith CN, Cheng DT, Stein EA, Helmstetter FJ. Amygdala and hippocampal activity during acquisition and extinction of human fear conditioning. Cogn Affect Behav Neurosci. 2004;4(3):317–25.
8. Neumann DL, Waters AM, Westbury HR. The use of an unpleasant sound as the unconditional stimulus in aversive Pavlovian conditioning experiments that involve children and adolescent participants. Behav Res Methods. 2008;40(2):622–5.
9. Gazendam FJ, Kamphuis JH, Kindt M. Deficient safety learning characterizes high trait anxious individuals. Biol Psychol. 2013;92(2):342–52.
10. Milad MR, Quirk GJ. Neurons in medial prefrontal cortex signal memory for fear extinction. Nature. 2002;420(6911):70–4.
11. Milad MR, Pitman RK, Ellis CB, Gold AL, Shin LM, Lasko NB, et al. Neurobiological basis of failure to recall extinction memory in posttraumatic stress disorder. Biol Psychiatry. 2009;66(12):1075–82.
12. Kalisch R, Korenfeld E, Stephan KE, Weiskopf N, Seymour B, Dolan RJ. Context-dependent human extinction memory is mediated by a ventromedial prefrontal and hippocampal network. J Neurosci. 2006;26(37):9503–11.
13. Phelps EA, Delgado MR, Nearing KI, LeDoux JE. Extinction learning in humans: role of the amygdala and vmPFC. Neuron. 2004;43(6):897–905.
14. Graham BM, Milad MR. The study of fear extinction: implications for anxiety disorders. Am J Psych. 2011;168(12):1255–65.
15. Etkin A, Wager TD. Functional neuroimaging of anxiety: a meta-analysis of emotional processing in PTSD, social anxiety disorder, and specific phobia. Am J Psych. 2007;164(10):1476.
16. Milad MR, Orr SP, Lasko NB, Chang Y, Rauch SL, Pitman RK. Presence and acquired origin of reduced recall for fear extinction in PTSD: results of a twin study. J Psychiatr Res. 2008;42(7):515–20.
17. Blechert J, Michael T, Vriends N, Margraf J, Wilhelm FH. Fear conditioning in posttraumatic stress disorder: evidence for delayed extinction of autonomic, experiential, and behavioural responses. Behav Res Ther. 2007;45(9):2019–33.
18. Michael T, Blechert J, Vriends N, Margraf J, Wilhelm FH. Fear conditioning in panic disorder: enhanced resistance to extinction. J Abnorm Psychol. 2007;116(3):612.
19. Barrett J, Armony J. Influence of trait anxiety on brain activity during the acquisition and extinction of aversive conditioning. Psychol Med. 2009;39(02):255–65.
20. Sehlmeyer C, Dannlowski U, Schöning S, Kugel H, Pyka M, Pfleiderer B, et al. Neural correlates of trait anxiety in fear extinction. Psychol Med. 2011;41(04):789–98.
21. Soliman F, Glatt CE, Bath KG, Levita L, Jones RM, Pattwell SS, et al. A genetic variant BDNF polymorphism alters extinction learning in both mouse and human. Science. 2010;327(5967):863–6.
22. Chen Z-Y, Jing D, Bath KG, Ieraci A, Khan T, Siao C-J, et al. Genetic variant BDNF (Val66Met) polymorphism alters anxiety-related behavior. Science. 2006;314(5796):140–3.
23. Yu H, Wang Y, Pattwell S, Jing D, Liu T, Zhang Y, et al. Variant BDNF Val66Met polymorphism affects extinction of conditioned aversive memory. J Neuro. 2009;29(13):4056–64.
24. Felmingham KL, Dobson-Stone C, Schofield PR, Quirk GJ, Bryant RA. The brain-derived neurotrophic factor Val66Met polymorphism predicts response to exposure therapy in posttraumatic stress disorder. Biol Psychiatry. 2013;73(11):1059–63.
25. Zhang L, Benedek D, Fullerton C, Forsten R, Naifeh J, Li X et al. PTSD risk is associated with BDNF Val66Met and BDNF overexpression. Molecular psychiatry. 2013.
26. Dunsmoor JE, Åhs F, LaBar KS. Neurocognitive mechanisms of fear conditioning and vulnerability to anxiety. Front Hum Neurosci. 2011;5.
27. Indovina I, Robbins TW, Núñez-Elizalde AO, Dunn BD, Bishop SJ. Fear-conditioning mechanisms associated with trait vulnerability to anxiety in humans. Neuron. 2011;69(3):563–71.
28. Torrents-Rodas D, Fullana MA, Bonillo A, Caseras X, Andión O, Torrubia R. No effect of trait anxiety on differential fear conditioning or fear generalization. Biol Psychol. 2013;92(2):185–90.
29. Lissek S, Powers AS, McClure EB, Phelps EA, Woldehawariat G, Grillon C, et al. Classical fear conditioning in the anxiety disorders: a meta-analysis. Behav Res Ther. 2005;43(11):1391–424.
30. Dunsmoor JE, Campese VD, Ceceli AO, LeDoux JE, Phelps EA. Novelty-facilitated extinction: providing a novel outcome in place of an expected threat diminishes recovery of defensive responses. Biological Psychiatry. In press.
31. McEvoy PM, Mahoney AE. To be sure, to be sure: intolerance of uncertainty mediates symptoms of various anxiety disorders and depression. Behav Ther. 2012;43(3):533–45.
32. Whalen PJ. The uncertainty of it all. Trends Cogn Sci. 2007;11(12):499–500.
33. Grupe DW, Nitschke JB. Uncertainty and anticipation in anxiety: an integrated neurobiological and psychological perspective. Nat Rev Neurosci. 2013;14(7):488–501.
34. van der Heiden C, Muris P, van der Molen HT. Randomized controlled trial on the effectiveness of metacognitive therapy and intolerance-of-uncertainty therapy for generalized anxiety disorder. Behav Res Ther. 2012;50(2):100–9.
35. Dugas MJ, Robichaud M. Cognitive-behavioral treatment for generalized anxiety disorder: From science to practice. Taylor & Francis; 2007
36. Schiller D, Kanen JW, LeDoux JE, Monfils M-H, Phelps EA. Extinction during reconsolidation of threat memory diminishes prefrontal cortex involvement. Proc Natl Acad Sci. 2013;110(50):20040–5.
37. Delgado MR, Nearing KI, LeDoux JE, Phelps EA. Neural circuitry underlying the regulation of conditioned fear and its relation to extinction. Neuron. 2008;59(5):829–38.
38. Neumann DL, Waters AM. The use of an unpleasant sound as an unconditional stimulus in a human aversive Pavlovian conditioning procedure. Biol Psychol. 2006;73(2):175–85.
39. Spielberger CD, Gorsuch RL, Lushene R, Vagg P, Jacobs G. Consulting Psychologists Press, Inc. 2». Palo Alto (CA). 1983.
40. Meyer TJ, Miller ML, Metzger RL, Borkovec TD. Development and validation of the Penn State worry questionnaire. Behav Res Ther. 1990;28(6):487–95.
41. Bradley MM, Lang PJ. The international affective digitized sounds (2nd edition; IADS-2): affective ratings of sounds and instruction manual. Technical report B-3. Gainesville, Florida: Florida University; 2007.
42. Watson D, Clark LA, Tellegen A. Development and validation of brief measures of positive and negative affect: the PANAS scales. J Pers Soc Psychol. 1988;54(6):1063.
43. Buhr K, Dugas MJ. The intolerance of uncertainty scale: psychometric properties of the English version. Behav Res Ther. 2002;40(8):931–45.
44. Patton JH, Stanford MS. Factor structure of the Barratt impulsiveness scale. J Clin Psychol. 1995;51(6):768–74.
45. Smith SM. Fast robust automated brain extraction. Hum Brain Mapp. 2002;17(3):143–55.

46. Jenkinson M, Bannister P, Brady M, Smith S. Improved optimization for the robust and accurate linear registration and motion correction of brain images. Neuroimage. 2002;17(2):825–41.

47. Desikan RS, Ségonne F, Fischl B, Quinn BT, Dickerson BC, Blacker D, et al. An automated labeling system for subdividing the human cerebral cortex on MRI scans into gyral based regions of interest. Neuroimage. 2006;31(3):968–80.

48. Johnstone T, van Reekum CM, Urry HL, Kalin NH, Davidson RJ. Failure to regulate: counterproductive recruitment of top-down prefrontal-subcortical circuitry in major depression. J Neurol Sci. 2007;27(33):8877–84.

Current understanding of the bi-directional relationship of major depression with inflammation

Berhane Messay, Alvin Lim and Anna L Marsland[*]

Abstract

Consistent evidence links major depression and its affective components to negative health outcomes. Although the pathways of these effects are likely complex and multifactorial, recent evidence suggests that innate inflammatory processes may play a role. An overview of current literature suggests that pathways between negative moods and inflammation are bi-directional. Indeed, negative moods activate peripheral physiologic mechanisms that result in an up regulation of systemic levels of inflammation. Conversely, peripheral inflammatory mediators signal the brain to affect behavioral, affective and cognitive changes that are consistent with symptoms of major depressive disorder. It is likely that these pathways are part of a complex feedback loop that involves the nervous, endocrine, and immune systems and plays a role in the modulation of peripheral inflammatory responses to central and peripheral stimuli, in central responses to peripheral immune activation and in the maintenance of homeostatic balance. Further research is warranted to fully understand the role of central processes in this feedback loop, which likely contributes to the pathophysiology of mental and physical health.

Keywords: depression, negative affect, inflammation, inflammatory markers, cytokines

Background

Evidence shows an association of major depression with increased risk for adverse physical health outcomes. Indeed, depression, whether assessed as a continuum of symptoms or as the presence of a clinical syndrome, predicts the incidence and progression of diseases of aging, including cardiovascular, metabolic and neurode-generative diseases, as well as all-cause mortality [1-3]. Given the burden of these physical illnesses, it is not surprising that affective symptoms and disorders are more prevalent among the medically-ill than the general population [4,5], raising the possibility that associations between affective disorders and physical health are bi-directional in nature. It is also likely that lifestyle choices contribute to poorer health among individuals with depression [6]; however, to date, evidence suggests that behavioral factors contribute only minimally to depression-related variability in health risk. Thus, other mechanisms must also be operating. Accumulating evidence suggests that the immune system may play a role.

Main Text

Early studies show an association of depression with the down-regulation of functional parameters of the immune system (for example, decreased ability of NK cells to destroy tumor cells [7]). However, this immune suppression is not as 'global' as initially proposed. Indeed, recent attention has focused on the activation of innate, non-specific inflammatory mechanisms that also accompany depressed mood [8]. These differential immune responses to negative mood have been interpreted within an evolutionary context as a down-regulation of processes that take time and energy in favor of an up-regulation of processes that are immediately available to defend the organism [9]. Although adaptive and of potential health benefit in the short-term, growing evidence shows that chronic elevation of inflammation plays a role in the pathogenesis and course of numerous age-related physical health conditions, possibly

* Correspondence: marsland@pitt.edu
Department of Psychology, University of Pittsburgh, 3213 Sennott Square, 210 S. Bouquet St., Pittsburgh, PA 15260, USA

contributing to the co-morbidity of depression with chronic physical illness [10].

The inflammatory response is a non-specific immune reaction that is initiated when monocytes/macrophages are activated by pathogens or tissue damage to release pro-inflammatory cytokines, such as interleukin (IL)-6, IL-1β, and tumor necrosis factor (TNF)-α. These cytokines initiate a local and systemic inflammatory response, which includes the hepatic synthesis and release of acute phase proteins, such as C-reactive protein (CRP) and fibrinogen [11]. Peripheral pro-inflammatory cytokines also signal the brain, resulting in symptoms of sickness that typically accompany infectious disease, such as fever, depressed affect, suppressed appetite, increased sleep, and cognitive deficits [12,13].

Circulating levels of pro-inflammatory mediators are widely accepted as a marker of systemic levels of inflammation. However, caution should be taken in assuming these inflammatory mediators are immune-derived as many cells produce these signaling proteins, including adipocytes and endothelial cells [14]. Regardless of source, circulating levels of IL-6 are relatively stable over extended periods [15], are positively related to age [16], and predict risk for a range of age-associated diseases [17]. Consistent evidence also shows that individuals with major depressive disorder have higher levels of circulating markers of inflammation than non-depressed individuals. For example, two recent meta-analyses concluded that increased plasma levels of TNF-α, IL-6, IL-1, and CRP accompany major depression [18,19].

Available data suggest that relationships between pro-inflammatory cytokines and depressed mood are bi-directional. In support of immune-to-brain pathways, sickness symptoms mediated by increases in circulating pro-inflammatory cytokines are consistent with symptoms of depression including fatigue, sleep disturbances, anxiety, negative mood, anhedonia, and loss of appetite [20]. Indeed, the experimental or clinical administration of cytokines or endotoxins results in a range of symptoms of depression [21]. For example, clinical administration of the pro-inflammatory cytokine interferon (IFN)-α in the treatment of cancer or chronic infection induces symptoms of major depressive disorder in 23% to 45% of all patients, with the degree of depression being positively related to dose and duration of treatment [22]. Epidemiologic evidence also shows that systemic inflammation predicts future risk for depressive symptoms and clinical episodes of depression in some [23-25], but not all longitudinal studies [26,27].

To examine the impact of peripheral inflammation on the central nervous system, recent attention has focused on whether immune-related patterns of brain activation are consistent with those that accompany clinical depression. Here, animal studies show that pro-inflammatory cytokines can penetrate the blood-brain barrier to stimulate the production of central pro-inflammatory cytokines by microglial cells in discrete brain regions that are involved in mood regulation and reward processing [20]. Recent human studies have employed randomized double-blind trials, exposing subjects to either immune stimulants (usually endotoxin) that generate low-grade systemic inflammatory responses or saline placebo and then comparing patterns of brain activation across the groups using functional magnetic resonance imagery. Using these methods, peripheral inflammation has been associated with negative mood states that are accompanied by increased activation of the subgenual anterior cingulate cortex (sgACC) and decreased connectivity of the sgACC with the amygdala, prefrontal cortex, nucleus accumbens, and superior temporal sulcus in response to emotional stimuli [28]. A similar pattern of heightened sgACC activity has been observed in response to IFN-α treatment [29] and during episodes of major depression, with activity returning to normative levels once symptoms remit [30]. Peripheral administration of endotoxin also reduces activity in the ventral striatum in response to a monetary reward task, a region of the brain implicated in the pleasurable effects of reward [31]. Taken together, these results raise the possibility that inflammation plays a role in the pathophysiology of the affective and anhedonic symptoms of depression [32].

In addition to immune-to-brain pathways, evidence also shows that negative mood states, stressful experiences, and antagonistic dispositions can activate peripheral physiologic pathways that modulate immune function. For example, negative moods are associated with activation of the hypothalamic-pituitary-adrenal (HPA) axis and the peripheral release of cortisol, along with increased activation of the sympathetic and decreased activation of the parasympathetic branches of the autonomic nervous system [33,34]. These physiologic responses modulate the activity of immune cells and are associated with increased production of pro-inflammatory cytokines [35] and levels of systemic inflammation [36]. Indeed, symptoms of depression have been positively associated with production of TNF-α by monocytes of healthy men and women [37,38]. Furthermore, some longitudinal studies show that symptoms of depression precede increases in systemic inflammation rather than result from them [26,39,27].

Conclusion

In sum, converging evidence supports reciprocal pathways linking inflammation and the disruption of mood. It is likely that these pathways are part of a complex feedback loop that involves the neuroendocrine and immune systems and plays a role in both the modulation of peripheral inflammatory responses to stimuli and the maintenance of homeostatic balance. Further research examining specific symptoms and the central processes involved in these circuits is warranted to fully understand the role of inflammation in the pathophysiology of depression and of associated health morbidity. Evidence suggests that examining the impact of peripheral inflammation on central processes that play a role in specific symptoms of depression may point to novel targets for future intervention. For instance, Motivala *et al.* [40] found that changes in sleep during depression shared a stronger association with peripheral proinflammatory cytokines than other symptoms. Further research is also warranted to examine whether age-related increases in systemic inflammation impact brain function and thus contribute to late-life depression.

Authors' contributions

BM conducted an up to date review of the relevant literature and wrote the initial draft of the manuscript. ALM edited the manuscript and made substantial revisions. AL read, contributed relevant research, and provided feedback on early and final versions of the manuscript. All authors read and approved the final manuscript.

Authors' information

ALM: Anna Marsland, Ph.D. is the Director of the Behavioral Immunology Laboratory and a member of the Biological and Health Psychology faculty at the University of Pittsburgh. Her expertise is in the field of psychoneuroimmunology. BM: Berhane Messay is a second year graduate student in the Clinical and Biological/Health Psychology Programs at the University of Pittsburgh. AL: Alvin Lim is a second year graduate student in the Biological/Health Psychology Program at the University of Pittsburgh.

Competing interests

The authors declare that they have no competing interests.

References

1. Wulsin LR, Singal BM: **Do depressive symptoms increase the risk for the onset of coronary disease? A systematic quantitative review.** *Psychosom Med* 2003, 65:201-210.
2. Eaton WW, Armenian H, Gallo J, Pratt L, Ford DE: **Depression and risk for onset of type II diabetes. A prospective population-based study.** *Diabetes Care* 1996, 19:1097-1102.
3. Evans DL, Charney DS, Lewis L, Golden RN, Gorman JM, Krishnan KR, Nemeroff CB, Bremner JD, Carney RM, Coyne JC, Delong MR, Frasure-Smith N, Glassman AH, Gold PW, Grant I, Gwyther L, Ironson G, Johnson RL, Kanner AM, Katon WJ, Kaufmann PG, Keefe FJ, Ketter T, Laughren TP, Leserman J, Lyketsos CG, McDonald WM, McEwen BS, Miller AH, Musselman D, et al: **Mood disorders in the medically ill: scientific review and recommendations.** *Biol Psychiatry* 2005, 58:175-189.
4. Koening HG: **Depression in hospitalized older patients with congestive heart failure.** *Gen Hosp Psychiatry* 1998, 20:29-43.
5. Katon WJ: **Clinical and health services relationships between major depression, depressive symptoms, and general medical illness.** *Biol Psychiatry* 54:216-226.
6. Fergusson DM, Goodwin RD, Horwood LJ: **Major depression and cigarette smoking: results of a 21-year longitudinal study.** *Psychol Med* 2003, 33:1357-1367.
7. Herbert TB, Cohen S: **Depression and immunity: a meta-analytic review.** *Psychol Bull* 1993, 113:472-486.
8. Irwin MR, Miller AH: **Depressive disorders and immunity: 20 years of progress and discovery.** *Brain, Behav Immun* 2007, 21:374-383.
9. Segerstrom SC, Miller GE: **Psychological stress and the human immune system: a meta-analytic study of 30 years of inquiry.** *Psychol Bull* 2004, 130:601-630.
10. Raison CL, Capuron L, Miller AH: **Cytokines sing the blues: inflammation and the pathogenesis of depression.** *Trends Immunol* 2006, 27:24-31.
11. Black PH, Garbutt LD: **Stress, inflammation and cardiovascular disease.** *J Psychosom Res* 2002, 52:1-23.
12. Maier SF, Watkins LR: **Cytokines for psychologists: implications of bidirectional immune-to-brain communication for understanding behavior, mood, and cognition.** *Psychol Rev* 1998, 105:83-107.
13. Dantzer R, O'Connor JC, Freund GG, Johnson RW, Kelley KW: **From inflammation to sickness and depression: when the immune system subjugates the brain.** *Nat Rev Neurosci* 2008, 9:46-56.
14. Mohamed-Ali V, Goodrick S, Rawesh A, Katz DR, Miles JM, Yudkin JS, Klein S, Coppack SW: **Subcutaneous adipose tissue releases interleukin-6, but not tumor necrosis factor-alpha, in vivo.** *J Clin Endocrinol Metab* 1997, 82:4196-4120.
15. Rao KM, Pieper CS, Currie MS, Cohen HJ: **Variability of plasma IL-6 and crosslinked fibrin dimers over time in community dwelling elderly subjects.** *Am J Clin Pathol* 1994, 102:802-805.
16. Kiecolt-Glaser JK, Preacher KJ, MacCallum RC, Atkinson C, Malarkey WB, Glaser R: **Chronic stress and age-related increases in the proinflammatory cytokine IL-6.** *Proc Natl Acad Sci USA* 2003, 100:9090-9095.
17. Ridker PM, Hennekens CH, Buring JE, Rifai N: **C-reactive protein and other markers of inflammation in the prediction of cardiovascular disease in women.** *N Engl J Med* 2000, 342:836-843.
18. Dowlati Y, Hermann N, Swardfager W, Liu H, Sham L, Reim EK, Lanctot KL: **A meta-analysis of cytokines in major depression.** *Biol Psychiatry* 2010, 67:446-457.
19. Howren MB, Lamkin DM, Suls J: **Associations of depression with C-reactive protein, IL-1, and IL-6: a meta-analysis.** *Psychosom Med* 2009, 71:171-186.
20. Miller AH, Maletic V, Raison CL: **Inflammation and its discontents: the role of cytokines in the pathophysiology of major depression.** *Biol Psychiatry* 2009, 65:732-741.
21. Reichenberg A, Yirmiya R, Schuld A, Kraus T, Haack M, Moraq A, Pollmächer T: **Cytokine-associated emotional and cognitive disturbances in humans.** *Arch Gen Psychiatry* 2001, 58:445-452.
22. Asnis G, De La Garza: **Interferon-induced depression in chronic hepatitis C: a review of its prevalence, risk factors, biology, and treatment approaches.** *J Clin Gastroenterol* 2006, 40:322-335.
23. Gimeno D, Kivimäki M, Brunner EJ, Elovainio M, De Vogli R, Steptoe A, Kumari M, Lowe GD, Rumley A, Marmot MG, Ferrie JE: **Associations of C-reactive protein and interleukin-6 with cognitive symptoms of depression: 12-year follow-up of the Whitehall II study.** *Psychosom Med* 2009, 39:413-423.
24. Milaneschi Y, Corsi AM, Penninx BW, Bandinelli S, Guralnik JM, Ferrucci L: **Interleukin-1 receptor antagonist and incident depressive symptoms over 6 years in older persons: the InCHIANTI study.** *Biol Psychiatry* 2009, 65:973-978.
25. Pasco JA, Nicholson GC, Williams LJ, Jacka FN, Henry MJ, Kotowicz MA, Schneider HG, Leonard BE, Berk M: **Association of high-sensitivity C-reactive protein with de novo major depression.** *Br J Psychiatry* 2010, 197:372-377.
26. Duivis HE, de Jonge P, Penninx BW, Na BY, Cohen BE, Whooley MA: **Depressive symptoms, health behaviors, and subsequent inflammation in patients with coronary heart disease: prospective findings from the heart and soul study.** *Am J Psychiatry* 2011, 168:913-920.
27. Stewart JC, Rand KL, Muldoon MF, Kamarck TW: **A prospective evaluation of the directionality of the depression-inflammation relationship.** *Brain, Behav Immun* 2009, 23:936-944.
28. Harrison NA, Brydon L, Walker C, Gray MA, Steptoe A, Critchley HD: **Inflammation causes mood changes through the alterations in subgenual cingulate activity and mesolimbic connectivity.** *Biol Psychiatry* 2009, 66:407-414.
29. Capuron L, Pagnoni G, Demetrashvili M, Woolwine BJ, Nemeroff CB, Berns GS, Miller AH: **Anterior cingulate activation and error processing during interferon-alpha treatment.** *Biol Psychiatry* 2010, 58:190-196.

30. Drevets WC, Savitz J, Trimble M: **The subgenual anterior cingulate cortex in mood disorders.** *CNS Spectr* 2008, **13**:663-681.
31. Eisenberger NI, Berkman ET, Inagaki TK, Rameson LT, Marshal NM, Irwin MR: **Inflammation-induced anhedonia: endotoxin reduces ventral striatum responses to reward.** *Biol Psychiatry* 2010, **68**:748-754.
32. Krishnan V, Nestler EJ: **The molecular neurobiology of depression.** *Nature* 2008, **455**:894-902.
33. al'Absi M, Bongard S: **Neuroendocrine and behavioral mechanisms mediating the relationship between anger expression and cardiovascular risk: assessment considerations and improvements.** *J Behav Med* 2006, **29**:573-591.
34. Suarez EC, Kuhn CM, Schanberg Sm, Williams RB Jr, Zimmermann EA: **Neuroendocrine, cardiovascular, and emotional responses of hostile men: the role of interpersonal challenge.** *Psychosom Med* 1998, **60**:78-88.
35. Marsland AL, Gianarod PJ, Prather AA, Jennings JR, Newmann SA, Manuck SB: **Stimulated production of proinflammatory cytokines covaries inversely with heart rate variability.** *Psychosom Med* 2007, **69**:709-716.
36. Miller GE, Stetler CA, Carney RM, Freedland KE, Banks WA: **Clinical depression and inflammatory risk markers for coronary heart disease.** *Am J Cardiol* 2002, **90**:1279-1283.
37. Suarez EC, Krishnan RR, Lewis JG: **The relation of severity of depressive symptoms to monocyte-associated proinflammatory cytokines and chemokines in apparently healthy men.** *Psychosom Med* 2003, **65**:362-368.
38. Suarez EC, Lewis JG, Krishnan RR, Young KH: **Enhanced expression of cytokines and chemokines by blood monocytes to in vitro lipopolysaccharide stimulation are associated with hostility and severity of depressive symptoms in healthy women.** *Psychoneuroendocrinology* 2004, **29**:1119-1128.
39. Deverts DJ, Cohen S, DiLillo VG, Lewis CE, Kiefe C, Whooley M, Matthews KA: **Depressive symptoms, race, and circulating C-reactive protein: the coronary artery risk development in young adults (CARDIA) study.** *Psychosom Med* 2010, **72**:734-741.
40. Motivala SJ, Sarfatti A, Olmos L, Irwin MR: **Inflammatory markers and sleep disturbances in major depression.** *Psychosom Med* 2005, **67**:187-194.

Permissions

The contributors of this book come from diverse backgrounds, making this book a truly international effort. This book will bring forth new frontiers with its revolutionizing research information and detailed analysis of the nascent developments around the world.

We would like to thank all the contributing authors for lending their expertise to make the book truly unique. They have played a crucial role in the development of this book. Without their invaluable contributions this book wouldn't have been possible. They have made vital efforts to compile up to date information on the varied aspects of this subject to make this book a valuable addition to the collection of many professionals and students.

This book was conceptualized with the vision of imparting up-to-date information and advanced data in this field. To ensure the same, a matchless editorial board was set up. Every individual on the board went through rigorous rounds of assessment to prove their worth. After which they invested a large part of their time researching and compiling the most relevant data for our readers.

The editorial board has been involved in producing this book since its inception. They have spent rigorous hours researching and exploring the diverse topics which have resulted in the successful publishing of this book. They have passed on their knowledge of decades through this book. To expedite this challenging task, the publisher supported the team at every step. A small team of assistant editors was also appointed to further simplify the editing procedure and attain best results for the readers.

Apart from the editorial board, the designing team has also invested a significant amount of their time in understanding the subject and creating the most relevant covers. They scrutinized every image to scout for the most suitable representation of the subject and create an appropriate cover for the book.

The publishing team has been an ardent support to the editorial, designing and production team. Their endless efforts to recruit the best for this project, has resulted in the accomplishment of this book. They are a veteran in the field of academics and their pool of knowledge is as vast as their experience in printing. Their expertise and guidance has proved useful at every step. Their uncompromising quality standards have made this book an exceptional effort. Their encouragement from time to time has been an inspiration for everyone.

The publisher and the editorial board hope that this book will prove to be a valuable piece of knowledge for researchers, students, practitioners and scholars across the globe.

List of Contributors

Patrick M Fisher
Center for Neuroscience, University of Pittsburgh, Pittsburgh, Pennsylvania 15260, USA
Center for the Neural Basis of Cognition, University of Pittsburgh, Pittsburgh, Pennsylvania 15260, USA

Julie C Price
Center for the Neural Basis of Cognition, University of Pittsburgh, Pittsburgh, Pennsylvania 15260, USA
Department of Radiology, University of Pittsburgh, Pittsburgh, Pennsylvania 15260, USA

Carolyn C Meltzer
Department of Radiology, Emory University, Atlanta, Georgia 30322, USA

Eydie L Moses-Kolko
Department of Psychiatry, University of Pittsburgh, Pittsburgh, Pennsylvania 15260, USA

Carl Becker
Department of Radiology, University of Pittsburgh, Pittsburgh, Pennsylvania 15260, USA

Sarah L Berga
Department of Gynecology & Obstetrics, Emory University, Atlanta, Georgia 30322, USA

Ahmad R Hariri
Department of Neuroscience & Psychology, Duke University, Durham, North Carolina 27710, USA
Institute for Genome Sciences & Policy, Duke University, Durham, North Carolina 27710, USA

Malin Gingnell
Department of Women's and Children's Health, Uppsala University, Uppsala, Sweden

Victoria Ahlstedt1, Elin Bannbers and Inger Sundström-Poromaa
Department of Women's and Children's Health, Uppsala University, Uppsala, Sweden

Johan Wikström
Department of Radiology, Oncology and Radiation Science, Uppsala University, Uppsala, Sweden

Mats Fredrikson
Department of Psychology, Uppsala University, Uppsala, Sweden

Joaquim Radua
Institute of Psychiatry, King's College London, De Crespigny Park, London, UK
Research Unit, FIDMAG-CIBERSAM, Sant Boi de Llobregat, Barcelona, Spain

David Mataix-Cols
Institute of Psychiatry, King's College London, De Crespigny Park, London, UK

Abdulrahman M El-Sayed
Department of Epidemiology, Mailman School of Public Health, Columbia University, 722 W. 168th Street, R521, New York, NY 10032, USA
College of Physicians and Surgeons, Columbia University, New York, NY, USA

Michelle R Haloossim
Department of Sociomedical Sciences, Mailman School of Public Health, Columbia University, 722 W. 168th Street, New York, NY 10032, USA

Sandro Galea
Department of Epidemiology, Mailman School of Public Health, Columbia University, 722 W. 168th Street, 1508, New York, NY 10032, USA

Karestan C Koenen
Department of Epidemiology, Mailman School of Public Health, Columbia University, 722 W. 168th Street, R720G, New York, NY 10032, USA

Tara S Peris
Division of Child and Adolescent Psychiatry,
UCLA Semel Institute for Neuroscience and
Human Behavior, 760 Westwood Plaza,
Room 67-439, Los Angeles, CA 90095, USA

Adriana Galván
Department of Psychology, University of
California, Los Angeles, USA
Brain Research Institute, University of
California, Los Angeles, USA

Anja Stuhrmann and Udo Dannlowski
University of Münster, Department of
Psychiatry, Albert-Schweitzer-Campus 1,
Building, A9, 48149 Münster, Germany

Thomas Suslow
University of Münster, Department of
Psychiatry, Albert-Schweitzer-Campus 1,
Building, A9, 48149 Münster, Germany
University of Leipzig, Department
of Psychosomatic Medicine and
Psychotherapy, Semmelweißstraße 10,
04103 Leipzig, Germany

Liat Levita
Present address: Department of Psychology,
University of Sheffield, Western Bank,
Sheffield S10 2TN, UK

Catherine Bois
Department of Psychology, University of
York, York YO10 5DD, UK
Department of Psychiatry, University of
Edinburgh, Edinburgh EH10 5HF, UK

**Andrew Healey, Emily Smyllie, Evelina
Papakonstantinou and Tom Hartley**
Department of Psychology, University of
York, York YO10 5DD, UK

Colin Lever
Department of Psychology, University of
Durham, Durham DH1 3LE, UK

Andrea Hermann and Rudolf Stark
Department of Psychotherapy and
Systems Neuroscience, Bender Institute of
Neuroimaging, Justus Liebig University, Otto-
Behaghel-Strasse 10H, Giessen 35394, Germany
Bender Institute of Neuroimaging, Justus
Liebig University, Giessen, Germany

**Verena Leutgeb, Wilfried Scharmüller and
Anne Schienle**
Department of Clinical Psychology, University
of Graz, Graz, Austria

Dieter Vaitl
Bender Institute of Neuroimaging, Justus
Liebig University, Giessen, Germany

**Stephanie Boehme, Alexander Mohr and
Wolfgang HR Miltner**
Department of Biological and Clinical
Psychology, Friedrich Schiller University
Jena, Am Steiger 3 // 1, Jena D-07743,
Germany

Michael PI Becker and Thomas Straube
Institute of Medical Psychology and Systems
Neuroscience, University of Muenster,
Von-Esmarch-Str. 52, Muenster D-48149,
Germany

**Kelimer Lebron-Milad, Mohammed R
Milad, Mohammed A Zeidan and Daphne
J Holt**
Department of Psychiatry, Harvard
Medical School & Massachusetts General
Hospital, 149 13th St, Charlestown, MA,
02129, USA

Brandon Abbs
Departments of Psychiatry and Medicine,
Harvard Medical School, Connors Center
for Women's Health and Gender Biology,
Brigham and Women's Hospital, 75 Francis
St., Boston, MA, 02120, USA

Jill M Goldstein
Department of Psychiatry, Harvard Medical School & Massachusetts General Hospital, 149 13th St, Charlestown, MA, 02129, USA
Departments of Psychiatry and Medicine, Harvard Medical School, Connors Center for Women's Health and Gender Biology, Brigham and Women's Hospital, 75 Francis St., Boston, MA, 02120, USA

Clas Linnman
Department of Psychiatry, Harvard Medical School & Massachusetts General Hospital, 149 13th St, Charlestown, MA, 02129, USA
P.A.I.N. Group, Department of Anesthesia, Children´s Hospital, Boston, MA, , USA

Ansgar Rougemount-Bücking
Department of Psychiatry, Harvard Medical School & Massachusetts General Hospital, 149 13th St, Charlestown, MA, 02129, USA
Department of Psychiatry, Centre Hospitalier Universitaire Vaudois and University of Lausanne, 7 rue Saint-Martin1003, Lausanne, Switzerland

Arash Javanbakht
Department of Psychiatry, University of Michigan, Ann Arbor, 1500 East Medical Center Drive, Ann Arbor, MI 48109, USA
Department of Psychiatry and Behavioral Neurosciences, Wayne State University, 540 E Canfield, Detroit, MI 48201-1998, USA

Israel Liberzon
Department of Psychiatry, University of Michigan, Ann Arbor, 1500 East Medical Center Drive, Ann Arbor, MI 48109, USA

Alireza Amirsadri, Klevest Gjini and Nash N Boutros
Department of Psychiatry and Behavioral Neurosciences, Wayne State University, 540 E Canfield, Detroit, MI 48201-1998, USA

Adam X Gorka, Spenser R Radtke and Ahmad R Hariri
Laboratory of NeuroGenetics, Department of Psychology and Neuroscience, Duke University, 417 Chapel Drive, Durham, NC 27708, USA

Jamie L Hanson
Laboratory of NeuroGenetics, Department of Psychology and Neuroscience, Duke University, 417 Chapel Drive, Durham, NC 27708, USA
Center for Developmental Science, University of North Carolina at Chapel Hill, 100 East Franklin Street, Suite 200 CB#8115, Chapel Hill, NC 27599, USA

Jasmeet P Hayes
National Center for PTSD, VA Boston Healthcare System, Boston, MA, USA
Neuroimaging Research Center, VA Boston Healthcare System, Boston, MA, USA
Department of Psychiatry, Boston University School of Medicine, Boston, MA, USA

Scott M Hayes
Neuroimaging Research Center, VA Boston Healthcare System, Boston, MA, USA
Department of Psychiatry, Boston University School of Medicine, Boston, MA, USA
Memory Disorders Research Center, VA Boston Healthcare System and Boston University School of Medicine, Boston, MA, USA

Amanda M Mikedis
National Center for PTSD, VA Boston Healthcare System, Boston, MA, USA
Neuroimaging Research Center, VA Boston Healthcare System, Boston, MA, USA

Thomas Straube, Judith Lipka, Andreas Sauer, Martin Mothes-Lasch and Wolfgang HR Miltner
Department of Biological and Clinical Psychology, Friedrich-Schiller- University, Jena, Germany

Brittany R Howell and Mar M Sanchez
Department of Psychiatry & Behavioral Sciences, Emory University, 101 Woodruff Circle, WMB Suite 4000, Atlanta, GA 30322, USA
Yerkes National Primate Research Center, Emory University, 954 Gatewood Road NE, Atlanta, GA 30329, USA

Kai M McCormack
Yerkes National Primate Research Center, Emory University, 954 Gatewood Road NE, Atlanta, GA 30329, USA
Department of Psychology, Spelman College, 350 Spelman Lane, Box 209, Atlanta, GA 30314, USA

Alison P Grand and Xiaodong Zhang
Yerkes National Primate Research Center, Emory University, 954 Gatewood Road NE, Atlanta, GA 30329, USA

Nikki T Sawyer
Department of Natural Sciences, Clayton State University, 2000 Clayton State Boulevard, Morrow, GA 30260, USA

Dario Maestripieri
Department of Comparative Human Development, University of Chicago, 5730 South Woodlawn Avenue, Chicago, IL 60637, USA

Xiaoping Hu
BiomedicalImaging Technology Center, Emory University, 1760 Haygood Drive, Room W232, Atlanta, GA 30322, USA

Francesco Amico and Danuta Lisiecka
Department of Psychiatry, Trinity College Dublin, College Green, Dublin 2, Ireland
Institute of Neuroscience, Trinity College Dublin, College Green, Dublin 2, Ireland

Angela Carballedo
Department of Psychiatry, Trinity College Dublin, College Green, Dublin 2, Ireland
Institute of Neuroscience, Trinity College Dublin, College Green, Dublin 2, Ireland
Adelaide and Meath Hospital incorporating the National Children's Hospital, Tallaght, Dublin 24, Dublin, Ireland

Andrew J Fagan and Gerard Boyle
St James's Hospital,Centre of Advanced Medical Imaging (CAMI), James's Street, Dublin 8, Dublin, Ireland

Thomas Frodl
Department of Psychiatry, Trinity College Dublin, College Green, Dublin 2, Ireland
Institute of Neuroscience, Trinity College Dublin, College Green, Dublin 2, Ireland
Adelaide and Meath Hospital incorporating the National Children's Hospital, Tallaght, Dublin 24, Dublin, Ireland
St James's Hospital, Centre of Advanced Medical Imaging (CAMI), James's Street, Dublin 8, Dublin, Ireland

Heide Klumpp
Mood and Anxiety Disorders Research Program, Department of Psychiatry (HK, DAF, KLP), University of Illinois at Chicago, 1747 W. Roosevelt Rd, Chicago, IL 60608, USA
Department of Psychology (HK, MKK, SAS, KLP), University of Illinois at Chicago, Chicago, IL, USA
Department of Psychiatry (HK, SAS, KLP), University of Illinois at Chicago, Chicago, IL, USA

Michael K Keutmann
Department of Psychology (HK, MKK, SAS, KLP), University of Illinois at Chicago, Chicago, IL, USA

Daniel A Fitzgerald
Mental Health Service (DAF, KLP), Jesse Brown VA Medical Center, Chicago, IL, USA

Stewart A Shankman
Department of Psychology (HK, MKK, SAS, KLP), University of Illinois at Chicago, Chicago, IL, USA
Department of Psychiatry (HK, SAS, KLP), University of Illinois at Chicago, Chicago, IL, USA

K Luan Phan
Mood and Anxiety Disorders Research Program, Department of Psychiatry (HK, DAF, KLP), University of Illinois at Chicago, 1747 W. Roosevelt Rd, Chicago, IL 60608, USA
Department of Psychology (HK, MKK, SAS, KLP), University of Illinois at Chicago, Chicago, IL, USA
Department of Psychiatry (HK, SAS, KLP), University of Illinois at Chicago, Chicago, IL, USA
Mental Health Service (DAF, KLP), Jesse Brown VA Medical Center, Chicago, IL, USA

Jayne Morriss, Anastasia Christakou and Carien M. van Reekum
Centre for Integrative Neuroscience and Neurodynamics, School of Psychology and Clinical Language Sciences, University of Reading, Earley Gate, Whiteknights Campus, RG6 6AH Reading, UK

Berhane Messay, Alvin Lim and Anna L Marsland
Department of Psychology, University of Pittsburgh, 3213 Sennott Square, 210 S. Bouquet St.,Pittsburgh, PA 15260, USA

Index

A

Activation Likelihood Estimation, 22, 28, 30-31, 133

Amygdala Reactivity, 1-6, 9-10, 12-13, 17, 19-21, 47, 52, 69, 178

Anterior Cingulate Cortex (acc), 1, 55, 92, 102

Anxiety Disorders, 13, 20, 26, 28, 31, 33-45, 47-48, 52-53, 72, 77, 79-80, 83, 90, 93, 98, 101, 110, 124-125, 130-131, 146-147, 152-153, 162, 164, 175, 178, 184-186, 192-193, 196

Anxious Adolescents, 49, 51

Attentional Load, 146-147, 149-153, 155

B

Brain Activation, 32, 68-69, 80-81, 83, 85, 87, 89-93, 95-99, 101, 134, 144, 151, 153-154, 175-176, 199

C

Childhood Maltreatment, 65, 70, 123-125, 127-131, 156, 162, 166-167

Cnv (contingent Negative Variation), 111

Cognitive Behavioral Therapy (cbt), 178

Cognitive Reappraisal, 81-91, 142

Conceptions, 170

Contextual Modulation, 48-49, 51, 53

Corticolimbic Circuit, 1-2, 13, 17

Corticolimbic Gray Matter, 123-124, 126

Corticolimbic Reactivity, 13, 15, 17, 19, 21

D

Dental Phobia, 82, 90-91

Differential Mapping, 22, 30

Diffusion Tensor Imaging, 156, 160, 166-169

Dorsomedial Prefrontal Cortex (dmpfc), 81

E

Early Life Stress, 123-124, 129, 156-157, 162, 167, 176

Electrophysiology, 111-112, 121-122

Emotion Regulation, 6, 55, 66-68, 81-84, 88, 90-91, 120, 133, 141-143, 178-179, 182, 184

Epigenetic Modifications, 33, 35-46

Erp Abnormalities, 111

F

Facial Emotion Processing, 54-55, 57-59, 61, 63-65, 67, 69

Fear Conditioning, 82, 101-105, 107, 109-110, 133-134, 185-186, 196

Fear Extinction, 21, 82, 90, 101-102, 107-110, 132, 185-189, 191-197

Functional Anomalies, 170-171, 173, 175, 177

Functional Connectivity, 20, 28, 54-56, 58, 63-64, 66, 68-69, 72, 145, 184

Functional Magnetic Resonance Imaging (fmri), 2, 92, 170, 178

G

Generalized Social Anxiety, 20, 100, 178-179, 181, 184

Genomic Expression, 33

H

High Cortisol, 156

Hippocampus, 21, 28, 36, 39-40, 56, 60, 63, 71, 73-80, 101-102, 104, 109-110, 123-132, 143-144, 161, 163, 165, 183

Histone Modification, 33

I

Inflammatory Markers, 198, 201

Information Processing (ip) Abnormalities, 111

Intolerance of Uncertainty, 185, 187, 189, 191, 193, 195-197

K

Kernel Density Analysis, 22, 28, 30

L

Lateral Orbitofrontal Cortex (lofc), 81

Luteal Phase-induced Negative Affect, 12

M

Magnetic Resonance Imaging, 1-2, 10, 14, 19-20, 22, 32, 54, 68-70, 80, 82-83, 92, 94, 99, 101, 109-110, 131, 133, 144, 146-147, 154, 166-167, 170, 176, 178, 184-185, 195

Major Depression, 36, 38, 45, 54-55, 57, 59, 61, 63-65, 67-70, 80, 131, 144, 157, 177, 197-201

Medial Prefrontal Cortex (mpfc), 1, 47, 101-102

Methylation, 33-37, 39-43, 45-46

Mmn (mismatch Negativity), 111-112

Mood Disorders, 33-34, 36, 38, 40, 43, 68, 70, 124, 157, 164-166, 168, 178, 200-201

Mpfc Activation, 47, 51, 108, 179

Mpfc Glutamatergic Neurons, 1

N

Neural Activity, 20, 55, 63, 66, 70, 100, 133, 135, 137, 139, 141, 143, 145

Neurocircuitry of Ptsd, 133

Neuroimaging, 1-2, 7-9, 11, 14, 20, 22-23, 25-32, 54-57, 59, 61, 63, 65, 67-70, 72-73, 77, 79-81, 90-91, 99-100, 133-136, 142-145, 147, 159, 166, 168-169, 171, 173, 181, 184, 196

Neutral Faces, 7, 11, 47-54, 58, 65-66, 100, 113, 116, 118, 121, 135, 146, 151, 173

Non-clinical Population, 73, 75, 77, 79

O

Orbitofrontal Cortex, 40, 54-55, 61-62, 66, 69, 81, 89, 91, 109-110, 124, 130-131, 136, 166, 177, 179, 184

P

Perceptual Load, 146-147, 150-154

Positron Emission Tomography (pet), 1

Potential Studies, 111, 113, 115, 117, 119, 121

Prefrontal Gray Matter, 123, 125, 127, 129, 131

Progesterone Sensitivity, 12

Psychiatric Disease, 170-171

Q

Quantitative Meta-analysis, 20, 133, 135, 137, 139, 141, 143, 145

R

Region of Interest, 6, 11, 22, 25, 30, 55, 59, 62, 98, 148, 151, 174, 184

Rhesus Monkeys, 156-161, 163, 165-169

Risk Factor, 13, 67, 123, 170, 185

Rostral Anterior Cingulate (racc), 106

S

Salience Network, 133, 139, 143

Sensitivity to Punishment, 71-72, 75-76, 79

Sex Differences, 90, 101-109, 144, 168

Social Anxiety Disorder (sad), 92, 97, 99

Social Stimulation, 13, 15, 17, 19, 21

Specific Phobia, 13, 20, 32, 81-85, 87, 89-90, 93, 99-100, 142, 147, 152, 154, 196

Spider-phobic, 147, 149, 152-153

Stress Response Circuitry, 101, 108-109

Structural Mri, 70-71, 73, 78, 80, 125

Symptom Provocation, 28, 81-84, 86-87, 89-90, 92-93, 95-99, 134-142

T

Threat-related Stimuli, 1, 5, 99, 146-147, 155

Trait Anxiety, 10, 12, 14, 16, 19-21, 48, 71-73, 75, 79-80, 112, 117, 121, 123-131, 146, 148, 152, 185-187, 192-193, 195-196

Tumor Necrosis Factor (tnf)-a, 199

V

Ventromedial Prefrontal Cortex (vmpfc), 64, 185

Voxel-based Morphometry, 22, 31-32, 72, 126, 130-131

Printed in the USA
CPSIA information can be obtained
at www.ICGtesting.com
JSHW051326221024
72173JS00006B/1295